Respiratory therapy equipment

Respiratory therapy equipment

STEVEN P. McPHERSON, R.R.T.

Director, Respiratory Therapy
Tucson Medical Center
Tucson, Arizona

with 752 illustrations

THE C. V. MOSBY COMPANY

Saint Louis   1977

The C. V. Mosby Company
11830 Westline Industrial Drive, St. Louis, Missouri 63141

Library of Congress Cataloging in Publication Data

McPherson, Steven P   1946-
    Respiratory therapy equipment.

    Bibliography: p.
    Includes index.
    1. Inhalation therapy—Equipment and supplies.
I. Title. [DNLM: 1. Respirators. 2. Resuscitation—
Instrumentation.   WF26 M172r]
RM161.M23   615'.836   75-5602
ISBN 0-8016-3319-2

GW/CB/B   9   8   7   6   5   4   3   2   1

To those who were instrumental
in my being able to write this book.

My father   who taught me what a man is
My grandfather   who taught me what wisdom means
Dr. Donald F. Egan   who taught me to be a Respiratory Therapist
Dr. William F. Miller   who has taught me since

and

Lisa   who, at the age of 5, gave up her weekends
to correct my grammar and spelling

PREFACE

This book is written to provide students and clinicians with a single, comprehensive presentation of the principles of respiratory therapy equipment because adequate literature about the various types of such equipment and their function is not available. Equipment made possible respiratory therapy's evolution as a specialty in the allied health field, and it continues to serve as its essential foundation. In the words of Dr. W. F. Miller, "Let there be no doubt, respiratory therapy is a largely mechanical therapy."

Sound knowledge of mechanical concepts provides the capability for determining whether clinical problems are physiologic in nature, are caused by related medical problems, or arise from the apparatus used in treatment of the patient. Furthermore, such knowledge enables the clinician to provide an optimum therapeutic approach by regulating the physical and pharmacologic factors to fit the patient's individual requirements. Also, the ability to properly modify apparatus to meet special clinical requirements is one of the therapist's most critical responsibilities.

The approach taken in this text is to first review the principles of physics that must be comprehended to fully understand equipment function. The first chapters start with the simpler devices used in respiratory therapy. The principles described in these chapters are utilized to analyze component functions of more complex apparatus in later chapters.

This book will achieve its purpose if it assists clinicians to fulfill their responsibilities in providing expeditious, effective, and comprehensive care to patients with cardiopulmonary disorders. To paraphrase Dr. W. Curtis Wilcox, respiratory care of patients is founded on quality people, so we must be concerned about them and provide them with quality preparation.

Much credit is due those who have joined in this effort to provide respiratory therapists with a detailed examination of the equipment utilized in respiratory therapy. I want to acknowledge those who really put this book together under my supervision—Bud Spearman, R.R.T., for contributing to and editing the manuscript; Judy Roads Booth, C.R.T.T., for research and coordination; Paul Petrocci for artwork; Ann McPherson and Pat McMahan, R.R.T., for technical review; and Val Elston, Pam Sampsell, Linda Porter, Robin Bossov, and Marsha McCormick for typing.

Without the equipment companies' support and aid, this book would not have been possible.

A note of gratitude is also in order for the respiratory therapy staff, Mrs. Marie Booth, W. Curtis Wilcox, M.D., and the administration at Tucson Medical Center for their support.

Steven P. McPherson

ACKNOWLEDGMENTS

The following companies that supply respiratory therapy equipment made many of the figures and content possible:

Air Shields, Inc., Hatboro, Pennsylvania
Beckman Instruments, Inc., Irvine, California
Bendix Corporation, Davenport, Iowa
Bennett Respiration Products, Inc., Santa Monica, California
Bird Corporation, Palm Springs, California
Bourns, Inc., Life Systems Division, Riverside, California
Cairtron KDC Medical Sales, Anaheim, California
Chemetron HealthCare Systems, St. Louis, Missouri
Warren E. Collins, Inc., Braintree, Massachusetts
DeVilbiss Company, Somerset, Pennsylvania
J. H. Emerson Company, Cambridge, Massachusetts
Extracorporeal Medical Specialties, Inc., King of Prussia, Pennsylvania
Foregger Air Products, Allentown, Pennsylvania
Hudson Oxygen Therapy Sales Company, Temecula, California
Inspiron, Division of C. R. Bard, Inc., Upland, California
Isolette, Warminster, Pennsylvania
Jones Medical Instruments Corporation, Oak Brook, Illinois
LKB Medical, Rockville, Maryland
Laerdal Medical Corporation, Armonk, New York
Mine Safety Appliances Company, Pittsburgh, Pennsylvania
Mist-O-Gen Equipment Company, Oakland, California
Monaghan, Division of Sandoz-Wander, Inc., Littleton, Colorado
V. Mueller, Division of A.H.S.C., Chicago, Illinois
National Catheter Corporation, Argyle, New York
National Fire Protection Association, Boston, Massachusetts
National Welding Equipment Company, Richmond, California
North American Drager, Telford, Pennsylvania
O.E.M. Medical, Edison, New Jersey
Ohio Medical Products, Division of AIRCO, Madison, Wisconsin
Portex, Division of Smiths Industries, Wilmington, Massachusetts
Puritan-Bennett Corporation, Kansas City, Missouri
Respiratory Care, Inc., Arlington Heights, Illinois
Robertshaw Controls Company, Anaheim, California
Searle Cardio-Pulmonary Systems, Inc., Hayward, California
Shiley Laboratories, Inc., Santa Ana, California
Siemens Corporation, Union, New Jersey
Veriflo Medical Division, Richmond, California

CONTENTS

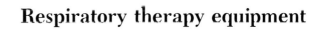

Respiratory therapy equipment

1 Gas physics

Since respiratory therapy has a great deal to do with gases, it is reasonable to consider some of the physics of gases and their effect on the apparatus that respiratory therapists utilize. In addition, a clear grasp of the physical characteristics of gases should be obtained to provide a strong foundation for the understanding of the equipment used daily in the clinical setting.

STATES OF MATTER

In our atmosphere, there are three states of matter: solids, liquids, and gases. The state of matter of a substance largely depends on the kinetic activity (motion) that the molecules of that substance possess. The degree of motion is most dependent on the temperature of those molecules (Fig. 1-1). Increased molecular velocity causes molecules to exert more force when they hit something because of their inertia, such as when they collide with each other (inertia [force] = mass × velocity²). This increased force on each other tends to move the molecules farther apart, causing expansion. If the molecules move far enough apart, they will change states of matter (solid to liquid or liquid to gas). The higher the temperature the molecule achieves, the faster it moves, and it is, then, more inclined to change its state of matter (Fig. 1-1). As the molecules of a solid gain heat, they tend to expand and, ultimately, become a liquid. As molecules in the liquid state absorb more heat, they tend to become a gas.

Lord Kelvin, a professor of physics at Glasgow University in the late 1800s, calculated absolute zero.[1] *Absolute zero* is the cessation of molecular kinetic activity (all molecules have come to a complete rest). Based on that calculation, he devised a method of conversion between the Celsius and Kelvin scales by adding 273 degrees to the Celsius value (°K = 273° + °C).

This is the succession of events that transpires when a substance is heated. As any substance is brought above absolute zero in temperature, its molecules begin to move. When a substance is still in its solid form, the molecules simply vibrate. As they gain more heat, their kinetic activity increases, and therefore their vibrational energy increases proportionally. At the melting point of a solid, the kinetic activity is high enough for the molecules to break free from their own mass attraction sufficiently to escape and to travel at random within the space of their containing vessel. The substance is now considered to be in the liquid state (Fig. 1-2). The *melting point* can be defined as *the temperature at which transition occurs from a solid to a liquid state*. The *freezing point* of that same substance would occur at the same temperature, but the transition would be in the reverse

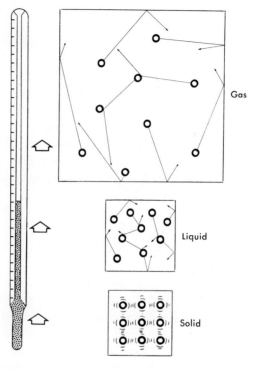

Fig. 1-1. Increased molecular heat causes increase in molecular motion and force. Result is tendency to expand and change to more fluidlike state of matter. Solid will change to liquid and liquid to gas as heat and molecular motion increase.

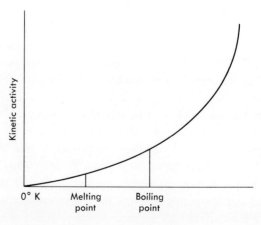

Fig. 1-2. As heat content of molecules increases above absolute zero, they start to move. When heat is sufficient to cause enough vibrational motion that molecules break free from each other, they change to liquid state. That temperature is *melting point.* As heat content increases further, molecules can gain enough force that they break free and travel around as individual gas molecules. That temperature at atmospheric pressure is considered *boiling point.*

fashion. As the temperature of the substance increases further, the molecules of the liquid gain more and more kinetic activity and then travel around more freely and exert more force. Ultimately they reach a point at which they can break free from the attraction of the liquid. At this point in temperature, the molecules all begin to convert to a gas (Fig. 1-2). That temperature at atmospheric pressure is considered to be its boiling point. The *boiling point* can be defined as *that point at which a transition occurs between a liquid and gaseous state at atmospheric pressure*. As substances change states of matter, there is progressively more noticeable expansion involved than is evident by merely heating the substance in the previous state. Thus the expansion appreciated when a substance changes from a solid to a liquid increases by a definitely smaller expansion factor than when that same substance converts from liquid to a gas (Fig. 1-1). For example, oxygen increases its volume 862 times as it converts from a liquid state to its gaseous state at room temperature.

Every substance known to exist has its own melting and boiling points. Table 1-1 lists some common examples.

Under certain conditions, molecules can completely bypass the liquid state. As the heat content increases and the molecules vibrate more vigorously, they may break loose below the melting point and then become free gas molecules. This process is called *sublimation* (Fig. 1-3). Solid carbon dioxide (dry ice) is the most common example of this process.

Table 1-1. Melting and boiling points and critical temperatures and pressures of gases common in respiratory therapy

Substance	Melting point	Boiling point at 1 atm	Critical temperature	Critical pressure	State at room temperature
Oxygen	−218.4° C −361.1° F	−182.96° C −297.4° F	−118.4° C −181.9° F	715.87 psig*	Gas
Nitrogen	−209.86° C −345.7° F	−195.80° C −320.36° F	−147.0° C −232.87° F	477.50 psig	Gas
Carbon dioxide	−78.4° C −108.4° F (Sublimation)	−78.4° C −108.4° F (Sublimation)	31.0° C 87.8° F	1057.4 psig	Liquid (and vapor)
Helium	272.1° F	−268.9° C −452.1° F	−267.9° C −450.3° F	18.5 psig	Gas
Hydrogen	−259.14° C −434.2° F	−252.78° C −423.0° F	−239.9° C −399.9° F	176.1 psig	Gas
Cyclopropane	−127.22° C −197.7° F	−32.694° C −27.15° F	124.7° C 256.0° F	780.3 psig	Liquid (and vapor)
Ethylene	−168.89° C −272.9° F	103.3° C −154.8° F	9.44° C 49.0° F	730.3 psig	Gas
Nitrous oxide	−90.8° C −131.3° F	−88.5° C −127.3° F	36.11° C 97.7° F	1039.3 psig	Liquid (and vapor)
Water	0° C 32.0° F	100.0° C 212.0° F	705.2° F 374.1° C	5484.5 psig	Liquid (and vapor)

*Pounds per square inch gauge.

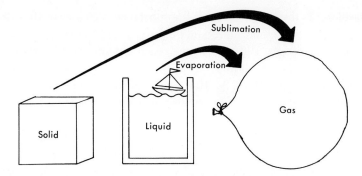

Fig. 1-3. Occasionally a molecule from a solid may vibrate loose and become a free vapor molecule. That process is called *sublimation.* Molecules of a liquid may become free vapor molecules below boiling point as they hit liquid surface. That is called *evaporation.*

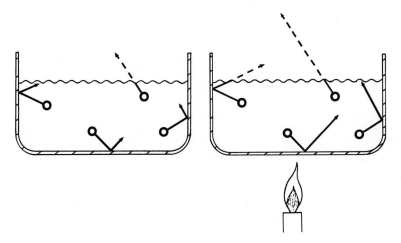

Fig. 1-4. As liquid molecules are heated, their velocity increases. They then hit surface more often and with more inertia, which increases their force and frequency of their escape as a vapor.

Occasionally some molecules of substances can break through the surface of the liquid and convert to free gaseous molecules below the boiling point. This phenomenon is called *evaporation* (Fig. 1-3) and is commonly seen in simple humidifying devices. The frequency with which this occurs is directly dependent on the liquid's temperature. The higher its temperature, the more force is exerted when the molecules hit the liquid's surface; therefore the molecules are more likely to escape. A measure of this force is called *vapor pressure.* It is that pressure which the molecules of the liquid exert as they hit the surface and escape. Vapor pressure increases with temperature as molecular velocity (force) increases (Fig. 1-4). The humidity content possible for a gas increases with a rise in its temperature. As the water molecules in the liquid state gain more velocity as their temperature increases, then they exert more force at the liquid surface, and more of them escape. Therefore more molecules of gaseous water (humidity) are present in the gas above the water's surface.

The forces opposing the molecule's escape are (1) mass attraction of the molecules for each other and (2) the pressure of the gas above the liquid's surface. A

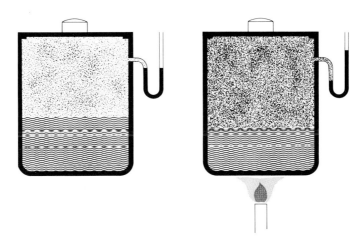

Fig. 1-5. Increased temperature causes liquid molecules to escape (evaporate) with more force. Once force is counterbalanced by gas and vapor pressure force above liquid surface, equilbrium exists, and no more liquid molecules can escape until a gas molecule returns to liquid. This pressure increase is related to vapor pressure or force with which liquid molecules escape to gas.

rise in temperature increases the velocity and force of the molecules hitting each other and moves them farther apart. The mass attraction is then decreased because of the increased distance between the molecules (Fig. 1-1). Therefore the molecules escape more easily and more frequently with a temperature rise. If the gas pressure above the liquid decreases, there is less opposing force for the molecules to escape, and they will do so more easily (Fig. 1-4). This concept explains why the boiling point of water, for example, is lower on Mt. Everest than at sea level; this occurs because the barometric pressure is lower, and the force (pressure) opposing the escape of molecules is decreased. If a liquid can be kept in a closed container, the force of the molecules trying to escape from the liquid will eventually reach an equilibrium with the water vapor pressure, and no more liquid molecules will escape (Fig. 1-5). In other words, the force of the molecules in the liquid is not sufficient to break loose from an increased opposing force resulting from the increased vapor pressure. Now, one water vapor molecule must accidentally hit the surface of the water and return to a liquid state before another liquid molecule can escape to become a gas or vapor molecule. So the forces of molecular mass attraction plus gas pressure and vapor pressure are in equilibrium. However, as the temperature of the liquid increases, the force of its molecules increases, resulting in reduced mass attraction. The vapor pressure, in turn, increases as a higher opposing force is necessary to equilibrate the molecules' escape from the liquid state. At its boiling point, the force of the molecules in the liquid equals the surrounding vapor pressure (atmospheric), and they may all escape. So, in essence, boiling point is that temperature at which the force exerted by the molecules of the liquid trying to escape equals the forces opposing escape (atmospheric pressure and mass attraction). As gas molecules are heated above the boiling point, their force increases, and the force (pressure) required to convert them back to a liquid also increases (Fig. 1-6).

Ultimately, a point would be reached at which the gaseous molecules could not be converted back to a liquid no matter what pressure was exerted on them. That

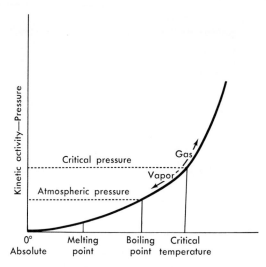

Fig. 1-6. Example of temperature and pressure effects on changes of states of matter of a substance.

point would be considered critical temperature. *Critical temperature* could be defined as the temperature above which a gas cannot be converted to liquid at any applied pressure. The pressure required to convert a gas back into a liquid at its critical temperature is called its *critical pressure*. Besides the boiling point and critical temperature, the pressure exerted on the gas is also a critical factor in deciding whether the majority of molelcules will remain as a gas or convert back to a liquid. In essence, a high enough pressure at a given point somewhere between the critical temperature and boiling point can be reached to overcome the kinetic activity of the gas molecules sufficiently to convert them back into the liquid state. Therefore as the temperature of a substance rises above its boiling point toward its critical temperature, the pressure necessary to change it to a liquid increases proportionally. Then, finally, as the gas passes its critical temperature, no amount of pressure is sufficient due to the heat content and the kinetic activity of the gas molecules to convert it back into a liquid.

As a technical point, there is a basic difference between the terms *gas* and *vapor*. Gas is above its critical temperature. Therefore, a true gas cannot be converted back to a liquid with any given amount of pressure, but a vapor can.

Throughout history, several leading men of their time contributed significant information that, in total, contributed to the kinetic theory of gases. Among these were Robert Boyle, Jacques Charles, Joseph Gay-Lussac, John Dalton, Thomas Graham, Amedeo Avogadro, and others.[1] Any gas that fits this theory is considered to be an ideal gas.[1] Although the gases used in respiratory therapy are real and not ideal gases and deviate to certain degrees from the theory, the concept is one that should be well understood. The composite of ideas of these men and the kinetic theory, therefore, consider the behavior of gases by making several points.

First, gases are composed of small molecules. *The space between these molecules is large in comparison to their diameter.* On the average, the distance between molecules is approximately 300 times that of their own diameter.[1]

The second point of the theory is that *molecules of a gas are in constant and random motion.*[1] They travel in straight lines until they collide with something

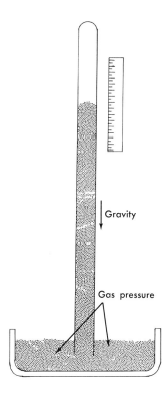

Gravity

Gas pressure

Fig. 1-7. Liquid barometer opposes forces of gas pressure exerted on liquid surface with that of gravity, forcing liquid in column downward. Equilibrium is reached, and then fluctuations in one force, such as increased gas pressure, will be reflected on the other force (by rise in liquid level) so that new equilibrium of force is reached.

else: another molecule, the side of a container, or any object in their path. At that point, they rebound off that article and resume a straight, free path.

The third point is that *molecular collisions are completely elastic in nature.*[1] Molecules do not gain or lose force with collisions. In essence, what happens is that the charges of the electrons and their outer shells, both being negative, repel each other in the same way as the like poles of a magnet, and the molecules never really hit each other.

The fourth point of the kinetic theory is that *kinetic energy, or kinetic activity, increases in direct proportion to the molecules' temperature* (absolute or Kelvin) as mentioned earlier.[1]

The fifth and final point is that *molecules of an ideal gas do not attract or repel* each other but travel freely around.[1]

GAS PRESSURE MEASUREMENT

The force of gas molecules hitting things because of their kinetic activity causes gas pressure. There are various types of apparatus utilized to measure gas pressure. Examples are the mercury and aneroid barometers. They basically form some type of equilibration of forces between the molecular gas pressure force and a mechanical or weight force. The mercury barometer utilizes the weight of a column of mercury to equilibrate with the kinetic activity (force) of the molecules hitting the surface of a mercury reservoir (Fig. 1-7). A column is completely filled with mercury and erected with its open end below the surface in the mercury reservoir. The mercury in the column attempts to return to the reservoir due to gravity, but the reservoir has submitted on it the force of gas molecules hitting its surface. The gas molecules' force pushes the mercury up the column from the reservoir. When the force of gravity on the weight of mercury in the column equals the gas pressure force, equilibrium exists and the gas pressure can be measured. This pressure is measured by (1) height of the mercury column (mm Hg), or (2) the dimensions of the column of mercury could be utilized to calculate the gas pressure force in terms of weight per area such as grams per square centimeter.

An aneroid barometer equilibrates gas pressure force with mechanical force or the expansion force of an evacuated metal container (Fig. 1-8).

An increase in the atmospheric gas pressure on the surface of the metal container tends to compress it. The change in the container's dimensions is recorded by means of the gearing mechanism, which changes an indicator's location on a recording dial. Likewise, a reduction of gas force surrounding the container allows the metal container to re-expand toward its normal shape.

Pressure is defined as force per unit area, and there are various ways of measuring this force. One way is that force can be recorded in a form of the height of a column as in the mercury barometer; therefore it can be recorded in millimeters of mercury pressure or centimeters of water pressure. The force could also be weight per unit area such as pounds per square inch, grams per square centimeter, etc.

The *Bourdon gauge* is another mechanism measuring this pressure. It consists of a coiled tube and a gear mechanism on which an indicator is attached (Fig. 1-9). As the gas pressure within the Bourdon tube increases, its force is exerted on the top of the inside of the tube to a larger degree due to the larger surface area there. This increasing pressure tends to straighten the tube, causing the indicator to rotate to a new location on a dial due to a gearing mechanism.

All of the following are equal in terms of force measured:

$$
\begin{aligned}
1 \text{ atm} &= 760 \text{ mm Hg} \\
&= 29.921 \text{ in Hg} \\
&= 33.93 \text{ ft } H_2O \\
&= 1034 \text{ cm } H_2O \\
&= 1034 \text{ gm/cm}^2 \\
&= 14.7 \text{ lb/in}^2
\end{aligned}
$$

The following conversion factors provide a mechanism to convert from one set of values to another. They can be obtained by dividing one value at atmospheric pressure by another, for example:

$$\frac{1034 \text{ cm } H_2O}{760 \text{ mm Hg}} = 1.36 \text{ cm } H_2O/\text{mm Hg}$$

$$1 \text{ mm Hg} = 1.36 \text{ cm } H_2O = 0.019 \text{ lb/in}^2$$

$$1 \text{ cm } H_2O = 0.0142 \text{ lb/in}^2 = 0.735 \text{ mm Hg}$$

$$1 \text{ lb/in}^2 = 51.70 \text{ mm Hg} = 70.34 \text{ cm } H_2O$$

Two factors used to convert from one pressure to another should be memorized by respiratory therapists. The first is *1.36 cm of water pressure for each millimeter of mercury*. That same numerical value can be utilized to convert from millimeters of mercury to centimeters of water or vice versa. If one needs to know how many centimeters of water pressure are equivalent to x number of millimeters of mercury,

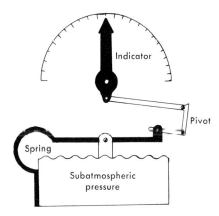

Fig. 1-8. Aneroid barometer opposes pliable strength of evacuated metal box with gas pressure. As gas pressure increases, box is forced to contract. Spring is pulled down, causing lever to pivot and move indicator to higher value on scale.

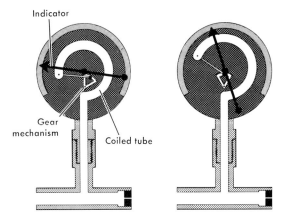

Fig. 1-9. As increase in gas pressure is transmitted up coiled, flattened Bourdon tube, it tends to straighten (rise) due to surface area on outer side of coiled tube being larger than on inside. Tube straightens and rises, causing gearing mechanism to rotate indicator to higher point on gauge.

then using the factor 1.36 times x will reveal that value. If the conversion is from centimeters of water pressure to millimeters of mercury, then the answer is obtained by simply dividing the number of centimeters of water pressure by 1.36:

EXAMPLE:

$$20 \text{ mm Hg} \times 1.36 \text{ cm H}_2\text{O/mm Hg} = 27.2 \text{ cm H}_2\text{O}$$
$$27.2 \text{ cm H}_2\text{O} \div 1.36 \text{ cm H}_2\text{O} = 20 \text{ mm Hg}$$

The other numerical conversion value is *70.34 cm of water pressure per pound per square inch*. Conversion from one unit of measurement to the other can be accomplished in the same fashion as just described:

EXAMPLE:

$$0.5 \text{ psi} \times 70.34 \text{ cm H}_2\text{O/psi} = 35.17 \text{ cm H}_2\text{O}$$
$$35.17 \text{ cm H}_2\text{O} \div 70.34 \text{ cm H}_2\text{O/psi} = 0.5 \text{ psi}$$

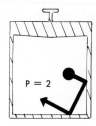

Fig. 1-10. Gas molecules hitting surface exert force measured as gas pressure. This molecule hits sides twice, exerting abstract pressure of 2.

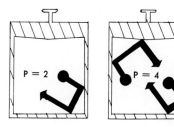

Fig. 1-11. If second gas molecule is added to container, *right*, both molecules hit twice, exerting total pressure of 4.

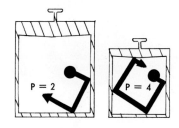

Fig. 1-12. If volume of container is reduced to half, *right*, gas molecule needs to travel only half as far to hit sides; therefore it must hit twice as often to exert pressure of 4.

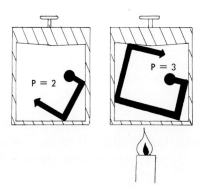

Fig. 1-13. Increased heat content of gas molecule increases velocity, making it hit more times and exert pressure of 3.

CHARACTERISTICS OF GASES

As a gas molecule hits something, it exerts a force. Described previously was the method of measuring that force in terms of gas pressure. Assume that each time a gas molecule hits something, such as the side of a container, it exerts a pressure of 1, using an abstract value for pressure. In the first example shown in Fig. 1-10, the gas molecule collides twice; therefore the pressure of the gas on that container is 2. If another gas molecule is placed in that container and they each hit the container twice, then the total gas pressure exerted on the container will be 4

(Fig. 1-11). Referring back to the original example in which the one gas molecule hits twice, the volume of the container is decreased to half. The gas molecule now has only half as far to travel before it hits something, in this case, the sides of the container (Fig. 1-12). Therefore in the same amount of time or in the same amount of distance traveled, the gas molecule will now hit four times, exerting a gas pressure of 4, double the previous value. Looking back to the original example again of the gas molecule hitting twice and exerting the pressure of two, heat is now added (Fig. 1-13). Since the molecule is now at a higher temperature, it will possess a higher kinetic activity, thus traveling at a higher velocity. It will travel further, therefore, in a given amount of time, and in this example it will hit the container three times rather than twice as it did before heat was added. Therefore the gas pressure was raised to 3 by increasing the molecular speed.

GAS LAWS

The phenomena just described were first observed, described, and recorded by several men and are now considered to be gas laws. Robert Boyle was among the first to do this. He described the relationship between volume and pressure in his paper "The Spring of Air" in 1660.[2] *Boyle's law* can be described as follows: "If the temperature and mass remain constant, the volume of the gas varies inversely with its pressure." The symbol for Boyle's law is, therefore, simply PV. In the example described previously, the gas molecule hit the sides of the container twice and exerted the pressure of 2. By decreasing the volume to half, the molecule traveled less distance before it collided with the sides of the container. The molecule then hit four times (as in Fig. 1-12), and the pressure increased to four. Therefore, when the volume was decreased to half, the result was twice the pressure. This example simplified the application of what Boyle discovered. Utilization of Boyle's law in calculations can be accomplished by the equation $P_1V_1 = P_2V_2$. As an example of applying this equation, given 1000 cc of a gas at one atmosphere of pressure, what is the new volume if subjected to two atmospheres of pressure? The problem would be computed as follows:

$$P_1V_1 = P_2V_2$$

$$V_2 = \frac{P_1V_1}{P_2}$$

$$V_2 = \frac{(1 \text{ atm}) (1000 \text{ cc})}{2 \text{ atm}}$$

$$V_2 = \frac{1000}{2}$$

$$V_2 = 500 \text{ cc}$$

Another example that fits into everyday clinical use would be finding the volume difference, per unit of pressure change, within a closed container. This problem involves setting up some known values. Assume that the first pressure (P_1), atmospheric pressure, is defined in terms of centimeters of water pressure; P_1, therefore, would be 1034 cm H_2O pressure. One unit of pressure change would be equal to 1034 cm H_2O pressure + 1 cm H_2O pressure, or 1035 cm H_2O pressure (P_2). If V_1 is specified as 1000 cc, the problem can then be set up in this fashion:

GIVEN: 1000 cc of a gas at 1034 cm of water pressure

FIND: Volume 2 as the pressure is increased to 1035 cm of water pressure

$$P_1V_1 = P_2V_2$$

$$V_2 = \frac{P_1V_1}{P_2}$$

$$V_2 = \frac{(1034 \text{ cm } H_2O \text{ pressure}) (1000 \text{ cc})}{1035 \text{ cm } H_2O \text{ pressure}}$$

$$V_2 = \frac{1,034,000}{1035}$$

$$V_2 = 999.03 \text{ cc}$$

$$V_2 \cong 999 \text{ cc}$$

The above calculation determined that V_2 is 999 cc. If that value is subtracted from V_1, the volume change can be determined:

$$1000 \text{ cc} - 999 \text{ cc} = 1 \text{ cc}$$

The pressure change or the differences between P_1 and P_2 are as defined:

$$1035 \text{ cm } H_2O \text{ pressure} - 1034 \text{ cm } H_2O = 1 \text{ cm } H_2O \text{ pressure}$$

The base volume utilized in the equation was 1 liter (1000 cc). Therefore the volume change per unit of pressure change was:

$$1 \text{ cc/L/cm } H_2O \text{ pressure}$$

This calculation finds practical application in the use of volume ventilators. *Tubing compliance* is, basically, a combination of (1) circuitry volume or the gas's compressibility with it (as just calculated) and (2) the elasticity of the tubing. Tubing elasticity is a minor factor in comparison to that of compressibility. Normally, the *compression factor* or tubing compliance factor for volume ventilators is reasonably close to the actual volume of their circuitry. Therefore, there will be a 1 cc/cm H_2O per liter of circuitry volume pressure change (compression factor), as just cal-

Table 1-2. Pressure-volume conversion factors*

Cylinder size	Conversion factor
E	$\dfrac{622.0 \text{ liters}}{2200 \text{ psi}} = 0.28 \cong 0.3$
G	$\dfrac{5260.0 \text{ liters}}{2200 \text{ psi}} = 2.39 \cong 2.4$
H-K	$\dfrac{6600.0 \text{ liters}}{2200 \text{ psi}} = 3.0 = 3.0$

*Boyle's law indicates the relationship between pressure and volume. Pressure-volume conversion factors for the various sizes of cylinders are obtained simply by dividing the full contents volume by its full pressure to get a volume factor per pressure (liters per psig). As an example, E cylinders are filled to a standard filling pressure of 2200 psig, at which 622 liters of gas have been pumped into them. If the cylinder pressure is divided into the volume contained, the conversion factor can be found as volume per pressure (liters per psig). For example:

$$\frac{622 \text{ liters}}{2200 \text{ psig}} = 0.28 \cong 0.3 \text{ L/psig}$$

culated above. If a ventilator had 3 liters of volume in its circuitry, it would have a compressibility factor of approximately 3 cc/cm H_2O.

Other calculations based on Boyle's law that find use clinically are the pressure-volume conversion factors for gas cylinders of different sizes, found in Table 1-2.

The French mathematician and physicist, Jacques Charles, described the expansion of gas in 1778.[2] This later became known as *Charles' law*. His law can be described as follows: "If the pressure and mass remain constant, the volume of a gas varies directly with the changes in absolute (Kelvin) temperature." The symbol for Charles' law can be expressed as V/T. Referring back to the previous basic example of a gas molecule hitting the sides of a container twice and exerting a pressure of 2, the container is made out of a flexible substance that has the ability to expand. Heat applied to the container causes the temperature within to increase, and the increased force of the gas molecule causes the container itself to expand. Therefore, even though the gas molecule is traveling faster, it now has to travel farther to hit the sides of the container. It hits only twice and exerts a pressure of 2 (Fig. 1-14). Calculations utilizing Charles' law can be accomplished by the formula:

$$\frac{V_1}{T_1} = \frac{V_2}{T_2}$$

An example of utilizing that formula: Given 1000 cc of gas at 27° C, what temperature would be required for that gas to occupy a 500 cc volume? The problem would be set up as follows:

$$\frac{V_1}{T_1} = \frac{V_2}{T_2}$$

$$T_2 = \frac{T_1 V_2}{V_1}$$

$$T_2 = \frac{(27° + 273°)\,(500 \text{ cc})}{1000 \text{ cc}} = \frac{150,000}{1000} = 150° \text{ K}$$

$$T_2 = 150° \text{ K} - 273° = -123° \text{ C}$$

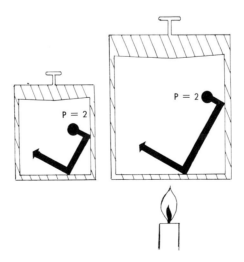

Fig. 1-14. If container is able to expand, increased velocity and force of gas molecule due to increased heat would enlarge container, and gas molecule's pressure would be maintained at 2.

An important factor in calculations involving temperatures of gases is the conversion of degrees of Celsius (centigrade) to Kelvin or Fahrenheit to Rankin. This is done by *adding 273° to Celsius values to obtain Kelvin scale* and by *adding 460° to Fahrenheit values to obtain Rankin temperatures.* At the end of the calculation, the temperature is converted back to its previous scale by subtracting the appropriate conversion number.

An example that is applicable to clinical situations: Given 1000 cc of a gas at room temperature (72° F), what volume would it occupy at body temperature (99° F)? Setting up the equation would be as follows:

$$\frac{V_1}{T_1} = \frac{V_2}{T_2}$$

$$V_2 = \frac{V_1 T_2}{T_1} = \frac{(1000 \text{ cc}) (99° + 460°)}{72° + 460°} = \frac{(1000) (559°)}{532}$$

$$\frac{559,000}{532} = 1050.75 \text{ cc}$$

(Volume change = $V_2 - V_1$ = 1050.75 − 1000 cc = 50.75 cc)

From this calculation, it is easily noted that the expansion of the gas, owing to the temperature change, actually resulted in an increase in volume of 50.75 cc. This would be similar to the expansion that occurs when a gas at room temperature is delivered from a volume ventilator to a patient. One could take this calculation one step further beyond the volume change noted and simply divide the temperature change into the volume change to obtain a factor:

$$\frac{50.75 \text{ cc}}{99° - 72°} = \frac{50.75}{27°} = 1.88 \text{ cc/° F/L}$$

Therefore for each degree Fahrenheit rise in temperature, one can expect each liter of gas to expand 1.88 cc.

Charles went on to describe more about gas characteristics, but the real credit for explaining the relationship of pressure and temperature of a gas goes to Joseph Louis Gay-Lussac. He reported his law in 1809, although even he admitted that Charles actually described it first.[1] This became known as *Gay-Lussac's law* and can be described as follows: "If the volume and mass remain constant, the pressure exerted by gas varies directly with the absolute (Kelvin) temperature." The symbol for Gay-Lussac's law can be expressed as P/T. By returning again to the simple example utilized in the study of characteristics of gases, the gas molecule hits the container twice and exerts a pressure of 2. By the addition of heat, the velocity and kinetic activity of the gas molecule increases, the molecules hit more often, and in this case, exert a gas pressure of 3 (Fig. 1-15). Therefore as the temperature of the gas is increased, its pressure increases as well. Calculations based on Gay-Lussac's law can be accomplished by the utilization of the equation

$$\frac{P_1}{T_1} = \frac{P_2}{T_2}$$

A practical example in respiratory therapy: Given a cylinder with a pressure of 2400 psig at 70° F, what would the content's pressure be if that cylinder were warmed to 110° F? Calculations would be as follows.

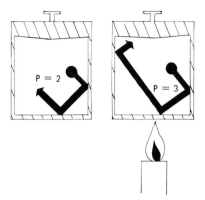

Fig. 1-15. Increased heat content of gas molecule increases its velocity, making it hit more times and exert pressure of 3.

$$\frac{P_1}{T_1} = \frac{P_2}{T_2}$$

$$P_2 = \frac{P_1T_2}{T_1}$$

$$P_2 = \frac{(2400 \text{ psig})(110° + 460°)}{(70° + 460°)} = \frac{1,368,000}{530} = 2581.13 \text{ psig}$$

The three gas laws just described can be consolidated into a *combined gas law*. That could be expressed simply by the symbol PV/T. Derived from the combined gas law is the *universal gas law* equation,

$$\frac{P_1V_1}{T_1} = \frac{P_2V_2}{T_2}$$

Its algebraic derivatives are as follows:

$$P_2 = \frac{P_1V_1T_2}{V_2T_1}$$

$$V_2 = \frac{P_1V_1T_2}{P_2T_1}$$

$$T_2 = \frac{P_2V_2T_1}{P_1V_1}$$

The use of the universal gas law equation requires that pressure and volume units remain constant throughout the equation and that temperature values be converted to their absolute counterparts. An example of utilization of this equation: Given 100 ml of dry gas, measuring 37° C and 760 mm Hg pressure, what would its volume be at 60° C and 800 mm Hg pressure? The calculation would be as follows:

$V_1 = 100$ ml $\qquad\qquad$ $V_2 = ?$

$P_1 = 760$ mm Hg $\qquad\qquad$ $P_2 = 800$ mm Hg

$T_1 = 37° + 273° = 310°$ K $\qquad\qquad$ $T_2 = 60° + 273° = 333°$ K

$$V_2 = \frac{V_1 P_1 T_1}{P_2 T_1}$$

$$V_2 = \frac{100 \text{ cc} \times 760 \text{ mm Hg} \times 333° \text{ K}}{800 \text{ mm Hg} \times 310° \text{ K}}$$

$$V_2 = \frac{25,308,000}{248,000}$$

$$V_2 = 102 \text{ ml}$$

John Dalton, in 1802, described in one of his papers certain information that is now considered *Dalton's law of partial pressure.* His law can be best described as follows[2]:

1. The total pressure of a gaseous mixture is equal to the sum of the partial pressures of the constituent gases.
2. The partial pressure of each gas in the mixture is the pressure it would exert if it occupied the entire volume alone.
3. The partial pressure exerted by each constituent gas is proportional to its volumetric percentage of the mixture.

As an example of Dalton's law, if ten gas molecules were within a confined space and each hit the container once, they would exert a total gas pressure of 10. If two of those molecules were oxygen and the other eight were nitrogen, then their effect could be analyzed in terms of pressure (Fig. 1-16). First, if the two oxygen molecules were removed from the gas mixture, the pressure would drop to 8. There would now be only eight molecules remaining, each hitting the side of the container once. If the two oxygen molecules were placed in that same volume by themselves, each would only collide once and exert a total pressure of 2. Their partial pressure is, in essence, the same as their percentages in the mixture multiplied by the total gas pressure. For example, oxygen makes up 2/10 or 20% of the gas mixture; 20% of the total pressure of 10 is 2. A practical example of Dalton's law is as follows: Oxygen

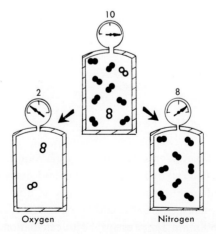

Fig. 1-16. In top container, ten molecules (two oxygen and eight nitrogen) are responsible for exerting total pressure of 10. If constituent gases are segregated into containers of equal volume, individually they exert pressure equivalent to their percentage of total (that is, 20% of 10 = 2 and 80% of 10 = 8). (Modified from McIntosh, R., Epstein, H. G., and Mushin, W.: Physics for the anaesthetist, Oxford, England, 1968, Blackwell Scientific Publications, Ltd.)

makes up approximately 20.95% of the atmosphere. If that percentage is multiplied by the total atmospheric barometric pressure, the partial pressure that oxygen exerts in the environment could be found:

$$760 \text{ mm Hg pressure} \times 0.2095 = 159 \text{ mm Hg pressure}$$

This value, 159 mm Hg, would be the partial pressure of oxygen at sea level. A derivative of Dalton's law can be utilized to calculate alveolar gas partial pressures. The equation, in a simplified, clinically useful form, would be

$$P_{AO_2} = (P_B - P_{H_2O}) F_{IO_2} - \frac{P_{aCO_2}}{0.8}$$

where P_B is barometric pressure. Utilization of this equation to calculate normal alveolar P_{O_2} for a normal individual at sea level breathing room air would be

$$P_{AO_2} = [(P_B - P_{H_2O}) F_{IO_2}] - \frac{P_{aCO_2}}{0.8}$$

$$P_{AO_2} = [(760 \text{ mm Hg} - 47 \text{ mm Hg}) 0.2095] - \frac{40 \text{ mm Hg}}{0.8}$$

$$P_{AO_2} = (713)(0.2095) - 50$$

$$P_{AO_2} = 149 - 50$$

$$P_{AO_2} = 99 \text{ mm Hg}$$

where

$$
\begin{aligned}
P_{AO_2} &- \text{Partial pressure of alveolar oxygen} \\
P_{H_2O} &= \text{Partial pressure of water vapor in the} \\
&\quad \text{respiratory tract} \\
F_{IO_2} &= \text{Fraction of inspired oxygen} \\
P_{aCO_2} &= \text{Partial pressure of arterial carbon dioxide} \\
0.8 &= \text{Respiratory exchange ratio}
\end{aligned}
$$

To calculate values for other (1) inspired oxygen concentrations, (2) barometric pressures, and (3) P_{CO_2}'s, their values can simply be substituted into the same equation.

DIFFUSION

Diffusion of gas plays a major role in respiratory therapy. Diffusion of gases is actually an intermolecular mingling that occurs within fluids.[3] Diffusion can be classified into two types: (1) that which occurs in a gaseous medium and (2) that of gas molecules in a liquid medium. In terms of equipment, the category most commonly found is that of diffusion in a gaseous medium.

Diffusion can be defined as an intermolecular mingling that occurs as a result of fluid molecules randomly bouncing off each other, producing a homogeneous mixture. This occurs as the result of the previously discussed phenomenon of the gas molecules traveling in random paths, rebounding off objects or themselves with complete elastic recoil with no energy loss. Ultimately, if there is a high concentration of gases in one area, simple diffusion occurs as a result of their rebounding off each other, and the mixture finally contains uniform levels of all gas molecules at any point within the container (Fig. 1-17).

Fick's law describes the rate of gaseous diffusion in terms of a concentration

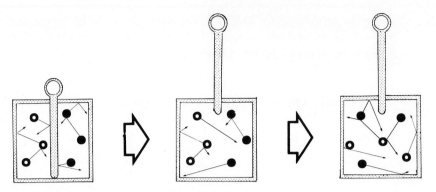

Fig. 1-17. Diffusion is intermolecular mingling that results from gas molecules colliding and pushing each other around until homogeneous mixture results. This is shown here starting at left and moving toward right.

gradient.[3] The law states that *the rate of the diffusion of gases in a gaseous medium is proportional to the gradient of their concentration.* Therefore the higher the concentration gradient from one area to another, the faster the gases will diffuse (Fig. 1-18). Calculation of gas diffusibility in a gaseous medium is rare clinically, although the mechanisms involved are important. Some common examples of diffusibility are (1) helium diffusing through porous substances, such as disposable masks, or (2) diffusion of carbon dioxide through tent canopies keeping its content to a minimum.

The diffusion of gases in a liquid medium requires other considerations. *Henry's law* describes the weight of a gas dissolving in a liquid.[4] His law reads as follows: *The weight of a gas dissolving in a liquid at a given temperature is proportional to the partial pressure of the gas.* In essence, the higher the partial pressure of the given gas, the more it will dissolve. Each gas has its own solubility coefficient, which is actually a measurement of the quantity of gas that will dissolve, per millimeter of mercury pressure, into a liquid. The solubility coefficient of oxygen is 0.023 ml/ml plasma at 37° C and 760 mm Hg, and the solubility coefficient of carbon dioxide is 0.510 mm/ml plasma at 37° C and 760 mm Hg. As noted, the solubility of carbon dioxide far exceeds that of oxygen. In fact, it is approximately nineteen times more soluble in plasma than oxygen. *Graham's law* takes Henry's law one step further; it states: *The rate of diffusion of a gas through a liquid medium is directly proportional to the solubility of the gas and inversely proportional to the square root of its density or its gram molecular weight.*[4] In essence, the more soluble a gas is, or the lower its density is, the more diffusible it is. The diffusibility of carbon dioxide is compared to that of oxygen as follows:

$$\text{Diffusibility of CO}_2 \cong \frac{\text{Sol coef CO}_2 \times \sqrt{\text{gmw O}_2}}{\text{Sol coef O}_2 \times \sqrt{\text{gmw CO}_2}}$$

$$\cong \frac{0.510 \times \sqrt{32}}{0.023 \times \sqrt{44}}$$

$$\cong \frac{0.510 \times 5.657}{0.023 \times 6.663}$$

$$\cong \frac{19}{1}$$

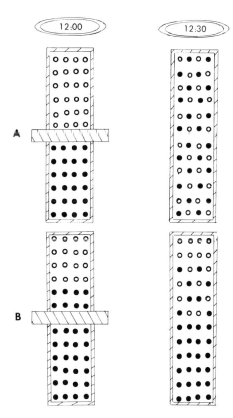

Fig. 1-18. Rate of diffusion. The higher the concentration gradient of gas is, the more rapidly diffusion occurs. In **A**, concentration gradient is higher, so diffusion occurs more quickly than in **B**.

The end product demonstrates that *carbon dioxide is nineteen times more diffusible in liquid medium than is oxygen*. The major factor concerned with the higher diffusion capability of carbon dioxide relates more specifically to the solubility of the gas. If solubility is removed as a factor, carbon dioxide's diffusibility would actually be slightly less than that of oxygen.

$$\text{Diffusibility of } CO_2 \cong \frac{\sqrt{\text{gmw } O_2}}{\sqrt{\text{gmw } CO_2}}$$

$$\cong \frac{\sqrt{32}}{\sqrt{44}}$$

$$\cong \frac{5.657}{6.663}$$

$$\cong 0.849$$

Although the diffusion of gases in a liquid medium deals more with the physiologic aspects of respiratory therapy than the equipment aspects, it needs to be well understood by the respiratory therapist.

GAS FLOW

The physics involved in gas flow are similar to those of diffusion. In diffusion, it was the molecules hitting each other that pushed them around the container until the mixture was evenly dispersed with constituent gases. Gas flow, on the other hand, is movement of a gas volume from one place to another in relation to time. This motion of gases is not of the individual molecular activity, but rather that of the whole group of molecules from one location to another (Fig. 1-19). *Gas flows from one place to another in response to a pressure gradient.* In essence, what occurs is that the gas molecules in the area of high pressure are closer together, hit each other more often, and, therefore, exert more force on each other. When there is a communicating path to an area of lower pressure (where the molecules are farther apart and exert less force on each other), the gas molecules simply flow or push each other out from the area of high force to the area of low force (Fig. 1-20).

In considering the flow of gases with the use of respiratory therapy equipment, there are two factors of concern relating to the flow of a given gas. The first factor is that of the *pressure gradient* itself. The higher the pressure gradient, the higher the flow across a set size opening or restriction. Fig. 1-21 indicates such a situation. In the first illustration there is a pressure of 2 on one side and a second pressure of 0 on the other. The second example shows a pressure of 4 on one side of an orifice and 0 on the other. In both examples, the orifice is the same. The pressure gradient was doubled in the last example; therefore the flow was doubled also. A Bourdon regulator, described in Chapter 3, utilizes this principle.

The larger the port size between two different pressures (gradient), the higher the gas flow will be. An example of this is shown in Fig. 1-22. The pressure gradient in both examples is the same since the pressures are 2 and 0 on the two sides of each respective orifice. Flow in the first example is indicated by the symbol Y, and in the second example, where the orifice size is twice that of the first example, the flow is double. Thus the larger the area is through which the molecules can travel, the more molecules that can get through in a given amount of time. This *linear* relationship between pressure gradients and orifice size is not true for low-pressure systems, but concepts presented here for changing flows do apply. A clear understanding of the two mechanisms related to gas flow is extremely important, since many types of apparatus control flow by using one or both of those factors. A Thorpe tube flowmeter utilizes this principle.

Bernoulli described the flow of fluid through a tube, and one of his theorems later became known as *Bernoulli's principle.*[4] It is as follows: *As the forward velocity of a gas increases, its lateral pressure decreases with a corresponding increase in forward pressure.* The motion (flow) of the gas causes a transfer in the force that the molecules exert. Fig. 1-23 indicates a gas molecule contained within a small volume. The gas molecule travels around the container and hits all sides, exerting a total pressure of 5. This gas molecule is then released and allowed to flow through a tube. In this example, the gas flows first through a reasonably large tube and changes its direction of impact to a more forward one. The velocity of the molecule is still the same as in the container, but it now travels to the side or to the right through the tube with a higher relative forward speed than it does laterally. The result is that the molecule hits the sides of the tube less often than in the previous example, and the lateral pressure will drop. Similarly, the amount that the lateral pressure is decreased is transferred to the forward pressure, which rises proportionately. In the next example, the tube is narrowed even further. The gas molecule now travels at a higher

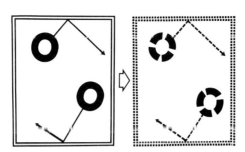

Fig. 1-19. Flow is movement of volume of gas to new location, usually based on time factor. Molecules retain their individual motion and group of molecules is relocated, as depicted by moving volume on left to its new position on right.

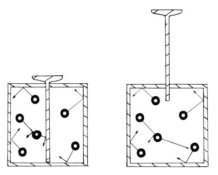

Fig. 1-20. Flow of gas results from difference in force (pressure) between one area and another. This is commonly referred to as *pressure gradient:* gas flows from area of high force (pressure) to area lower in force (pressure). Molecules in area of high pressure are closer together, exerting greater force on each other, and literally pushing each other to low-force area. In this example, high-force area is on left so that molecules are pushed to right.

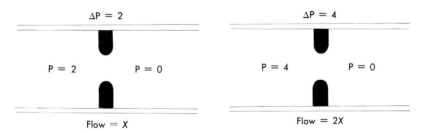

Fig. 1-21. Flow across orifice of fixed size is directly related to pressure gradient. Pressure gradient in bottom example is double that of top one, and flow is double as well.

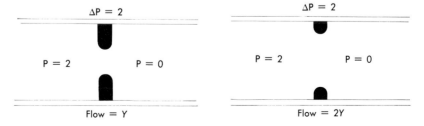

Fig. 1-22. At set pressure gradient, flow is directly related to orifice size. Bottom example has orifice twice as big as top, and flow is doubled as well.

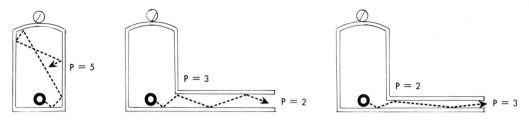

Fig. 1-23. Example of static and dynamic gas pressures (see text).

forward velocity than it did in the previous example, therefore hitting the sides of the tube less often than before. As a direct result, the lateral pressure drops even further, and the forward pressure increases in a corresponding manner.

Thus it is seen that as gas flow meets a restriction, the molecules must travel faster in a forward direction than they did previously. An analogy to this phenomenon would be an example of four lanes of traffic each containing cars traveling at 25 mph. If that highway narrowed to one lane, each car would have to travel four times as fast, or 100 mph, for them to all pass through in the same amount of time. This same phenomenon occurs with gases. More specifically, they alter the dispersion of their velocity so that it is higher in a forward direction than it is laterally. The kinetic activity of gas molecules normally disperses their speed of travel in all directions uniformly as the molecules rebound off each other. However, once they begin to flow, even though their individual velocity is still the same, it is directed toward the direction of flow and less toward other directions. This directional change occurs most significantly at a narrowing or restriction just as with the lane reduction from four to one in the example of cars.

Fig. 1-24, the *jet*, a device commonly found in numerous types of respiratory therapy apparatus, is an example of the application of Bernoulli's principle. As gas travels to the jet's restriction, there is an increase in its forward velocity as its lateral pressure drops. If the lateral pressure drops below atmospheric pressure, that device can then be utilized to entrain fluid. The fluid could be air, as in a simple oxygen/air dilution system, or it could be a liquid, as in a nebulizer. There are two factors that affect the degree of fluid uptake by a jet. They are (1) *jet orifice size* and (2) *the size of the entrainment ports*. Using the pressure before the jet, the smaller a jet is, the higher the forward velocity is of the gas passing through it. Therefore the lateral pressure will be lower. In response to the lowered lateral pressure, the pressure gradient that exists from the atmospheric surroundings to the subatmospheric pressure at the jet increases, and air entrainment (or liquid uptake in the case of a nebulizer) will be higher. If that device were powered by oxygen and used to entrain air, the total gas flow from the apparatus with a smaller jet would be higher than that of a similar unit using a larger jet because of the added volume of air entrained. In addition, the oxygen concentration would be lower (Fig. 1-25). The second factor is the size of the entrainment ports. At a set jet size, the pressure gradient from the surrounding atmospheric to lateral subatmospheric pressure near the jet would remain reasonably constant at a certain flow. The entrainment or fluid uptake could then be altered by changing the port size through which the entrained fluid will travel (Fig. 1-26). The larger the port size, the larger the quantity of fluid entrained.

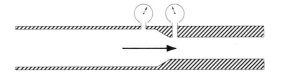

Fig. 1-24. As gas flow meets narrowing or restriction, direction of molecules changes to more forward, so that same number get through in given amount of time. As a result, they hit sides less frequently; therefore lateral pressure drops.

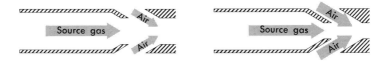

Fig. 1-25. *Right,* smaller restriction causes greater increase in forward velocity of gas, resulting in lower lateral pressure and larger quantity of air entrained through ports.

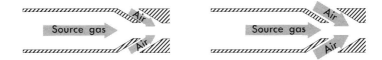

Fig. 1-26. Same orifice size in jet provides (1) same forward velocity, (2) same lateral subatmospheric pressure, and therefore, (3) same pressure gradient (atmospheric to subatmospheric) for air entrainment. Entrainment port size on right is larger, therefore, more air will be entrained at set pressure gradient.

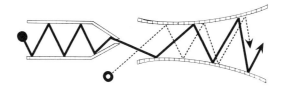

Fig. 1-27. Objective of Venturi tube is to allow entrainment, increasing flow, and to restore lateral pressure toward prerestriction pressure. In this example, molecules hit sides just as frequently before restriction as they do after entrainment in later portion of tube.

Also, if the air entrainment device were powered by oxygen, then the total gas flow from the apparatus would be increased, and the oxygen concentration would be lowered.

As flow through a jet increases, the forward velocity increases proportionally. In response to the increased forward velocity, the lateral pressure drops lower, entraining more air. As a result of increased jet oxygen flow, the entrainment of air increases proportionally, maintaining a constant oxygen delivery percentage.

Venturi described the addition of a tube to a jet (Bernoulli's principle) that could expand its versatility.[2] *Venturi's principle* is as follows: *The addition of a tube gradually increasing in diameter, not exceeding 15 degrees, in the direction of flow from the jet orifice will restore the lateral pressure of the gas toward prerestriction pressure.*[4] The advantage of using a tube of this nature is to attempt to restore the gas pressure, after fluid uptake, back toward its original lateral pressure before the restriction of the jet. As stated, this is accomplished by a tube that gradually increases in diameter (Fig. 1-27), which allows the gas to expand, slows down its forward

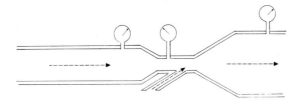

Fig. 1-28. Ideal Venturi restores lateral gas pressure to its prerestriction value after air entrainment, which increases total flow.

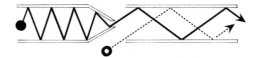

Fig. 1-29. Pitot tube is designed to maintain high forward velocity after air entrainment, therefore, to maintain high forward pressure.

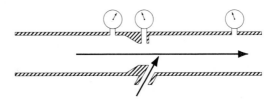

Fig. 1-30. By retaining high forward velocity and forward pressure after air entrainment, molecules of mixture comprised of source gas and entrained air hit side less frequently. Ideally, they exert low lateral pressure similar to that at restriction (jet) so that forward pressure is maximum.

velocity, and resumes an increased lateral pressure. Most Venturis are not totally effective in restoring gas pressure back to its prerestriction value, although some do an adequate job (Fig. 1-28). The advantages of a device of this nature would be for use in apparatus in which the end pressure from the unit is of ultimate importance, such as in ventilators. The total flow through the device can be increased by air entrainment, and by the addition of the Venturi tube to the jet, the lateral pressure can be restored.

Pitot tubes are finding more use in respiratory therapy apparatus. They were originally employed with flow-metering devices similar to those used in airplanes to estimate air speed. *The Pitot principle* is as follows: *An open-ended tube is faced in the direction of flow from the jet orifice so that the end pressure is equal to the total head pressure due to air velocity.* The Pitot tube design objective is the reverse of that of a venturi. Its objective is not to restore lateral pressure toward its prerestrictive value but rather *to maintain a high forward velocity;* therefore low lateral pressure will result. Fig. 1-29 indicates an example of a Pitot tube. Its design with a straight tube accommodates the increased volume of gas entrained and keeps the mixture of gases flowing forward at a velocity similar to that of the restriction velocity (Fig. 1-30). The advantages of this type of device is that any restrictions or resistance placed downstream from the unit will not alter fluid uptake as significantly as would happen with a Venturi. The Pitot tube is now finding increased use in the

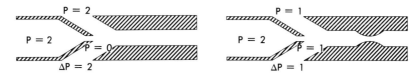

Fig. 1-31. Resistance to flow through jet, as in bottom example, causes backup of molecules behind restriction, called *back pressure*. Result is increase in lateral pressure at jet and reduction in pressure gradient (ΔP) for air entrainment.

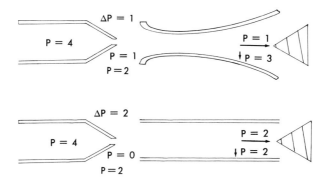

Fig. 1-32. Resistance to flow from Venturi is reflected back to jet, resulting in increase in lateral pressure at jet and reduced entrainment, *top*. Because of Pitot tube's design features, it is affected less by back pressure.

construction of nebulizers. Since the forward pressure is high from the tube, baffle placement can be close to acquire small particles without jeopardizing the quantity of air or liquid uptake. Another use of this unit is in oxygen entrainment devices in which there is moderate resistance downstream. Its function would be to decrease the effect of resistance and therefore stabilize alterations in oxygen concentration.

Resistance placed downstream to either a Venturi or Pitot tube acts to oppose the flow from them. The resistance causes the pressure to increase before this resistance area, causing a drop in the pressure gradient for gas to flow from the jet and out the tube (Fig. 1-31). *A Venturi's purpose is to entrain air and restore the delivered (lateral) pressure to a high value even though fluid entrainment may decrease with resistance* (as in ventilators). *A Pitot tube attempts to retain fluid entrainment at a high level and is not attempting to restore lateral pressure* (as in a nebulizer or entrainment device). A Pitot tube attempts to buffer the effect of resistance by absorbing the increased pressure within the tube. The altered pressure gradient is then between the tube and the resistance, rather than between the area after the jet and the tube as in the Venturi (Fig. 1-32). Therefore, when resistance is applied, the Venturi design delivers pressure with flow jeopardized, whereas a Pitot tube's design delivers flow at a compromise of pressure.

AVOGADRO'S LAW

Avogadro determined that *equal volumes of a gas at the same pressure and temperature contain the same number of molecules. Avogadro's number* was reported as being 6.02×10^{23} *molecules per gram molecular weight (gmw) of a gas at normal temperature and pressure.*[4] One gram molecular weight of a gas is its molecular weight multiplied by one gram. As an example, the molecular weight of oxygen is 32, and one gram molecular weight would be 32 grams. The molecular weight of nitrogen is 28, and one gram molecular weight of nitrogen would be 28 grams. Avogadro determined that *at normal temperature and pressure, one gram molecular weight of a gas occupies 22.4 liters.* Therefore one gram molecular weight of a gas contains 6.02×10^{23} molecules and occupies 22.4 liters. Loschmit determined that 2.68×10^{19} molecules of gas were present in a cubic centimeter of gas.[1]

Density of a gas is based on Avogadro's observations. Even though equal volumes of different gases contain the same number of molecules, their *mass* varies. An oxygen molecule is substantially heavier than a helium molecule, so oxygen weighs more or has more mass per volume than would helium. *Density* is simply *a measurement of mass per unit of volume.* The mass is normally reflected in the form of weight due to gravitational pull. Based on Avogadro's observations, a standard method of measuring gas densities would be utilizing the gram molecular weight and 22.4 liters (the volume a gram molecular weight occupies). If the gram molecular weight of a gas were simply divided by the volume 22.4 liters, the density could be determined in grams per liter.

EXAMPLE:

$$\text{Density (grams per liter)} = \frac{\text{Molecular weight}}{22.4 \text{ liters}}$$

Following are calculations of densities of some common gases:

$$\text{D } O_2 = \frac{\text{gmw}}{22.4} = \frac{32}{22.4} = 1.43 \text{ gm/L}$$

$$\text{D } N_2 = \frac{\text{gmw}}{22.4} = \frac{28}{22.4} = 1.25 \text{ gm/L}$$

$$\text{D He} = \frac{\text{gmw}}{22.4} = \frac{4}{22.4} = 0.1785 \text{ gm/L}$$

$$\text{D } CO_2 = \frac{\text{gmw}}{22.4} = \frac{44}{22.4} = 1.965 \text{ gm/L}$$

Specific gravity, on the other hand, is a *comparison of gas densities.* The objective is a comparison of one gas and density to all others. Usually specific gravities are calculated in terms of the density of oxygen, hydrogen, or air to obtain a specific gravity. For respiratory therapy, specific gravities based on that of air are probably the most useful. As an example, if the respiratory therapist would like to know how much lighter or heavier oxygen is than air, he or she can take the two densities of these gases and simply divide them. Using air as a base, its density can be divided into oxygen, and the abstract value obtained will indicate the weight or density of oxygen as compared to air (specific gravity, abbreviated *gr*).

EXAMPLE:

$$\text{Specific gravity of } O_2 = \frac{\text{Density of } O_2}{\text{Density of air}} = \frac{1.43 \text{ gr/L}}{1.28 \text{ gr/L}} = 1.12$$

The above calculation would indicate that the density or mass per volume of oxygen is approximately 112% of air's density. Therefore we would expect that a given volume of oxygen would weigh 112% as much as the same volume of air.

Viscosity is another factor important in terms of fluid motion. *Viscosity* is largely dependent on density but takes into account an additional factor not determined in density, which is *the frictional motion of a fluid.*[4] Water, for example, flows much more quickly than does blood because the frictional resistance to its flow is much less. *Temperature* is one factor of viscosity. The higher the temperature, the lower the viscosity. The common example of molasses in January gives an indication that at a low temperature, the viscosity due to the thickness of molasses is high, so it does not flow easily. If that same molasses were warmed up, such as in July, the viscosity would be much lower, and the molasses would flow much more easily. Other fluids, including gases, exhibit this same phenomenon. Temperature is just as major a factor on them as it is on any substance. In addition, viscosity of a gas most closely relates to its *density.* The higher the density a gas possesses, the higher its viscosity.

POISEUILLE'S LAW

Poiseuille stated the law that indicates the degree of resistance for fluid flow through a tube. His law is as follows: *The resistance or pressure gradient to fluid flow through a tube is directly related to the length and flow and inversely related to the viscosity of the fluid and the radius to the fourth power.* Poiseuille's law could be expressed as a formula as follows[4]:

$$n = \frac{\Delta P \pi r^4}{8\, l \dot{V}}$$ where n = Viscosity ΔP = Pressure gradient
r = Radius l = Length
$\dot{V}$ = Flow rate

Calculation of resistance to gas flow is not commonly done clinically, but Poiseuille's law can provide considerable insight into what can occur in the apparatus that is utilized. A more simplified version of Poiseuille's law would be as follows[4]:

$$\Delta P = \frac{\dot{V}}{r^4}$$

This describes the interrelation between three factors that have frequent clinical considerations. *Flow rate*, for example, if lowered, will also lower the resistance and therefore the pressure gradient across the tube. As an example, if the flow rate were dropped to half, the resistance would drop to half as well, and so would the pressure gradient required. *Radius*, however, if it were decreased to half of its previous value, would increase the resistance to the fourth power or sixteen times. Table 1-3 indicates alterations in the three factors necessary to acquire increased or decreased resistance to flow.

Table 1-3. Poiseuille's law*

Factor	Effect on resistance caused by decrease in factor	Effect on resistance caused by increase in factor
$\dot{V}$	↓	↑
l	↓	↑
r^4	↑	↓
n	↓	↑

*Decreased resistance is accomplished by decreased flow rate ($\dot{V}$), decreased length (l), increased r^4, or lower viscosity (n) of the gas. Radius has the greatest effect based on its exponent.

Two other factors of Poiseuille's law are of occasional clinical value, as well. These are *length* and *viscosity*. As the length of tubing increases, there is a proportional increase in resistance. Viscosity, in terms of clinical application, is restricted to utilizing helium-oxygen mixtures to reduce ventilatory resistance.

REYNOLD'S NUMBER

Reynolds devised a formula that calculates a numerical value. This value can indicate the presence of laminar or turbulent flow through a tube.[3] The major factors in his calculation are *flow, density,* and *viscosity,* which have a direct relationship to type of flow, and *diameter,* which would have an inverse relationship. The calculation of Reynolds' formula is rarely done clinically; however, an understanding of its principles provides insight into practical application. The magic *number for Reynolds' formula is 2000.* If the calculation is performed and the *value obtained is lower than 2000, the flow through that tube will be laminar.* If the calculation is performed and the *number resulting is over 2000, the flow through the tube will be turbulent.* The consideration of laminar versus turbulent flow that is most important in clinical application of flows is that laminar flow requires far less pressure gradient (or effort, depending on whether the patient or the apparatus is moving the gas) than does turbulent flow to move a given amount of gas. Therefore a laminar flow requires less energy or less peak pressure to accomplish the same end. Following is the formula for calculating Reynolds' number:

$$\frac{\text{Critical velocity (cm/sec)} \times \text{Diameter (cm)} \times \text{Density (gm/cm}^3)}{\text{Viscosity (Poise)}}$$

If the number is over 2000, flow will convert to turbulent, and the resistance and pressure gradient across that tube will increase significantly.

REFERENCES

1. Quagliano, J. V.: Quagliano chemistry, Englewood Cliffs, N.J., 1963, Prentice-Hall, Inc.
2. McPherson, S. P., and Roads, J. S.: History of respiratory therapy. (To be published.)
3. McIntosh, R., Epstein, H. G., and Mushin, W.: Physics for the anaesthetist, Oxford, England, 1968, Blackwell Scientific Publications, Ltd.
4. Egan, D. F.: Fundamentals of respiratory therapy, ed. 3, St. Louis, 1977, The C. V. Mosby Co.

2 Primary systems: cylinders and piping systems

Respiratory therapy employs apparatus utilized at the bedside and in most instances some type of gas source. The gas source and its system are considered to be *primary equipment*, and all apparatus used from the source outlet is considered to be *secondary equipment*. Somehow, primary systems tend to escape the everyday recognition of the respiratory therapist. However, understanding the normal function of this equipment is equally as important as understanding the apparatus used on a daily basis. If the cylinders, piping systems, or bulk systems were to fail, the respiratory therapist could potentially be rendered nearly helpless if he did not have a clear understanding of the mechanisms involved to enable him to respond quickly and effectively to the problem.

CYLINDERS

Since cylinders have been in use since 1888, when Liquid Carbonics and General Dynamics introduced the first medical cylinder, this chapter will examine these first, in terms of supplying clinical gas requirements.[1] Table 2-1 provides an outline of the preparation of the various gases that find medical use.[2,3] Once prepared, these gases are either placed in cylinders or transported in bulk to the user's site. The first aspect to be discussed is the construction and design of the cylinder container.

Oxygen is received as an inexpensive product in an expensive package. A cylinder may currently cost from $35 to $50 depending on its size, yet the cost of its contents may be from as low as $2 to $5. The reasons that this package is so expensive are somewhat obvious. For medical gases, the package must be able to withstand reasonably high pressures; therefore its strength must be such as to provide optimum safety both for those handling the cylinders and for the consumer, that is, the patient. Cylinders are constructed from seamless, high-quality steel that is either stamped into shape from a steel plug or simply spun into shape from hot steel. Type 3AA cylinders are produced from heat-treated steel and type 3A are not.[4] The type 3 cylinders were manufactured from low-carbon steel and are no longer produced.

Cylinder marks and codes

Federal regulation regarding the construction of cylinders used in transport of gases was originally under the jursidiction of the Interstate Commerce Commission

Table 2-1. Preparation methods of common gases

Gas	Method
Air	Compressed or made synthetically from purified components (nitrogen and oxygen)
Carbon dioxide	500° C, $C + O_2 = CO_2$. Combustion of coal, coke, natural gas, oil, etc. (1000° C, $2C + O_2 = 2 CO$) By-product gases from ammonia plants, lime kilns, etc. Fermentation process Gas wells, springs
Cyclopropane	Reduction of water solution of trimethylenechlorobromide with zinc as catalyst at 200° F Progressive thermal chlorination of propane
Ethylene	High-temperature coil cracking of propane or ethane and propane Catalytic decomposition of ethyl alcohol
Helium	Natural gas wells (some containing as high as 2% helium) Fractional distillation—small amounts
Hydrogen	Cracking operations using petroleum liquid or vapors Electrolysis Steam over heated, spongy iron reduces steam to hydrogen and iron oxide Steam and incandescent coke or coal Dissociation of ammonia
Nitrogen	Fractional distillation
Nitrous oxide	Thermal decomposition of ammonium nitrate into nitrous oxide and water
Oxygen	Fractional distillation of liquid air

(ICC), as of the 1948 (June 25) Interstate Commerce Act. On April 1, 1967, all safety regulations were transferred to the jurisdiction of the Department of Transportation, and on December 3, 1968, this change was officially recorded in the Federal Register, making it known to the public.[4] As of January 1, 1970, all new cylinders are marked with "DOT," as opposed to the previous "ICC" marking. Currently all transport of gases comes under the jurisdiction of the Department of Transportation's subdivisions (Fig. 2-1).[2] Transportation of gases by rail is governed by the Federal Railroad Administration (FRA).[4,5] Water transport lies within the authority of the United States Coast Guard (USCG), and road transport is

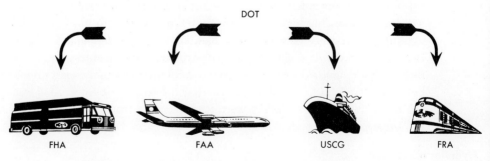

Fig. 2-1. Department of Transportation and its subdivisions. FHA regulates highway transport, FAA regulates air transport, USCG regulates water transport, and FRA regulates rail transport of cylinder gases.

under the control of the Federal Highway Administration (FHA).[4,5] Air conveyance is regulated by the Federal Aviation Administration (FAA) in cooperation with the International Air Transport Association, of which all major airlines are members.[2,5]

State regulations vary widely, and municipal agencies may also have regulations, although most of these are directed toward storage facilities.[2]

The Department of Transportation regulations outline acceptable cylinder construction. Some DOT regulations are made by the Bureau of Explosives, a private organization.[4] Table 2-2 indicates the different sizes of cylinders in common medical use, as well as the contents' weight, volume, and pressure to be used with the various medical gases.

Specifications for cylinders and their construction are as follows:

1. The steel utilized in cylinders must meet chemical and physical requirements of the Department of Transportation (in Canada it must meet the specifications of the Board of Transport Commissioners for Canada).[2]
2. Hydrostatic retest pressures are to be five thirds of service pressure on ICC 3A or 3AA cylinders and tested every 5 years (unless followed by a "★," which requires a retest every 10 years) to determine the expansion characteristics of the cylinder.[5]
3. Cylinders must contain a pressure release to prevent explosion, approved by the Bureau of Explosives (DOT regulation).[4]
4. Cylinders can be filled to 10% higher than the maximum filling pressure as marked.[5]
5. Internal and external visual examination must be made at the time of retest.[5]
6. A "+" must follow the stamped hydrostatic test date to indicate that the cylinder complied with requirements of the retest.[5]

Cylinder markings primarily reflect the regulations mentioned above, with a few additional markings as follows (Fig. 2-2):

1. The "ICC-" or "DOT-" followed by "3A" or "3AA" indicates the type of steel ("3A" indicates high-carbon or medium-manganese steel, and "3AA" indicates heat-treated steel).[5]
2. Following the "3A" or "3AA" is the service pressure of the cylinder (which may be filled in excess by 10%).[5]
3. The original hydrostatic test date is indicated as well as subsequent ones along with the tester's mark.
4. The "+" indicates that the visual, leak, and expansion checks were within acceptable limits.[5]
5. A manufacturer's mark is usually located in close proximity to those just mentioned. (The one in Fig. 2-2 is that of Harrisburg Steel, which manufactures the majority of medical gas cylinders in the United States).
6. An ownership serial number is usually found on the cylinder. It commonly indicates cylinder size, owner's initials, and a serial number. (The one in Fig. 2-2 is from a Puritan Compressed Gas Corporation "E" cylinder).
7. The country in which the cylinder is manufactured is indicated on the cylinder with a stamp, usually close to the neck (for example, "Made in USA").

Additional marking is required regarding the cylinder's contents and is usually done in the form of a label or stencil.[2] The following regulations were compiled

Table 2-2. Common cylinder sizes and gases used in respiratory therapy*

Cylinder sizes	Gas		Carbon dioxide	Cyclo-propane	Ethylene	Helium	Nitrous oxide	Oxygen	Helium-oxygen mixtures	Carbon dioxide mixtures
	Cylinder pressure at 70° F (psig†)		840	80	1250	1650 to 2000	745	1800 to 2400	1650 to 2000	1500 to 2200
D	Contents weight (lb)		4.0	3.3	2.0	0.1	4.0	1.0	—	—
	Gas volume at 70° F	Cu ft	33.0	30.0	26.6	10.6	34.5	12.6	11.0	12.6
	and 14.7 psia‡	Liters	934.0	848.0	752.0	300.0	975.0	356.0	310.0	356.0
E	Contents weight (lb)		6.6	—	3.3	0.2	6.6	2.0	—	—
	Gas volume at 70° F	Cu ft	56.0	—	44.0	17.0	57.0	22.0	18.0	22.0
	and 14.7 psia	Liters	1585.0	—	1245.0	480.0	1610.0	622.0	510.0	622.0
G	Contents weight (lb)		50.0	—	28.0	1.5	56.0	16.0	—	—
	Gas volume at 70° F	Cu ft	425.0	—	372.0	146.0	485.0	186.0	150.0	186.0
	and 14.7 psia	Liters	12,000.0	—	10,500.0	4130.0	13,750.0	5260.0	4250.0	5260.0
H-K	Contents weight (lb)		—	—	—	—	64.0	20.0	—	—
	Gas volume at 70° F	Cu ft	—	—	—	—	557.0	244.0	—	—
	and 14.7 psia	Liters	—	—	—	—	15,800.0	6900.0	—	—

*From the Standard for Nonflammable Medical Gas Systems (NFPA 56 F), Boston, 1973, National Fire Protection Association.
†Pounds per square inch gauge.
‡Pounds per square inch absolute.

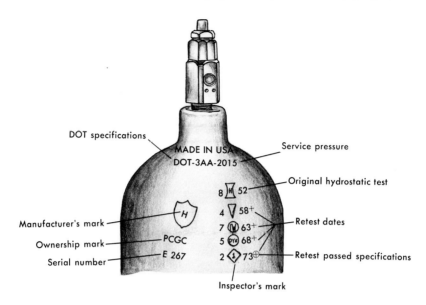

DOT specifications

MADE IN USA
DOT-3AA-2015

Service pressure

Original hydrostatic test

8 ⍢ 52

4 ▽ 58⁺

Manufacturer's mark

7 ⍥ 63⁺

Retest dates

Ownership mark

PCGC

5 ⍥ 68⁺

Serial number

E 267

2 ⍥ 73⊕

Retest passed specifications

Inspector's mark

Fig. 2-2. Cylinder markings. (Courtesy Bennett Respiration Products, Inc., Santa Monica, Calif.)

by the Compressed Gas Association and approved by the American Standards Association.[2]

1. The content's material must be identified in the language of the country where it is filled, or the international symbol or formula for the material must be utilized (Table 2-3).
2. Labels should be included to alert the user to hazards[2] (Fig. 2-3).
3. Labels should be of such design as to not conflict with DOT labels or colors.
4. Labels should be on a conspicuous location on the cylinder.
5. Precautionary measures and instructions in case of accidental exposure or contact with the contents should be included, if necessary (Fig. 2-3).
6. An indication of the content's high pressure should be made on the label.

The Compressed Gas Association (CGA) designed a color coding system for medical gases, which was later published by the United States Department of Commerce as a recommendation of the Bureau of Standards.[6] The color codes were designed primarily for anesthesiology. Originally, the reason that midshoulder

Table 2-3. International symbols for gases

Gas	*Symbol*
Air	Air
Carbon dioxide	CO_2
Carbon monoxide	CO
Cyclopropane	C_3H_6
Ethylene	C_2H_4
Ethylene oxide	C_2H_4O
Helium	He
Hydrogen	H_2
Nitrogen	N_2
Nitrous oxide	N_2O
Oxygen	O_2

O_2

LIQUID OXYGEN

WARNING!

Accelerates combustion
Keep oil and grease away
Extremely cold liquid
May cause burns

Avoid contact with skin, eyes, and clothing
Avoid spills

H_2

HYDROGEN

FLAMMABLE

Keep away from heat, flame, and sparks

C_4H_6

CYCLOPROPANE

FLAMMABLE

Keep away from heat, flame, and sparks

C_2H_4

ETHYLENE

FLAMMABLE

Keep away from heat, flame, and sparks

O_2

OXYGEN

WARNING!

Accelerates combustion
Keep oil and grease away

Fig. 2-3. Cylinder labeling of hazards.

height was chosen as the dividing point on the cylinder for color change was that when two colors were required, the anesthesiologist could easily see both colors as he looked down on the anesthetic apparatus from above.[6] All medical gas cylinders still follow that method of color division except for chrome cyclopropane cylinders, which have a color-coded label.[6] Color codes are only guides, and the label is still the primary means of identification. If the label is missing or illegible or if the color and label conflict, the cylinder should not be used. (Table 2-4 lists the medical gas color codes.) Helium-oxygen and carbon dioxide–oxygen mixtures are commonly divided into two categories of color coding, each based on the percentage of gases contained. In carbon dioxide–oxygen mixtures in which the carbon dioxide is greater than 7%, the cylinder is predominantly gray with the balance

Table 2-4. Medical gas color codes

Gas	Color
Oxygen	Green*
Carbon dioxide	Gray
Nitrous oxide	Light blue
Cyclopropane	Orange
Helium	Brown
Ethylene	Red
Carbon dioxide and oxygen	Gray and green
Helium and oxygen	Brown and green

*The international color code for oxygen is white

green, and if the carbon dioxide is less than 7%, then the predominant color is green. If helium is over 80% in a helium-oxygen mixture, then the predominant color is brown and the rest is green. Helium would be 80% maximally in all mixtures used as a life-supportive gas, and, in this case, the predominant color should be green.

CYLINDER VALVES

The valves on cylinders containing medical gases are usually of two types[7] (Fig. 2-4). The *direct-acting* valve, the first type, is basically a sophisticated needle valve.[8] Two fiber washers and a Teflon packing normally prevent gas leakage around the threads. The name *direct-acting* comes from the arrangement of movements in the valve wheel. These movements are directly reflected in the valve seat, since it is one piece moved by threads. The valve is capable of withstanding high pressures and is used on cylinders in which the content's gas pressure is high (above 1500 psi).

The second type of valve is the *diaphragm* type.[8] The stem that replaces the wheel on the direct-acting type is separated from the valve seat and spring by two diaphragms, one of steel and the other copper. When the stem is turned and, therefore, raised due to the threading, the diaphragms can be pushed upward with the stem by the valve seat and spring. This type of valve has the following advantages: (1) the valve seat does not turn and, therefore, is resistant to scoring, which could cause leakage; (2) no stem leakage can occur due to the diaphragm; and (3) the stem need only be turned part of a rotation, not turned two turns to open, as in the direct-acting type. Therefore the diaphragm type is preferable, generally, where the pressures are relatively low (under 1500 psi) and where no leaks can be allowed, such as with flammable anesthetics.

The outlet on the cylinder valve must be indexed for the specific gas it contains. Early work was done with indexing by the CGA and was later refined and adopted in 1949 by the American Standards Association.[9] *American Standard indexing* includes a system for large cylinders and one for small cylinders.[9]

Large cylinder valve outlets and connections are indexed by thread type, thread size, right- or left-handed threading, external or internal threading, and the nipple-seat design.[9] Fig. 2-5 lists the American Standard connections for gases commonly used in respiratory therapy.[9] The first number, such as "903," is the diameter in inches of the threaded outlet of an oxygen cylinder. The next number after the dash gives the number of threads per inch. A threaded oxygen cylinder outlet,

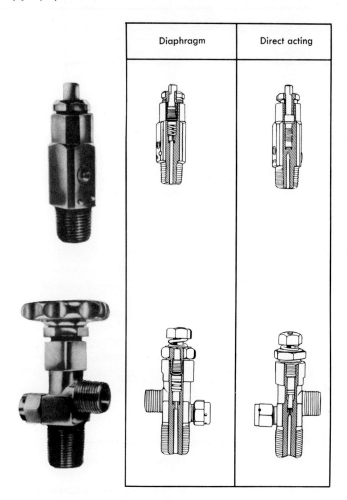

Fig. 2-4. Diaphragm and needle valves for cylinder. *Top,* diaphragm valve for lower-pressure gases. *Bottom,* needle valve (direct-acting) for higher-pressure gas cylinders. (Courtesy Ohio Medical Products, Madison, Wis.)

for example, has fourteen threads per inch. The letters following this indicate the type of thread used, that is, whether they are right-hand (RH) or left-hand (LH). Usually left-handed threads are indicated as such by a groove cut around the hexagonal inlet nut.

Small cylinders with post-type valves receive a different American Standard indexing called the *Pin Index Safety System* (PISS). In these cylinders' valves, the indexing is accomplished by the exact placement of two pins and two holes to receive the pins in the post valve. Fig. 2-6 shows eight of the ten possible pin combinations, numbered from left to right. Air is assigned combinations 1 and 5.

The Compressed Gas Association designed thread and nipple indexing for low-pressure (under 200 psig) devices called the *Diameter Index Safety System* (DISS). The diameter index for low-pressure devices is similar in design to the American Standard for high-pressure outlets, since the CGA was involved in designing both. Table 2-5 lists the connections commonly associated with respiratory therapy, and Fig. 2-7 shows an example of the Diameter Index Safety System.

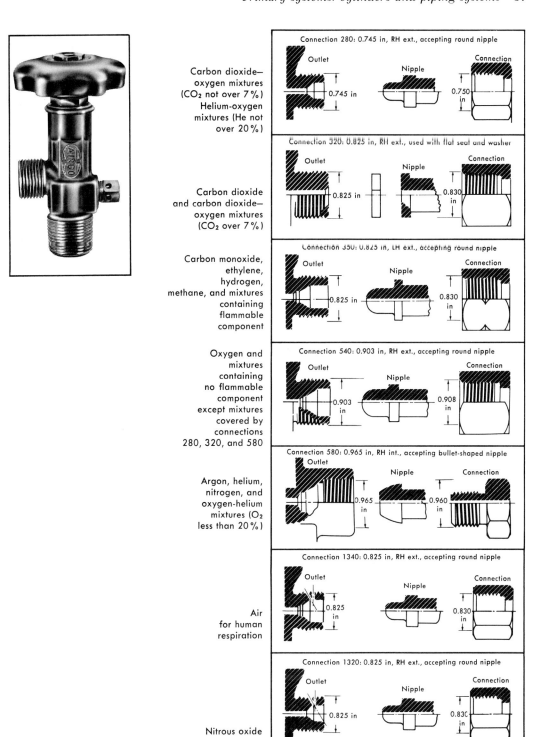

Carbon dioxide—
oxygen mixtures
(CO_2 not over 7%)
Helium-oxygen
mixtures (He not
over 20%)

Carbon dioxide
and carbon dioxide—
oxygen mixtures
(CO_2 over 7%)

Carbon monoxide,
ethylene,
hydrogen,
methane, and mixtures
containing
flammable
component

Oxygen and
mixtures
containing
no flammable
component
except mixtures
covered by
connections
280, 320, and 580

Argon, helium,
nitrogen, and
oxygen-helium
mixtures (O_2
less than 20%)

Air
for human
respiration

Nitrous oxide

Fig. 2-5. American Standard connections. Diameter indexing of large cylinder valves is accomplished by thread type and size, right- or left-handed threads, external or internal threading, and nipple-seat design. (Courtesy Ohio Medical Products, Madison, Wis.)

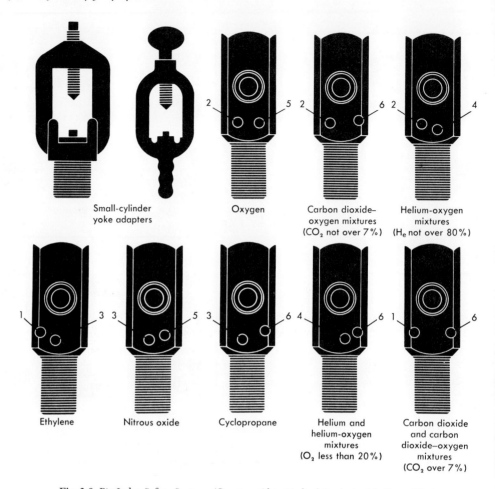

Fig. 2-6. Pin Index Safety System. (Courtesy Ohio Medical Products, Madison, Wis.)

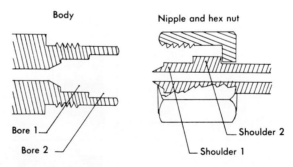

Fig. 2-7. Diameter Index Safety System. (From Egan, D. F.: Fundamentals of respiratory therapy, ed. 3, St. Louis, 1977, The C. V. Mosby Co.)

The Food and Drug Administration (FDA) requires that the purity of gases be at least at a certain level, and this must be indicated on the label as well. Table 2-6 lists these purity requirements as listed in the *United States Pharmacopeia* (USP) or *National Formulary* (NF); usually all manufacturers exceed these purity levels significantly. The FDA also requires that the name of the manufacturer,

Table 2-5. Connections commonly used in respiratory therapy

Connection number	Gas	Connection number	Gas
1020	Unassigned	1120	Unassigned
1040	N_2O	1140	C_2H_4
1060	He	1160	Air
	He/O_2 ($O_2 < 20\%$)	1180	He/O_2 (He 80% or less)
1080	CO_2	1200	O_2/CO_2 (CO_2 7% or less)
	O_2/CO_2 ($CO_2 > 7\%$)	1220	Suction
1100	$(CH_2)_3$	1240	O_2 (standard)

Table 2-6. USP gas purities

Gas	Purity
Nitrous oxide	97%
Cyclopropane	99%
Oxygen	99%
Carbon dioxide	99%
Helium	95%
Hydrogen	99.9%
Nitrogen	99%
Ethylene	99%*

*National Formulary.

packer, or distributor be included on the label as well as an accurate statement as to its content (usually the volume in liters at 70° F).[6] A statement of cautions in its administration must also be on the label.[6] Storage, internal transportation, and use of these cylinder gases require considerations to ensure optimum safety for patients and personnel. Most recommendations for cylinder gas safety are from either the CGA or the National Fire Protection Agency (NFPA), although state and municipal authorities may have regulations with which to comply also.[2] The NFPA[13] and CGA[6] recommendations for cylinders are as follows:

A. Storage
   1. Cylinders should not be stored in an area where the temperature exceeds 125° F.
   2. No flames should have the potential of coming in contact with the cylinders.
   3. The storage area must be permanently posted.
   4. Cylinders must be grouped by content.
   5. Full and empty cylinders must be segregated in the storage area.
   6. Storage rooms must be dry, cool, and well ventilated.
   7. The storage facility should be fire resistant where practical.
   8. Below-ground storage should be avoided.
   9. Cylinders must not be stored near flammable substances.
   10. Those gases supporting combustion must be stored in a separate location from those that are combustible.
   11. Cylinders should never be stored in the operating room.
   12. Large cylinders must be stored in an upright position.

13. Cylinders must be protected from being cut or abraded.
14. Cylinders must be stored to protect them from extreme weather to prevent rusting, excessive temperatures, and accumulations of snow and ice.
15. Cylinders should not be exposed to continuous dampness or corrosive substances to prevent rusting of the cylinder and its valve.
16. Cylinders must not be stored where readily combustible materials, such as oil and grease, may come in contact with them.
17. Cylinders should be protected from tampering.
18. Valves should be kept closed on empty cylinders at all times.
19. Cylinders must be stored with protective caps in place.

B. Transporting
1. If protective valve caps are supplied, they should be utilized whenever cylinders are in transport and until they are ready for use.
2. Cylinders must not be dropped, dragged, slid, or allowed to strike each other violently.
3. Cylinders must be transported on an appropriate cart secured by a chain or strap.

C. Use
1. Before connecting equipment to a cylinder, be certain that connections are free of foreign materials.
2. Turn valve outlet away from personnel and crack cylinder valve to remove any dust or debris from cylinder valve outlet.
3. Cylinder valve outlet connections must be American Standard or CGA pin indexed, and low-pressure connections must be CGA diameter indexed.
4. Cylinders must be secured at the administration site and not to any movable objects or heat radiators.
5. Outlets and connections must be tightened with only appropriate wrenches and must never be forced on.
6. Equipment designed for one gas should not be utilized on another.
7. Never use medical cylinder gases where contamination by back flow of other gases may occur.
8. Regulators should be off as the cylinder is turned on, and the cylinder valve should be opened slowly.
9. Before equipment is disconnected from a cylinder, the cylinder valve should be closed and the pressure released from the device.
10. Cylinder valves should be closed at all times except when they are in use.
11. Transfilling of cylinders is hazardous and must not be done.
12. Cylinders may be refilled only if permission is secured from the owner.
13. Cylinders must not be lifted by the cap.
14. *Never lubricate* valve outlets or connecting equipment (oxygen and oil under pressure causes an explosive oxidation reaction).
15. Flame testing for leaks must not be done (usually a soap solution is utilized).

16. When in use, open valve fully and then turn it back a quarter to a half turn.
17. Replace cap on empty cylinders.
18. Position the cylinder so that the label is clearly visible.
19. Check label *before* use; it should always match the color code.
20. A NO SMOKING sign must be posted at the administration site and should contain at least the minimum text, as indicated in Fig. 2-8. It must be legible from a distance of 5 feet and must be displayed in a conspicuous location.
21. Inform all occupants of the area of the hazards of smoking and of the regulations.
22. No sources of open flames shall be permitted in the area of administration.
23. Equipment connected to cylinders containing gaseous oxygen should be labeled: OXYGEN—USE NO OIL.
24. Equipment designated for use with a specific gas must be clearly and permanently labeled accordingly.
25. Enclosures intended to contain patients must have the minimum text regarding NO SMOKING (as indicated in Fig. 2-9), and the labels must be located (a) in a position to be read by the patient and (b) on two or more opposing sides visible from the exterior.
26. Cylinder carts must be of a self-supporting design with appropriate casters and wheels, and those intended for use in surgery must be grounded.
27. High-pressure oxygen equipment must not be sterilized with flammable agents (for example, alcohol and ethylene oxide), and the agents used must be oil-free and nondamaging.
28. Polyethylene bags must not be used to wrap sterilized high-pressure oxygen equipment, because polyethylene when flexed releases pure hydrocarbons that are severely flammable.
29. Oxygen equipment exposed to pressures of less than 60 psi may be sterilized with either nonflammable mixture of ethylene oxide and carbon dioxide or with fluorocarbons.
30. Cold cylinders must be handled with care to avoid hand injury due to tissue freezing caused by rapid gas expansion.

CAUTION OXYGEN IN USE No smoking No open flames	CAUTION OXYGEN IN USE Keep flames away No smoking No electrical appliances

Fig. 2-8. Minimum text for oxygen sign.   **Fig. 2-9.** Minimum text for oxygen enclosure label.

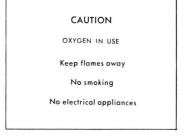

31. Cylinders must not be handled with oily or greasy hands, gloves, or clothing.
32. Cylinder contents must be identified before use by reading the label, which should not be defaced, altered, or removed.
33. Safety-relief mechanisms, noninterchangeable connections, and other safety features shall not be removed or altered.
34. Control valves on equipment must be closed both before connection and when not in use.

LIQUID GAS SYSTEMS

After the invention of *fractional distillation of liquid air* by Dr. Karl von Linde in 1907, the purchase of gases by health-care institutions became more economically feasible.[1] Linde's procedure provided for both liquefying air and dividing it into its main components, oxygen and nitrogen, in the liquid state.[1] Since that time, the use of liquefied gas in hospitals has become popular. The reasons are twofold: (1) liquid oxygen shipped in bulk is far less expensive than gas that is pumped into cylinders and then transported and (2) the space requirements for a liquid gas reservoir are far less than its volumetric equivalent in cylinder gas. For example, as oxygen converts from its liquid to a gaseous state at room temperature, it expands approximately 862 times.[10] Therefore, to store an equal amount of gas in cylinders, the space occupied by the cylinders would have to be 862 times greater than that of the liquid reservoir. The procedure for fractional distillation of liquid air, as follows, should be well understood by respiratory therapists.

1. *Air is dried and filtered.* Air is drawn through scrubbers to remove all dust and impurities. The air is then cooled to near freezing to remove all water.
2. *Air is compressed to 200 atm.* The air is then compressed, which causes the gas to heat up.
3. *Compressed air is cooled to room temperature.* To cool the gas back to room temperature, waste nitrogen is passed in coils around it.
4. *Gas is expanded to 5 atm.* Since the most efficient way to cool a gas is to expand it, the great drop in pressure drops the gas to a low temperature.
5. *Liquid air is obtained.* The temperature obtained by expanding the gas is below the critical temperature of nearly all of the gases in air, and they turn to a liquid.
6. *Liquid air is transferred to a distilled column.* The liquid air is trapped off into a distilling column for separation of the gases.
7. *Liquid air is warmed to boil off other gases.* As the liquid air is warmed, various gases boil off as their individual boiling points are reached until just below the boiling point of oxygen, where the warming is ceased, only liquid oxygen remains.

Nitrogen: $-320.4°$ F at 1 atm
Oxygen: $-297.3°$ F at 1 atm

8. *Distillation process is repeated.* The liquid is then recooled by expansion, and the process is repeated until the liquid oxygen is at least 99% pure with no toxic impurities.

9. *Pure liquid oxygen is obtained.* Although 99% pure is the standard, most medical oxygen exceeds that in purity.

10. *Liquid oxygen is drawn off to cold converters.* The liquid oxygen is then transferred to cold converters where it is delivered to hospitals and storage tanks and transferred as a gas to cylinders.

From this one process, the two major gases employed in liquid gas systems in hospitals are acquired. Oxygen is certainly the most widely used commercial gas, and nitrogen is the second. The following discussion of liquid gas reservoirs will pertain primarily to oxygen; however, the concepts relate to reservoirs for nitrogen as well.

The structure of bulk liquefied-gas reservoirs is regulated by several agencies. These are the recommendations made by the National Fire Protection Association and the American Society of Mechanical Engineers (ASME) regarding the structure of the bulk unit.[11] The Bureau of Explosives outlines regulations for pressure releases.[4,9] The storage container for liquefied oxygen is structured in a similar fashion to a large thermos bottle (Fig. 2-10). Several layers of insulation and, usually, a layer of near-vacuum are utilized to retard external heat transfer into the cold liquid.[10] A pressure release serves to allow some of the gas on top of the liquid to escape if the contents are warmed, thus releasing the pressure within. This release of gas allows the gas within the container to expand, thus lowering its temperature (Gay-Lussac's law); this maintains the gas under pressure between its boiling point and its critical temperature, so that the majority of the reservoir's contents will be maintained in a liquid state (Fig. 2-10).

All storage vessels and transport units are constructed principally the same as above, since they are attempting to accomplish the same purpose. At the site of usage, a vaporizer or vaporizing column is attached to the unit, through which gas is extracted from the liquefied gas reservoir. This vaporizer acts similarly to a large radiator so that heat can be absorbed from the environment into the gas, thus

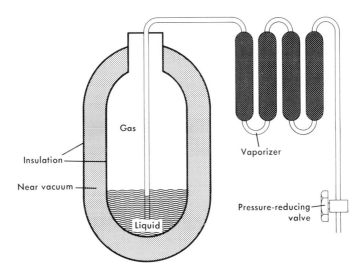

Fig. 2-10. Liquid oxygen is drawn off bulk storage container and passes through vaporizer.

allowing it to warm toward room temperature and expand. Once this temperature and expansion stability has been accomplished, the gas can pass through a pressure-reducing valve, which will drop its pressure to a desired level (normally 50 psig for hospitals); it is then piped to different administration sites as necessary. Bulk oxygen systems are considered to include the assembly of equipment on the vessel up to the point where the gas passes through a pressure-reducing valve and starts to enter the piping system at working pressure.[11] A *bulk oxygen system* (liquid and/or gas) is defined as *more than 13,000 cubic feet of oxygen (NTP) connected, ready for use, or 25,000 cubic feet or more of oxygen (NTP) that is on hand at the site.*[11] The structure of a bulk oxygen system should meet the following specifications acording to the NFPA[11]:

1. Containers that are permanently installed should be mounted on noncombustible supports and foundations.

2. Liquid oxygen containers should be constructed from materials that meet the impact test requirements of paragraph UG-48 of the ASME Boiler and Pressure Vessel Codes, Section VII. Containers operating above 15 psi must be designed and tested in accordance with the ASME Boiler and Pressure Vessel Code, Section VII, and the insulation of the liquid oxygen container must be of noncombustible material.

3. All high-pressure gaseous oxygen containers must comply with the construction and test requirements of ASME Boiler and Pressure Vessel Code, Section VIII.

4. Bulk oxygen storage containers must be equipped with safety-release devices as required by ASME Code IV and ICC specifications.

5. Isolation casings on liquid oxygen containers shall be equipped with suitable safety-release devices. These devices must be designed or located so that moisture cannot either freeze the unit or interfere in any manner with its proper operation.

6. The vaporizing columns and connecting pipes shall be anchored and/or sufficiently flexible to provide for expansion and contraction due to temperature changes. It must also have a safety-release device to properly protect it.

7. Any heat supplied to oxygen vaporizers must be done in an indirect fashion, such as with steam, air, water, or water solutions that do not react with oxygen. If liquid heaters are utilized to provide the primary source of heat, the vaporizer must be electrically grounded.

8. All equipment composing the bulk system must be cleaned to remove oxidizable material before the system is placed into service.

9. All joints and connections in the tubing should be made by welding or by use of flanged, threaded slip, or compressed fittings, and any gaskets or thread seals must be of suitable substance for oxygen service. Any valves, gauges, or regulators placed into the system must be designed for oxygen service.

10. Storage containers, piping valves, and regulating equipment must be protected against physical damage and tampering.

11. Any enclosure containing oxygen control of operating equipment must be adequately ventilated.

12. The location shall be permanently posted to indicate OXYGEN—NO SMOK-ING—NO OPEN FLAMES or an equivalent warning.
13. All bulk systems must be regularly inspected by qualified representatives of the oxygen supplier.
14. Weeds and tall grass must be kept back 15 feet of any bulk oxygen container. The bulk oxygen system must be appropriately located so that its distance provides maximum safety for other areas surrounding it. These minimum distances for location of a bulk oxygen system near the following structures (shown in Fig. 2-11) are:
    a. 50 feet from any combustible structure.
    b. 25 feet from any structure that consists of fire-resistant exterior walls or buildings of other construction that have sprinklers.
    c. At least 10 feet from any opening in the adjacent walls of fire-resistant structures.
    d. 50 feet from flammable, liquid storage above ground that is less than 1000 gallons in capacity, or 90 feet from these storage areas if the quantity is in excess of 1000 gallons.
    e. The bulk oxygen system must be located at least 15 feet from an underground, flammable liquid storage that is less than 1000 gallons, or 30 feet from one in excess of 1000 gallons capacity. The distance from the storage containers for oxygen to the filling and vent connections for the flammable liquid storage must be at least 50 feet.
    f. An oxygen system must be located at least 25 feet from combustible, gas storage above ground that is less than 1000 gallons capacity, or 50 feet from the storage of over 1000 gallons capacity.
    g. If combustible, liquid storage is below ground, it must be at least 15 feet from the bulk system, and the distance to the vent or filling connections must be at least 40 feet.
    h. If flammable gas storage is in the vicinity and is less than 5000 cubic feet NTP, it must be at least 50 feet from the bulk oxygen system; if the flammable gas quantity is in excess of 5000 cubic feet NTP, it must be located at least 90 feet from the oxygen system.
    i. The oxygen system must be located at least 25 feet from solid materials that burn slowly (coal and heavy timber).
    j. The oxygen system must be at least 75 feet away in one direction and 35 feet away at an approximately 90° angle from confining walls unless they are made from a fire-resistant material and are less than 20 feet high. (This is to provide adequate ventilation in the area in case venting occurs.)
    k. Places of public assembly must be at least 50 feet from the oxygen system.
    l. Areas occupied by nonambulatory patients should be at least 50 feet from the oxygen system.
    m. Public sidewalks must be 10 feet from an oxygen system.
    n. The oxygen system must be located at least 5 feet from any adjoining property line.
    o. The unit must be accessible by a mobile transport unit that fills the supply system.

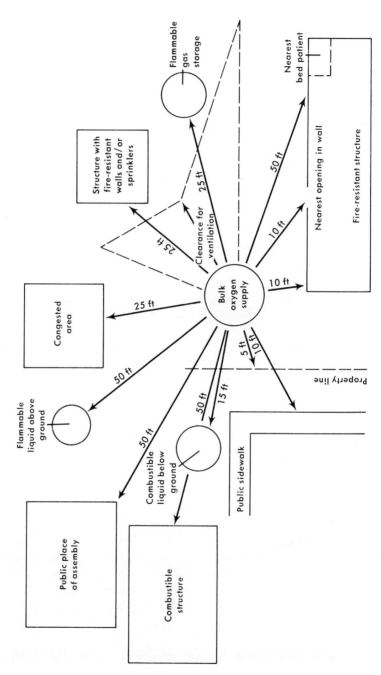

Fig. 2-11. Relative minimum distances between bulk oxygen supply system and various structures.

The specifications just listed were designed by the NFPA to provide maximum protection for all those in the vicinity of a bulk oxygen system, so that medical needs can be met in the safest possible manner.

SUPPLY SYSTEMS

Supply systems can be comprised of either cylinders that contain gaseous oxygen or of liquefied reservoirs (as previously described in this chapter). These can be placed into either one of two types of system, *continuous* or *alternating*.

The *continuous type* (Fig. 2-12) is designed so that there is a main supply reservoir(s) that is refilled periodically. Under normal operating conditions, this *primary source* always supplies the system with gas. A *reserve supply* is attached and should contain at least an average day's supply of oxygen in case the primary supply becomes exhausted.

The *alternating type* of supply system (Fig. 2-13) employs two sources to provide gas to the piping system. Only one *bank* of the manifold operates at a time, and it is considered the primary source. Once the primary source is exhausted, the *secondary source* automatically switches in to become the primary source or supply. The empty bank is simply refilled or replaced. A reserve supply may be attached to supply the system in the event that both the primary and secondary supplies become exhausted. A reserve supply does not normally operate except as a backup system where a secondary supply source is utilized in normal operating conditions.

If cylinders are employed to form the supply source(s), there are a few requirements to be met:

1. There must be at least two cylinders per bank in a *manifold*.[12] Therefore the smallest manifold would be four cylinders, comprising two banks of two cylinders each.

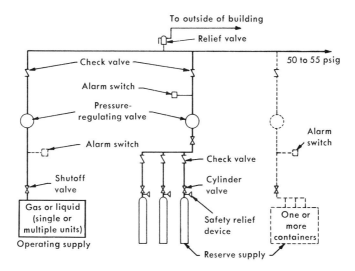

Fig. 2-12. Continuous supply system has one supply that provides gas to system and is refilled periodically. Reserve does not normally function except in emergencies. (Reproduced by permission from Standard for nonflammable medical gas systems [NFPA No. 56F], Boston, Mass., 1973, copyright National Fire Protection Association.)

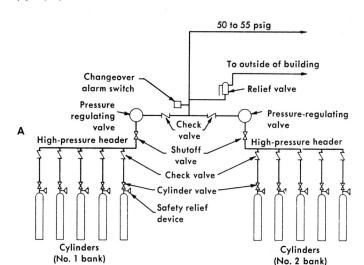

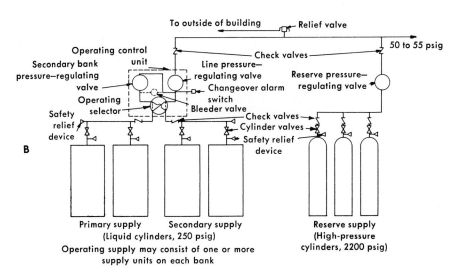

Fig. 2-13. Alternating supply system is composed of primary and secondary supply, **A,** which alternate to charge piping system. Unit may also have reserve supply, **B,** in case both should fail. (Reproduced by permission from Standard for nonflammable medical gas systems [NFPA No. 56F], Boston, Mass., 1973, copyright National Fire Protection Association.)

2. Each lead from the cylinder must contain a *check valve.*[12] This is to prevent back flow of gas into the cylinder in the event that one cylinder in the bank should have its pressure release ruptured, therefore exhausting that cylinder. If the check valves are not placed in the leads, the whole bank could shortly be exhausted, eliminating it as a supply source.

3. Standard connections of either DISS or American Standard, depending on their pressure, must be utilized in the connection of cylinder units to their respective connections.[12]

Other specifications from the NFPA[12] for a supply system that must be met are:

1. Each bank of the manifold must have its own pressure-reducing valve.

2. In the alternating-source system, the secondary supply must switch in automatically when the primary source becomes exhausted.

3. Other arrangements in the system are permissible provided they have equivalent safeguards.

4. A manual shutoff must be located upstream from each line reducing valve, and a shutoff or check valve must be located downstream.

5. Central supply systems must be contained in an enclosure containing a gate or door that may be locked.

6. No other items may be stored in this enclosure except disconnected, empty cylinders awaiting removal.

7. Ordinary electrical fixtures must be at least 5 feet above the floor to prevent physical damage.

8. When the supply system enclosure is located near sources of heat (furnaces, incinerators, boiler rooms, etc.), the enclosure must be constructed to properly protect the supply system from heat.

9. Open electrical conductors and transformers shall not be located near a supply system.

10. Supply systems shall not be located adjacent to oil storage tanks.

11. Smoking is prohibited in the supply system areas.

12. If located in the hospital, the room containing the supply system (more than 1500 cubic feet of gas) must have walls with a fire rating of at least an hour, and the room must not connect directly with locations of anesthetics or flammable-materials storage. The room must be vented to the outside.

13. If the capacity of the supply is less than 1500 cubic feet, it may be located in a room that is not vented to the outside. The doors must have louvers at the top and bottom, and the room must not connect directly with areas of flammable storage or usage (including locations of anesthetics).

PIPING SYSTEMS

To provide distribution of gas from a central source, a piping system is employed. There are certain structural requirements for piping systems to provide maximum safety as outlined by the NFPA[12]:

1. The piping system must be capable of delivering 50 psig to all the station outlets at its maximum flow rate.

2. Pressure-regulating devices must be capable of maintaining minimum, dynamic delivery pressure of 50 psi at maximum delivery line flow.

3. A pressure-release device must be placed downstream of the pressure-reducing valve in the piping system and be set at 50% above the normal line pressure. All pressure-release devices must close automatically when excessive pressure has been released. If the capacity of the total system is greater than 1500 cubic feet, this pressure release must be vented to the outside. All pressure-release valves must be designed specifically for oxygen service and shall be of brass or bronze.

4. The pipe used must be seamless type K or L (ASTMB-8) copper tubing or standard-weight brass pipe. Copper tubing should be hard-tempered for exposed conditions and soft-tempered for underground or concealed usage. Pipe size must be sufficient to maintain proper delivery volumes as well as conforming to good engineering practices.

5. Gas piping should not be supported by other pipes nearby, and must only be

supported by proper devices (pipe hooks, metal pipe strands, bands, or hangers) of suitable size and strength.

6. Fittings utilized for connecting the copper tubing must be copper, brass, or bronze and must be made especially for solder or brazing at the connection. If brass piping is used, it must be assembled with fittings of screwed brass, bronze, or brazed copper.

7. Buried piping must be adequately protected against such elements as frost, corrosion, and physical damage.

8. Oxygen piping may be placed in the same tunnel or trench with fuel gas pipe lines, electrical lines, or steam lines if they are separated, and providing there is good natural or forced ventilation. Oxygen pipelines must not be placed in areas where they could be exposed to oil contact.

9. Oxygen pipelines installed in combustible walls or partitions must be protected against physical damage by insulation such as another pipe or conduit.

10. Oxygen risers may be installed in pipe shafts as long as suitable protection is provided and if they do not come in contact with oil. Oxygen risers cannot be located in elevator shafts.

11. Oxygen pipelines should not be exposed in rooms storing combustible material, kitchens, laundries, or other areas of special hazard. If the installation of piping in such areas is unavoidable, it must be protected by an enclosure that would prevent the escape of oxygen within the room, should leaks occur in the piping. Pipes that are exposed and may encounter physical damage must be provided with suitable protection.

12. The gas content of pipelines must be readily identifiable by appropriate labeling with the name of the gas contained. The labeling must appear on the pipe at intervals of not more than 20 feet and at least once in each room and/or story that the pipeline traverses.

13. Piping systems for gases must not be utilized as a grounding electrode for electrical appliances.

The above regulations pertain directly to those installing piping systems but should also be understood by respiratory therapy personnel to prevent potential errors. If the system is not properly constructed and if adequate protection is not supplied for the piping, the system could malfunction sufficiently to jeopardize patients. At that point, the respiratory therapist will become involved rather quickly. Also, if the piping is not of sufficient size to accommodate high gas flows for some equipment, it will become nearly useless.

The design of a piping layout is also of importance to respiratory therapy personnel. *The zoning* of the system must be adequate to isolate all areas independently if maintenance is required or if a fire occurs. Adequate zoning provides for fast isolation of an area with little chance of a problem spreading to other areas of the hospital. There are other design regulations suggested by the NFPA[12] that must be met as well.

1. All shutoff valves that are readily accessible to other than authorized personnel must be installed in large boxes with frangible windows large enough to permit manual operation of these valves.

2. These valves must be labeled as follows:

CAUTION—OXYGEN VALVES

DO NOT CLOSE EXCEPT IN EMERGENCY

THIS VALVE CONTROLS THE OXYGEN SUPPLY TO (AREA AFFECTED)

3. The *zone valve* in the main oxygen supply line in any location must be accessible to be shut off easily in an emergency situation.
4. Every riser from the main line must be supplied with a zone valve adjacent to the riser connection.
5. Patient outlets must not be supplied directly from the riser unless supplied through the manual shutoff valve located in the same story in which the outlet is located.
6. A zone valve must be placed on each branch that supplies a patient unit. This zone valve must be easily operable from the standing position and must be located in the main corridor of the area that it serves. Zone valves must be placed so as to shut off the supply of oxygen to only the designated branch and not to alter oxygen flow to the rest of the system.
7. A zone valve must be located either outside or inside each anesthetizing location for every oxygen or nitrous oxide line and be so located as to be readily accessible at all times in an emergency situation. They must be so arranged that shutting off one valve does not affect any of the other operating rooms or anesthetizing locations. These valves must be safeguarded against physical damage and labeled:

OXYGEN—DO NOT CLOSE

8. Shutoff valves are not required for outlets immediately outside of an anesthetizing location, providing these lines terminate with female members of approved noninterchangeable, quick-connect couplers for oxygen or nitrous oxide.

Fig. 2-14 indicates the proper zoning of a typical hospital. It should be remembered that each patient area must be zoned and that each operating room's valves must be arranged so that closing one valve will not affect the operation of the pipeline elsewhere.

After a piping system is installed, it must be checked to indicate potential leaks and to assure that no crossing of lines occurred. The procedure from the NFPA[12] used for testing the system is as follows:

1. Prior to being erected, all piping valves and fittings, except those expressly designed for oxygen service by the manufacturer and sealed prior to being received, shall be cleaned thoroughly to remove oil, grease, and other readily oxidizable materials. This can be accomplished by washing the pipe in a hot solution of sodium carbonate or trisodium phosphate (in a proportion of 1 pound to 3 gallons of water). THE USE OF ORGANIC SOLVENTS SUCH AS CARBON TETRACHLORIDE IS PROHIBITED. Care must then be taken to prevent recontaminating the system before final assembly; all tools used in assembling the pipes must be free of oil and grease.
2. All joints for the piping system, except those of (a) an approved brass-flair

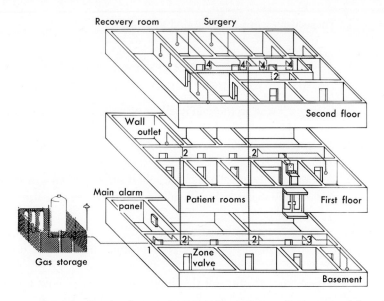

Fig. 2-14. Zone valves must be placed at *1*, entrance to hospital, *2*, each riser, *3*, each branch supplying an area, and *4*, each operating room. (Courtesy Bennett Respiration Products, Inc., Santa Monica, Calif.)

type, (b) gas tubing fittings, or (c) those on valves or on equipment requiring screw connections, must be brazed with silver alloy or a similar high-melting-point, brazing metal. Care must be exercised in applying the flux to avoid leaving any excess on the inside of the completed joints. The outside of a tube fitting must be cleaned with hot water after assembly.

3. Screw connections used on valves must be sealed with (a) soft solder, or (b) litharge and glycerine, or (c) an approved oxygen luting or sealing compound.

4. After the installation of the piping, but prior to the installation of the outlet valves, the line must be blown clear by means of oil-free dry air or nitrogen.

5. After installation of the station outlet, each section of the pipeline must be submitted to a test pressure of one and a half times the maximum working pressure, but not less than 150 psig, with oil-free dry air or nitrogen, and the following considerations must be made:

    a. The test pressure must be maintained until each joint has been examined for leakage. (This is done by means of applying soapy water to the joint or by an equally effective means of leak detection that is safe for use with oxygen.)

    b. Visual inspection of each brazed joint is recommended to make sure that the alloy is closed completely around the joint and that the hardened flux has not just formed a temporary seal that holds the test pressure (all flux should be removed for clear, visible inspection of brazed connections, and all leaks must be repaired and the sections retested).

    c. After the testing of each individual pipeline system is completed, all the associated piping systems must be subjected to a 24-hour standing-pressure test at one and a half times the maximum working pressure, but not less than 150 psig. The test gas must again be oil-free and must consist of either dry air or nitrogen. After the pipeline systems are filled with the test gas, the supply valve and all outlet valves are closed, and the source of test gases is discontinued. The system must remain leak free for the next 24 hours. The only allowable pressure alterations are those due to temperature changes surrounding the piping system during that period.

d. To determine that no cross connection to other pipeline systems exist, all systems must be reduced to atmospheric pressure and each system checked independently with oil-free, dry air or nitrogen. Then, with the appropriate adapters matching the outlet labels, each individual station outlet of all the systems must be checked to determine that the test gas is being dispensed only to the appropriate outlets. This system is then disconnected from the source test gas, and each other system must be tested independently in the same fashion.

6. Once the pressure testing has been completed, the appropriate gas supply should be connected to that corresponding gas system and each system should then be purged, starting with the outlet closest to the supply source. Gas should be permitted to flow every outlet until each system is purged of the test gas used in the tests described above.

7. Each labeled oxygen outlet must then be tested using oxygen in the desired purity. This test must be made at any time that changes are made in a piping system.

STATION OUTLETS

The station outlet should be well understood by respiratory therapy personnel, since they utilize these devices daily.

Station outlets are one of two types. The first type, the older of the two, is the *Diameter Index Safety System* (DISS) outlet. The NFPA regulations[12] relating to these are as follows:

1. Each station outlet for oxygen and nitrous oxide must provide either a manually operated or an automatic shutoff valve.

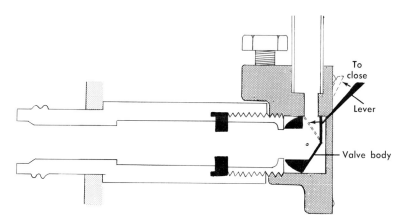

Fig. 2-15. DISS outlet, manual type. If lever is moved to left, valve body rotates to block incoming line, stopping gas flow. (Courtesy Bennett Respiration Products, Inc., Santa Monica, Calif.)

2. The station outlet must be legibly labeled with the name of the gas contained.
3. Manually operated valves must be equipped with a noninterchangeable connection complying with the DISS (CGA Pamphlet V-5).
4. Threaded outlets of this type must either be provided with a cap on a chain or be installed in a recessed box equipped with a door to protect the outlet when not in use. Station outlets in patients' rooms shall be either located approximately 5 feet above the floor or recessed to avoid physical damage to the valve or control equipment.
5. Each oxygen delivery line that services an anesthetic device through a yoke must have a backflow check valve installed in the line immediately adjacent to the yoke insert. Each check valve must be designed to hold a minimum of 2400 psig.

Primarily because of the above regulations and the accumulated knowledge acquired by manufacturers, DISS outlets are designed in one of two fashions. There is either a manual shutoff valve to close the outlet when not in use (Fig. 2-15), or there

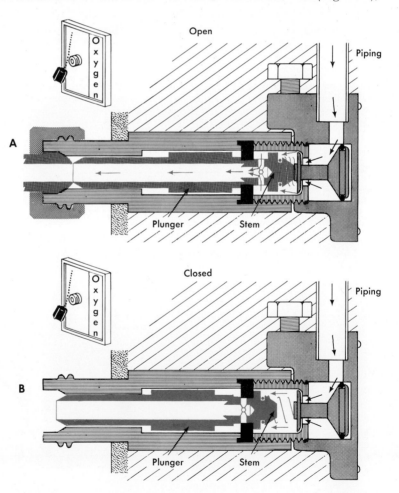

Fig. 2-16. DISS wall outlet. When equipment is attached to outlet, plunger is pushed to right, **A,** and gas is able to flow out of outlet. When equipment is removed, spring pushes plunger to left, seating it and stopping gas flow, **B.** (Courtesy Bennett Respiration Products, Inc., Santa Monica, Calif.)

is a spring-loaded plunger that automatically closes the outlet when the striker has been removed (Fig. 2-16).

The second type of outlet has become the most prevalent today and is designed to have noninterchangeable, quick-connect units for each gas. Fig. 2-17 indicates some common brands of quick-connect design.

Quick-connect outlets are subject to the same regulations as DISS outlets; the following additions from the NFPA[17] apply as well.

1. Each station outlet that is equipped with a female member of an approved quick-connect, noninterchangeable system for gas service must be so identified and provided with an automatic shutoff valve incorporated in such a manner that when the quick-connect is removed from the pipeline, the flow of gas must be automatically shut off until the male member is reattached.

2. Female members of the quick-connect couplers may be attached to manually operated shutoff valves.

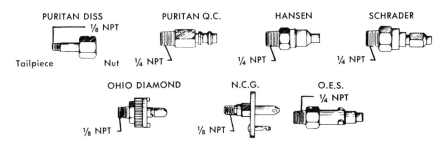

Fig. 2-17. Common brands of quick connects. (Courtesy Bennett Respiration Products, Inc., Santa Monica, Calif.)

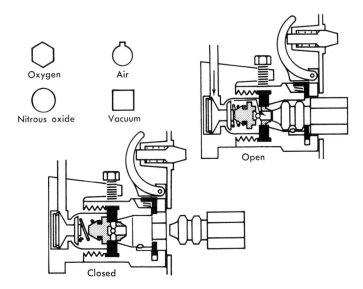

Fig. 2-18. An example of a quick-connect wall outlet. When male striker is placed into outlet, *top*, plunger is pushed back from its seat, and gas can flow out. Once striker is removed, spring pushes plunger to right against seat, stopping gas flow. (Courtesy Bennett Respiration Products, Inc., Santa Monica, Calif.)

A typical design for an automatic, quick-connect outlet incorporates a plunger that, when held forward by a spring, allows no gas to leave the outlet (Fig. 2-18). When the male quick-connect striker is inserted, the plunger is pushed backward, and gas is allowed to flow into the striker and on to the equipment to which it is attached. Once the male striker is removed, the spring reseats the plunger and closes the outlet. A manual shutoff valve can be substituted for the spring plunger unit.

Some outlets incorporate a second, automatic shutoff valve to facilitate the removal of the female quick-connect for maintenance (Fig. 2-19). The plunger for this secondary shutoff is pushed back against its spring when the female portion is in place, and gas can flow through. If the female coupling is removed, the spring pushes the secondary plunger forward, closing the outlet to gas flow.

COMPRESSORS

Since the atmosphere is man's normal environment for respiratory function, air is utilized as the basis for gas delivery in respiratory therapy. Generally, either air is compressed and piped to the site or compressed at the point of administration, rather than employing the use of air cylinders.

Compressors used to provide medical air are generally one of three types: the piston, diaphragm, and rotary units (Fig. 2-20).

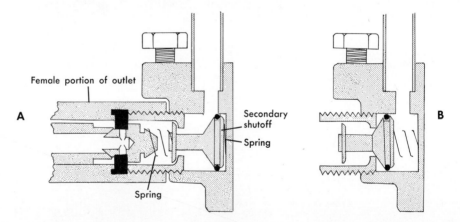

Fig. 2-19. While female coupling is in place, **A**, spring holds secondary shutoff to right, and gas passes by it freely. If female coupling is removed, **B**, spring to right of secondary shutoff pushes it to left, stopping gas flow. (Courtesy Bennett Respiration Products, Inc., Santa Monica, Calif.)

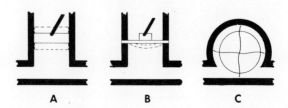

Fig. 2-20. Three types of compressors utilized in respiratory therapy: **A**, Piston. **B**, Diaphragm. **C**, Rotary. (Modified from The way things work, vol. 1, New York, 1967, Simon & Schuster, Inc.)

Piston compressors work similarly to a piston and cylinder in an engine, except that here the motion serves to compress gas. As the piston drops (Fig. 2-21), gas is drawn in through a one-way intake valve. On the upstroke, the intake valve closes, and gas leaves through an outflow (one-way) valve.

If carbon rings are used on the piston of the compressor, there should be an outflow filter to remove any carbon flakes that may be made. Carbon or teflon rings are commonly employed, and an oil lubrication must be avoided.

To power a respirator, the compressor must have (1) a high flow output, (2) usually have some type of reservoir to accommodate peak flow needs, and (3) pressure capabilities of nearly 50 psig. Larger, portable piston compressors generally have a double piston system; examples are the Bennett MC-1 and MC-2, Ohio High Performance Compressor, and the Timeter PCS-1 units. A small gas reservoir on these types of units is placed in a coiled tube to allow the hot, compressed gas to cool to room temperature. This removes some of the water content (humidity) so

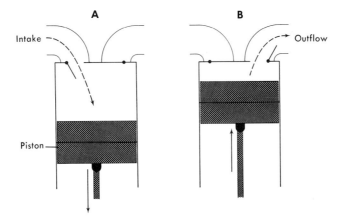

Fig. 2-21. Piston compressor. On downstroke, **A**, gas is drawn in one-way intake valve. On upstroke, **B**, gas is displaced out of one-way outflow valve.

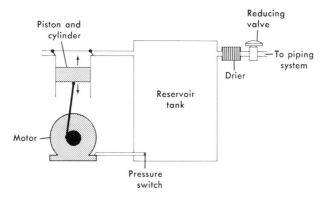

Fig. 2-22. Large compressor system for piping system. Compressor sends gas to reservoir at higher than line pressure. When preset pressure level is reached, pressure switch shuts compressor off. Gas leaves reservoir, passes through drier to remove moisture, and reducing valve reduces gas to desired line pressure. When reservoir pressure has dropped to near line pressure, pressure switch turns compressor back on.

that it will not enter into the attached device (for example, a respirator), which is powered by the compressor. There is usually a water drain near the compressor's outlet, and often a water trap is recommended at the device attached. Larger, portable piston compressors tend to be noisy, and therefore their cases are usually sound insulated.

The large units used for medical-air piping systems are frequently of the piston type. The limiting factor to their use consists of the noise and vibration they produce.

The higher the air demands for a system are, the larger the compressor required. To reduce wear on these larger compressors, a reservoir tank receives the compressed air and stores it at a higher pressure than needed in the piping system (Fig. 2-22). A drier removes humidity from the air, often by refrigeration, and a reducing valve on the reservoir outflow line reduces the air pressure to 50 psig or the desired working pressure. A pneumatic sensing unit turns the compressor off when the reservoir pressure has reached a preset high level and turns the compressor back on when the reservoir pressure drops, approaching 50 psig.

A large demand system may incorporate two alternating compressors to supply the reservoir and prolong compressor life and to allow maintenance on each compressor separately while the other one supplies the system.

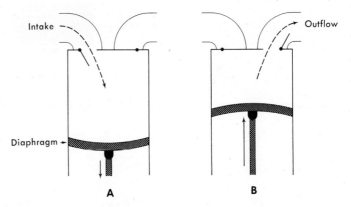

Fig. 2-23. Diaphragm compressor. On downstroke, **A**, diaphragm bows downward, drawing air in one-way intake valve. On upstroke, **B**, diaphragm bows upward, forcing gas out one-way outflow valve.

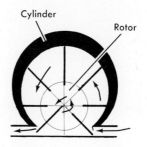

Fig. 2-24. Rotary compresor. As rotor turns counterclockwise, gas is drawn from right and is compressed as cylinder gets smaller; it is forced out left side. (Modified from The way things work, vol. 1, New York, 1967, Simon & Schuster, Inc.)

Diaphragm compressors substitute a flexible diaphragm for the piston (Fig. 2-23). On the downstroke, the diaphragm is bent downward and air enters the one-way intake valve. On the upstroke, the intake valve is closed and the compressed gas exits the outflow (one-way) valve. Examples of diaphragm compressors are the Air-Shields Diapump, the DeVilbiss small nebulizer compressor, and the unit used in the Porta Bird respirator from Bird Corporation.

Rotary compressors also find use in respiratory therapy. The rotor acts like a fan and pushes air from one area to another (Fig. 2-24). Low-pressure rotary compressors are employed in some ventilators, such as the Bennett MA-1 and the turbine units in the Ohio 560 and Critical Care Ventilators.

High-pressure units such as those used to supply medical air systems require a liquid sealant to provide efficiency in producing higher pressures. Oil cannot be employed as a seal with medical-air compressors, so water is usually used to provide this function.

Vacuum systems are devised similarly, using compressors. The compressors' intake supplies the reservoir tank with gas evacuation, producing a subatmospheric pressure (vacuum). Compressors providing vacuum cannot also be utilized for medical compressed air due to the possibility of gas contamination.

REFERENCES

1. McPherson, S. P., and Roads, J. S.: History of respiratory therapy. (To be published.)
2. Compressed Gas Association: Handbook of Compressed Gases, 1967, Reinhold.
3. Weast, R., editor: Handbook of chemistry and physics, ed. 49, 1968-1969, Chemical Rubber Company.
4. U.S. Department of Transportation: Personal correspondence.
5. Code of federal regulations: Title 49, Parts 1 to 199, October, 1973, U.S. Government Printing Office.
6. Compressed Gas Association: Characteristics and safe handling of medical gases, ed. 5, 1971.
7. Puritan Compressed Gas Corporation: Puritan medical gases, cylinder color chart, Puritan Compressed Gas Corporation.
8. Finch, G., Puritan Bennett Corporation: Personal correspondence.
9. Compressed Gas Association: American Standard, compressed gas cylinder valve outlet and inlet connections, 1965, Compressed Gas Association.
10. Union Carbide, Medical Products: How Linde USP oxygen is produced.
11. National Fire Protection Association: Bulk oxygen systems 1971, NFPA No. 50 (formerly No. 566), National Fire Protection Association.
12. National Fire Protection Association: Nonflammable medical gas systems 1970, NFPA No. 56F (formerly 565), 1970, National Fire Protection Association.
13. National Fire Protection Association: Inhalation therapy 1968, NFPA No. 56B, 1968, National Fire Protection Association.

3 Gas administration devices

An estimated 60% to 90% of the respiratory therapist's daily activities include setup and maintenance of equipment that reduces pressure, measures flow, and administers gases. Therefore a clear understanding of these devices is vital for effective delivery of patient care. The first part of this chapter deals with reducing valves, flowmeters, and regulators. The second part deals with administration devices, including masks, cannulas, and catheters.

REDUCING VALVES

The simplest of the three kinds of gas delivery devices are *reducing valves*. A reducing valve can be defined as a device that reduces a high pressure to a lower

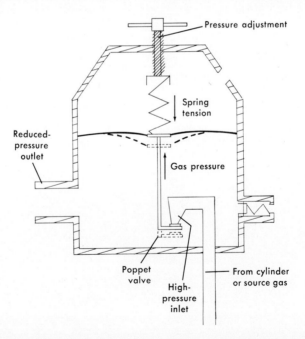

Fig. 3-1. Single-stage reducing valve functions due to opposition of two forces (gas pressure and spring tension). If the two forces are in equilibrium, diaphragm is straight and no gas enters bottom chamber. If bottom chamber's gas pressure is lower than spring tension, spring pushes downward, opening poppet valve and allowing gas to enter bottom chamber from cylinder. Gas will enter from cylinder until pressure in bottom chamber equalizes spring tension and pushes diaphragm up to straight position, closing poppet valve. (Modified from Bennett Respiration Products, Inc., Santa Monica, Calif.)

pressure. Commonly, reducing valves are utilized to reduce high pressures from cylinder gases to a lower working pressure, usually 50 psig. These devices are also employed in piping systems to drop the pressure from the bulk system to line pressure (again, usually 50 psig) and are also found in other devices that require pressure reduction, such as some ventilators. Fig. 3-1 outlines the typical structure of a *single-stage* reducing valve. The two forces that interplay, allowing the reducing valve to work, are (1) *spring tension* and (2) *gas pressure*. So that these forces oppose each other, a thin diaphragm is used to separate them. On the bottom of the diaphragm is gas pressure, which can be delivered to various apparatus, and on the top is a spring. When the two forces of spring tension and gas pressure are in equilibrium, the diaphragm is straight, and the poppet valve at the bottom closes the inlet from the cylinder (or other source). As gas pressure at the bottom drops, the spring tension is the dominant force and pushes the diaphragm downward. As a result, the poppet valve opens, allowing gas to flow into the bottom chamber of the reducing valve. Once enough gas has entered the bottom portion to cause a pressure rise equaling the spring tension, the diaphragm will again be straight, and the poppet valve will close. In this example, the spring tension would be set at the desired gas pressure, such as 50 psig.

The gauge on the reducing valve (Fig. 3-2) is a simple Bourdon gauge, as described in Chapter 1. As gas pressure rises within the Bourdon tube, the coiled tube tends to straighten, rotating an indicator by means of a gearing mechanism to indicate a higher pressure.[1,2] Conversely, a pressure drop results in less force on the outer side of the coiled tube and causes the coiled tube to regain its own shape (toward a more coiled position). The needle then drops on the scale, indicating a lower gas pressure; in this case, in the cylinder.

Reducing valves may incorporate a *poppet-closing spring*, as in Fig. 3-3, which helps overcome the pressure against the poppet from the cylinder gas pressure. The poppet spring tension is usually sufficient to oppose only the gas pressure attempting to push the poppet valve open. In this example, the reducing-valve

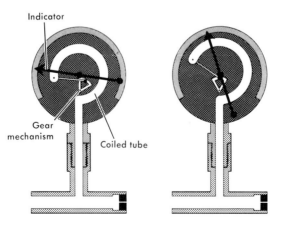

Fig. 3-2. Bourdon gauge. As gas force increases within coiled tube, tube tends to straighten or move upward. This motion is reflected through gearing mechanism as higher pressure (or flow as in case of Bourdon regulator) by indicator. (Modified from MacIntosh, R. R., Mushin, W. W., and Epstein, H. G.: *Physics for the anaesthetist,* ed. 3, Oxford, England, 1963, Blackwell Scientific Publications, Ltd.)

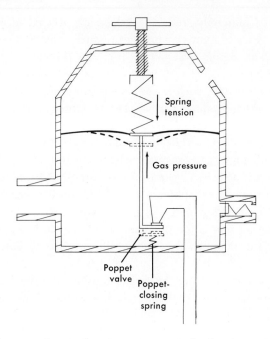

Fig. 3-3. Typical single-stage reducing valve. As gas pressure in chamber drops, center top spring pushes diaphragm assembly downward, opening poppet valve. As gas pressure in chamber equals top center-spring tension, diaphragm is pushed up, and small poppet spring closes poppet valve to gas flow.

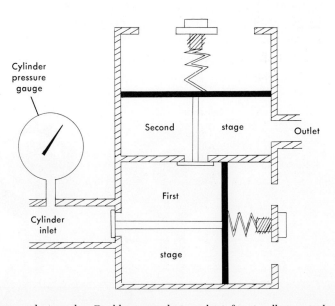

Fig. 3-4. Multistage reducing valve. Double-stage reducing valve is functionally two single-stage reducing valves working in tandem. Gas enters first stage (first reducing valve), and its pressure is lowered. Gas then enters second stage (second reducing valve), and pressure is lowered to desired working pressure (usually 50 psig). Three-stage reducing valve would have one more reducing valve in series.

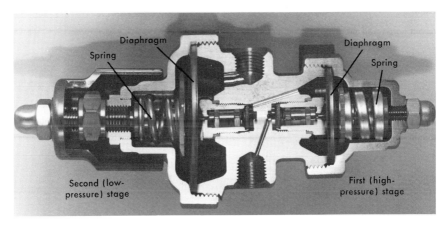

Fig. 3-5. National double-stage reducing valve. (Courtesy National Welding Equipment Co., Richmond, Calif.)

spring tension must overcome or equalize with not only the gas pressure but also the small poppet-closing spring as well:

Spring tension = Gas pressure + Closing spring tension

The *multistage* reducing valve is simply two or more single-stage reducing valves in series (Fig. 3-4). Gas enters the first stage, which is, in essence, a single-stage reducing valve. From there gas pressure is again lowered, this time by a second, single-stage reducing valve using a spring with less tension; this stage reduces the gas down to working pressure, and the gas can now be delivered to the apparatus attached. As seen in Fig. 3-4, the *double-stage* reducing valve is simply two single-stage reducing valves built together to work in series. A *triple-stage* reducing valve is actually three single-stage valves in series. Fig. 3-5 is a cross section of a National double-stage reducing valve. (Note the two diaphragms and the two springs, which adjust gas pressure in each stage.) There must always be a *pressure release* for each stage of a reducing valve. Fig. 3-6 displays the typical function of a pressure release on a reducing valve. A higher-pressure spring than the one used for the pressure control spring seats a disk or cylindrical pop-off. If a malfunction should allow the pressure in the reducing valve to rise and equal the pop-off tension, the plate simply moves from its seat and allows gas to escape around it to the atmosphere. Once the pressure has been restored to a lower level, the spring reseats the disk, and the reducing valve potentially returns to proper function. Normally, a pop-off is set at least 50% above the usual working pressure.

FLOWMETERS

Flowmeters control and indicate flow. The method of controlling flow operates on a reasonably simple principle. A flowmeter is designed to utilize a relatively constant pressure gradient (50 psi to atmospheric pressure) and adjust the size of the opening through which the gas can pass. As described in Chapter 1, if the pressure gradient is constant, the flow will increase proportionally with an increase in the orifice size through which it will pass. The orifice size changes are most often

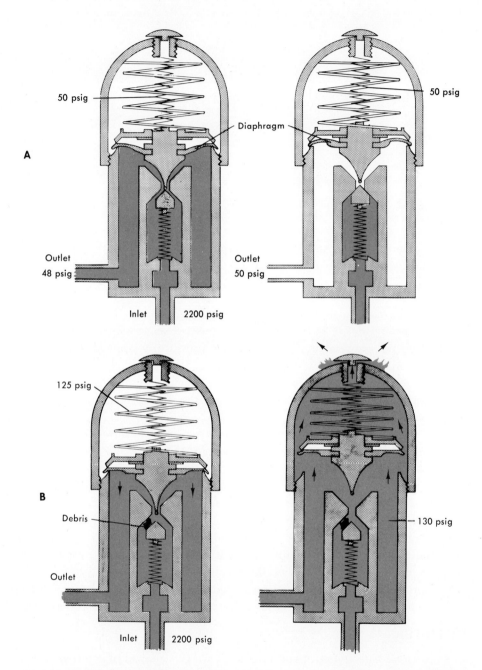

Fig. 3-6. A, Reducing valve with pressure release. If pressure rises above working pressure in compartment due to debris holding poppet valve open, **B,** gas pressure builds sufficiently to overcome outside spring, and excess gas pressure is released. (Courtesy Bennett Respiration Products, Inc., Santa Monica, Calif.)

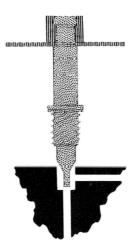

Fig. 3-7. Needle valve adjusts opening through which gas may pass due to pressure gradient across it.

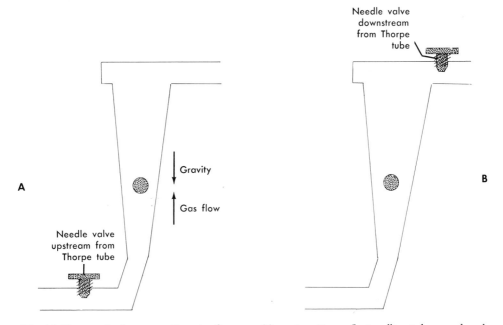

Fig. 3-8. Thorpe tube flowmeter. Opposing forces are (1) gravity acting on float, pulling it downward, and (2) force of gas molecules hitting bottom of float, pushing it upward; these forces reach equilibrium, and float remains stationary. If gas flow is increased, more force is exerted on bottom of float, and it is raised to new level, where more molecules can get past it, and equilibrium exists again. Back-pressure compensation depends primarily on location of needle valve (see text). **A,** Non–back-pressure-compensated Thorpe tube flowmeter. **B,** Back-pressure-compensated Thorpe tube flowmeter.

accomplished by manipulation of a threaded needle valve (Fig. 3-7). By turning a knob, the threads open or close the needle valve's orifice to a greater or lesser degree, and the flow is thereby increased or decreased respectively.

The most common type of flowmeter encountered in respiratory therapy is the *Thorpe tube*. The Thorpe tube (Fig. 3-8) incorporates a vertical tube of gradually increasing diameter. The ball float within it is the flow indicator. As gas flow through the unit increases, the number of molecules hitting the ball on the bottom also increases, pushing it higher. Now more gas is allowed to travel around the ball float due to the gradually increasing diameter of the Thorpe tube. Again, an opposition of forces is seen; in this case, they are (1) gravity pulling down on the ball float, and (2) molecules of the flowing gas pushing it up. Since gravity is a constant force, the flow through the tube increases the number of molecules hitting the bottom of the float and pushes the float upward. The float will rise until enough molecules can go around it so that an equilibrium again exists between gravity and the number of molecules hitting the bottom of the float.

Thorpe tubes can be *compensated* for back pressure, or they can be *non–back pressure compensated*. That is, when resistance (back pressure) is applied to the flowmeter's outlet, if the *indicated* flow is still accurate, the unit is said to be back pressure compensated.[3] The prime ingredient to denote the difference between them is the *location of the needle valve* (Fig. 3-8). If the needle valve is located upstream from the Thorpe tube, the pressure inside the Thorpe tube is basically atmospheric pressure. As resistance to flow downstream (distal) from the gas source is applied, the pressure within the Thorpe tube increases. This causes the density of the gas within the tube to increase as well, and at a given flow setting more gas molecules actually get by the ball than would at atmospheric pressure. This event occurs because the molecules are more dense, that is, they are closer together (Fig. 3-9). Once these gas molecules reach atmospheric pressure, they will expand, increasing the distance between them. Because the tube was calibrated when its internal pressure was atmospheric pressure, the reading on the scale will now reflect a lesser quantity of gas than is actually leaving the Thorpe tube. However, if the needle valve is placed downstream from the Thorpe tube, the Thorpe tube itself will always be subjected to approximately 50 psig (source gas), and its reading will not be affected by back pressure. Since back pressure cannot exceed source gas pressure (50 psig), it cannot alter the density of the gas in the tube. In a back-pressure-*compensated* flowmeter, *the needle valve is located downstream* from (after) the tube, and *the reading is accurate* even when subjected to back pressure. In a *non–back-pressure-compensated* flowmeter, *the needle valve is upstream* from (before) the Thorpe tube, and *in the presence of back pressure the actual flow out of the unit is higher than the reading indicates* (Fig. 3-11).

Another type of flowmeter is built similarly to the Thorpe tube and is called the *kinetic flowmeter*. The basic feature that differentiates it from the Thorpe tube is a *plunger* in place of the ball float (Fig. 3-10). It also has a tube of increasing diameter and can be compensated or not compensated for back pressure, relying again on the needle valve placement. In the kinetic flowmeter, as in the Thorpe tube, if the unit is back pressure compensated, its needle valve is located down-

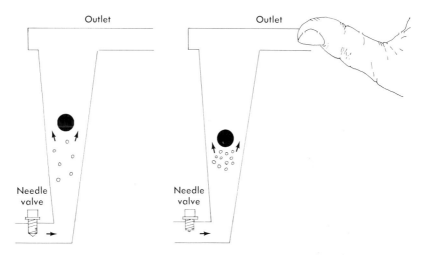

Fig. 3-9. Non–back-pressure-compensated Thorpe tube. If needle valve is located upstream from Thorpe tube, gas in tube is at and calibrated for atmospheric pressure. When resistance is posed, pressure within Thorpe tube increases above atmospheric pressure, and density of gas increases. As result of molecules being closer together, more of them get around float than at atmospheric pressure. Result is higher flow than indicated by float.

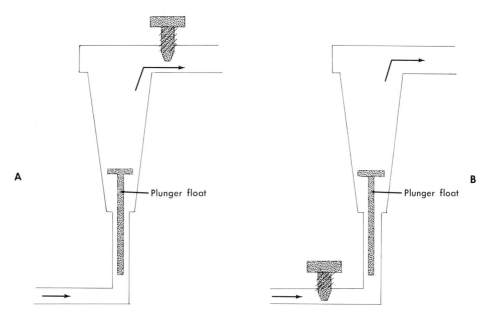

Fig. 3-10. Kinetic flowmeter. As with Thorpe tube flowmeter, needle valve placement dictates whether unit is back pressure compensated. **A,** If needle valve is downstream from tube, unit is back pressure compensated. **B,** If needle valve is upstream from tube, unit is non–back pressure compensated.

stream from the tube, and the unit will read lower than the actual flow if resistance is added (Fig. 3-11).

The ways in which a flowmeter, specifically the kinetic and the Thorpe tube types, can be checked to see if they are back pressure compensated follow.

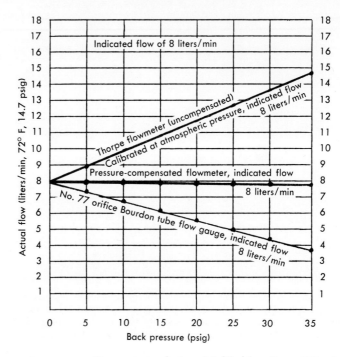

Fig. 3-11. Comparative accuracy of flow metering devices. (Modified from Bennett Respiration Products, Inc., Santa Monica, Calif.)

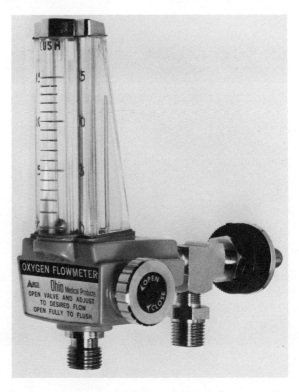

Fig. 3-12. Ohio back-pressure-compensated (Thorpe tube–type) flowmeter. (Courtesy Ohio Medical Products, Madison, Wis.)

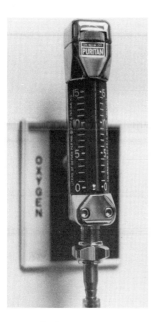

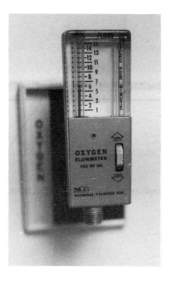

Fig. 3-13. Puritan back-pressure-compensated Thorpe tube flowmeter.

Fig. 3-14. NCG back-pressure-compensated (kinetic) flowmeter.

1. *Label.* If the unit is back pressure compensated, the label on the flowmeter will either indicate such by a statement or indicate that it was calibrated at 70° F, 50 psig (or desired pressure).
2. *Float.* If the needle valve is *closed* and the flowmeter is then plugged into the gas source, the float will jump in a back-pressure-compensated unit. This occurs because with the needle valve located downstream from the tube, the tube becomes charged with gas on plugging it into the wall outlet (gas source). Therefore the float will jump and then fall down to a zero reading when the pressure in the tube equals source pressure.
3. *Needle valve.* As a third check, the location of the needle valve will indicate whether the unit is compensated. If located downstream from the tube, the unit will be back pressure compensated. If located upstream, the unit will be non–back pressure compensated. However, looks can be deceiving, and the only way to tell for certain is by dismantling the unit.

Figs. 3-12 to 3-14 give examples of back-pressure-compensated flowmeters.

When a gas is utilized with a flowmeter other than the specified gas, the difference in gas density must be considered. For example, helium-oxygen mixtures are less dense than a 100% oxygen source. The gas molecules exert less force on the bottom of the float, making the reading lower than the actual flow. A mixture of 80% helium and 20% oxygen will deliver 1.8 times the indicated flow on an oxygen flowmeter, and a 70%-30% mixture delivers 1.6 times the indicated flow.[3]

REGULATORS

As previously described, reducing valves lower gas pressure to a specific working level. A flowmeter, by definition, would be a device that controls and measures flow. If the two devices, reducing valve and flowmeter, are incorporated into one unit, it then becomes a *regulator:* a device that reduces high-pressure gas to a safe working pressure as well as controls and measure flow. There are basically two types of regulators. The first type was the most common in the past and is the *Bourdon regulator.* The Bourdon regulator employs the simple principles described in Chapter 1, which regulate gas flow.[1,2] By utilizing a fixed orifice and altering the pressure gradient across it, flow can be adjusted. Most Bourdon regulators are structured as the one in Fig. 3-15. It is simply an adjustable reducing valve that adjusts the pressure that enters the chamber containing the fixed orifice. The higher the pressure is in that chamber, then the higher is the recording on the Bourdon gauge. This gauge's reading is calibrated as flow; when the pressure gradient is higher, the flow across the fixed-size orifice should also be higher. As long as the bottom end of the pressure gradient remains atmospheric pressure past the orifice, the flow indicated is accurate. Once a device with a built-in restriction has been attached to the regulator (Fig. 3-16), resistance occurs downstream from the reducing valve's orifice, and the indicated flow becomes inaccurate. In other words, as resistance to gas flow is imposed downstream from the Bourdon regulator, the pressure downstream from the Bourdon regulator's outlet is no longer atmospheric pressure. The result is a lowered pressure gradient and, therefore, lowered flow. The reading on the gauge will not reflect the change in actual flow, however, because the pressure it is actually sensing upstream from the restriction is still the same. Fig. 3-11 shows the relative accuracy of flowmetering devices. As resistance downstream is added to the Bourdon regulator, the flow leaving the unit is actually lower than the reading. In fact, when total occlusion of the outlet occurs, the *reading* is still unchanged (Fig. 3-16). An example of a Bourdon regulator is shown in Fig. 3-17.

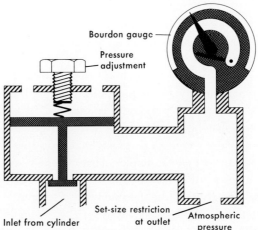

Fig. 3-15. Bourdon regulator. Adjustable reducing valve adjusts pressure exposed to set-size restriction. This same pressure is sensed by Bourdon gauge. If other side of set-sized restriction is at atmospheric pressure, result is adjustment of pressure gradient across restriction. Bottom end of gradient (if atmospheric pressure is constant), and prerestriction pressure changes reflected by Bourdon gauge would indicate pressure-gradient change. This pressure then indirectly indicates flow, and Bourdon gauge is calibrated in L/min.

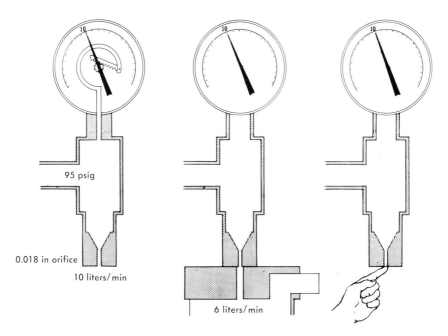

Fig. 3-16. Bourdon regulator with resistance downstream. If resistance is placed on Bourdon regulator, postrestriction pressure is no longer constant, as it will be somewhat higher than atmospheric. Pressure gradient is then decreased; since only prerestriction pressure and not actual pressure gradient is monitored, reading will be erroneously high. (Courtesy Bennett Respiration Products, Inc., Santa Monica, Calif.)

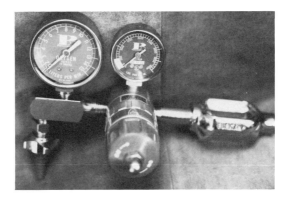

Fig. 3-17. Puritan Bourdon regulator.

The second type of regulator incorporates a reducing valve and a standard kinetic or Thorpe tube flowmeter. The accuracy of these units depends on the accuracy of the flowmeter attached. If the flowmeter is back-pressure compensated, the regulator will be accurate in the face of resistance. If the flowmeter is non–back-pressure compensated, then the reading will be lower than the actual flow when resistance is placed downstream. Two commonly used regulators are shown in Fig. 3-18.

In practical use, the regulators incorporating a back-pressure-compensated flow-

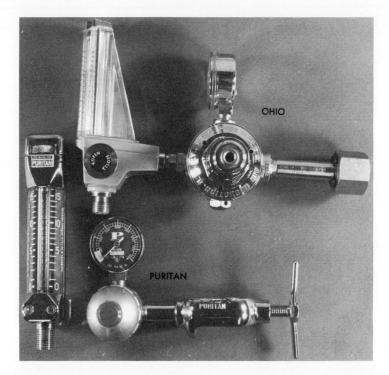

Fig. 3-18. Puritan and Ohio regulators (reducing valves with Thorpe tube flowmeters).

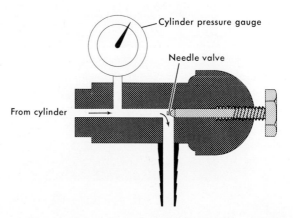

Fig. 3-19. Needle-valve regulator. Needle valve adjusts restriction through which gas must pass. As gas is removed from cylinder, pressure drops within it and flow continually diminishes due to declining pressure gradient.

meter are best unless they cannot be kept in the upright position, such as in some patient transport situations.

The Thorpe tube requires that it be in the vertical position for the reading to be accurately displayed. The Bourdon-type regulator is probably better in patient transport situations because it can be read in any physical position.

Although it is rarely found in modern hospitals, a device commonly called a *regulator* was frequently encountered in the past. It was actually only a simple needle valve connected directly to a high-pressure cylinder *without* a pressure-reducing valve (Fig. 3-19). The problem with this type of device is that, since cylinder pressure drops as gas is removed, the pressure gradient across the needle valve also decreases, and, therefore, the flow from the unit continually decreases. In addition, there is no flow-indicating device included to display what the flow being delivered actually is. Some definite problems could exist with this type of device. Therefore it has been replaced with other types of regulators such as those already described.

MASKS

Respiratory therapy was originally established for the administration of gases such as oxygen. Today, a large portion of the therapeutics delivered by respiratory therapy personnel still constitutes the administration of prescribed medical gases.

One of the first and still common types of oxygen administration devices employed in respiratory therapy is the *simple mask*. It is similar in design to the one invented by Ingenhouse, in 1789, and it is used today in a large variety of clinical situations (Fig. 3-20).[4] The simple mask is designed to provide a flow of gas into a cone-shaped piece that fits over the patient's nose and mouth. It has simple, open ports for exhalation from which a patient can also draw in some room air during inspiration if the flow of gas into the cone does not meet his peak inspiratory flow demands. In some instances, the cone can also act as a potential reservoir for accumulated, exhaled carbon dioxide if a minimal flow of gas is not maintained. Some variations of this mask incorporate a simple diluter to entrain room air as the oxygen flow enters the mask (Fig. 3-21), thus more adequately flushing the exhaled carbon dioxide from the mask. The oxygen-air mixture is not constant, since the oxygen flows used clinically allow some quantity of gas to be drawn in through the exhalation ports. This amount can be reduced by increasing the flow to the patient with the air-entrainment device attached. The oxygen percentages delivered through the simple mask can approach 35% to 55% when oxygen flow rates of 6 to 10 L/min are used for adults.[3]

The next type of mask employed in respiratory therapy is a *partial-rebreathing mask*. The face-piece structure is similar to that of a simple mask, but a reservoir bag has been added. Gas coming from the oxygen source is directed into the reservoir bag. When the patient inhales, he draws gas from both the bag and then, potentially, from the room through the exhalation ports (Fig. 3-22). As the patient exhales, the design of the unit allows for the first third of exhaled gas to go back into the bag. This third is the approximate portion of the inspired tidal volume that remains in the upper airways and is not exposed to respiratory gas exchange. Therefore the gas is reasonably high in oxygen percentage and low in carbon dioxide percentage. This gas is now mixed with what is in the reservoir bag as the patient exhales. This mixture is then inhaled by the patient in the next breath. This type of mask can be expected to deliver up to 60% oxygen.[3] The partial-rebreathing mask, as with all masks that have a reservoir bag, should have the gas flow into it adjusted so that the bag never completely collapses as the patient inhales.

The third type of mask found in medical-gas therapy is the *nonrebreathing mask*.

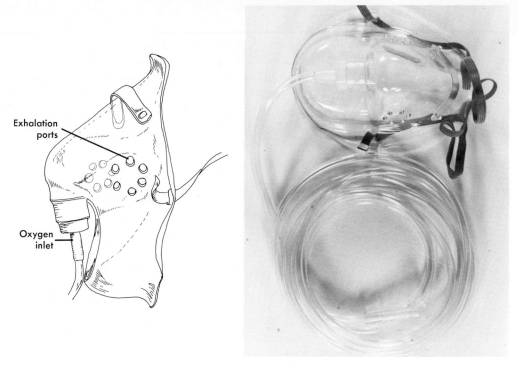

Fig. 3-20. Simple mask. Oxygen is delivered to cone-shaped facepiece from which patient both inhales oxygen and draws in room air through exhalation ports. On exhalation, gas exits exhalation ports.

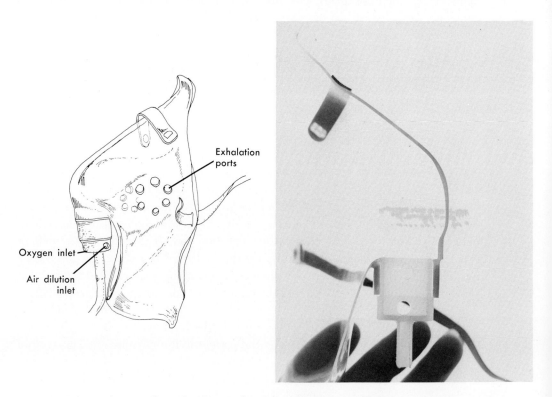

Fig. 3-21. Hudson simple mask. This simple mask incorporates simple diluter to entrain air, which increases total flow and maintains oxygen concentration at moderate level.

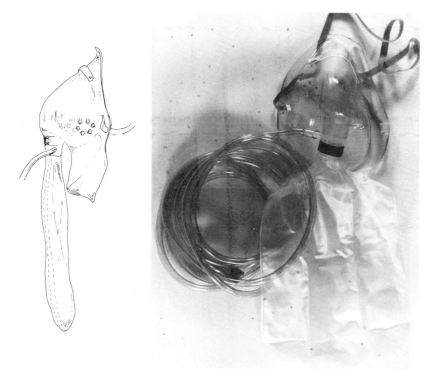

Fig. 3-22. Partial-rebreathing mask. Patient draws from reservoir bag as well as room. First portion of exhaled gas reenters bag, and remainder exits through exhalation ports.

Its structure is similar to the partial-rebreathing mask with the addition of two valve placements (Fig. 3-23). The first placement is a one-way valve between the reservoir bag and the mask. This allows gas flow to enter into the mask from the reservoir bag, but prevents gas flow back into the bag from the mask itself during the patient's exhalation as occurs in the partial-rebreathing mask. The second valve placement is at the exhalation ports. There are two one-way valves positioned so as not to allow gas to enter the mask from the room during the patient's inhalation but to allow gas to leave the mask on exhalation. When this type of mask fits the patient's face snugly, it can deliver 95% (plus or minus 5%) oxygen,[3] provided that the flow to the bag must be properly adjusted so that the bag never totally collapses as the patient inhales.

For completeness' sake, there is a fourth type of mask, the *rebreathing mask.* Although it is no longer used clinically in respiratory therapy, it was employed primarily as a resuscitation device at one time. It is still found today, although it is used nearly exclusively in administration of anesthetics. This type of unit consists of a cone-shaped mask without exhalation ports, which is connected directly to a bag without valves. The patient breathes into and from the attached bag (Fig. 3-24). In the administration of anesthetics, this unit has a carbon dioxide–absorbing agent, such as soda lime, placed between the mask and the bag. When the patient exhales back into the bag, the carbon dioxide from his expired gas is then absorbed. This keeps the concentration in the bag relatively high in oxygen and low in carbon

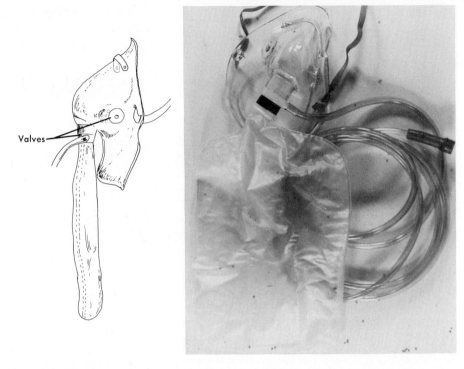

Valves

Fig. 3-23. Nonrebreathing mask. Patient can draw gas only from bag, and exhaled gas can exit only through exhalation ports, due to valves.

dioxide. When the volume of gas in the bag drops as oxygen is utilized by the patient, additional volume is added to the bag in the form of 100% oxygen.

Respiratory therapy has become more sophisticated in the delivery of its therapeutics; today, oxygen is often prescribed, as it should be, in terms of a specified concentration. There are several masks and adaptations of masks available on the market that allow for a set oxygen concentration to be delivered by a relatively simple principle. They are often called *Venturi masks*, although the name is not entirely appropriate, since they do not incorporate a true Venturi tube. Actually, these units work on a principle described by Bernoulli: a restriction, commonly called a *jet*, provides a low, lateral pressure past it and thus can entrain air (Chapter 1). By controlling the jet size or the air entrainment port size, a precise percentage of oxygen can be obtained, depending on the structure of the mask.

The important points to remember about *dilution-type masks* are:
1. The size of the entrainment ports and/or the jet dictate the percentage of oxygen attained by the mask.
2. As long as the total flow of gas from the unit exceeds the patient's peak inspiratory flow demands, the desired percentage will be delivered to the patient as he inhales.
3. The units cannot be subjected to significant resistance to gas flow, or the oxygen percentage to be delivered will increase.

Fig. 3-25 reviews the principles of air entrainment control described by Ber-

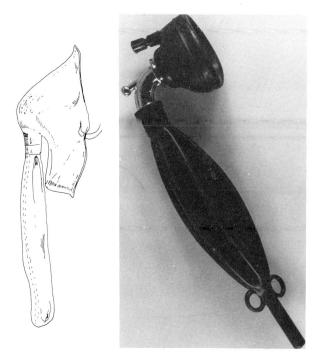

Fig. 3-24. Rebreathing mask. Patient breathes into and from bag. Under normal use, carbon dioxide–absorbing agent would be placed between bag and mask.

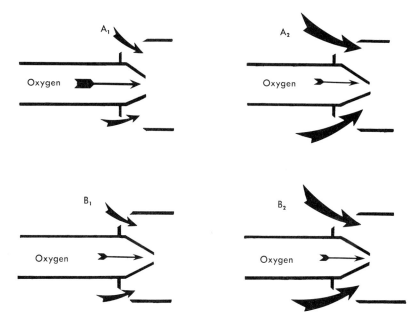

Fig. 3-25. Principles of entrainment control. A_1 and A_2 show relationship of smaller jet, A_2, entraining more air than larger jet, A_1, when both have identically sized entrainment ports. B_1 and B_2 show how, with same size jet, larger air entrainment ports, B_2, allow for increased air entrainment compared to B_1.

noulli's principle (discussed in Chapter 1). Several devices, such as the Ventimask, OEM's Venturi MixOMask, Inspiron's Accur Ox Masks, and Scott diluters alter jet size to obtain the oxygen percentage desirable. The units with smaller jet sizes produce lower oxygen mixtures because with a smaller jet size, the gas velocity through it is higher, and the lateral pressure beyond it is lower, causing more ambient air to be entrained. Also, with the increased amount of entrained air, the percentage delivered is lower, and the total gas flow becomes higher.

Other units, like Hudson's Multi-Vent, include a constant jet size and alter the entrainment-port size, as did Alvin Barach with his original "mix mask" in 1941.[4] With a constant flow through the jet, there will be a constant lateral subatmospheric pressure; thus the pressure exerted at the entrainment port will be a constant gradient (from atmospheric to the generated, lateral, negative pressure). Enlarging the port size will provide a larger area through which gas can pass; this is similar to opening the needle valve on a flowmeter to increase the area available for gas to flow through. Here, the results are an increased flow of air into the unit, a lower oxygen percentage, and a higher total gas flow to the patient.

Two pieces of apparatus that have been used for some period of time and that deliver relatively low oxygen concentrations (up to 50%) are the *nasal catheter* and the *cannula*. Oxygen catheters are placed into one of the two nares of the patient and then inserted straight back posteriorly until they come to rest in the pharynx, just behind the uvula. The purpose of this device is to provide a flow of oxygen into the oral pharynx, utilizing this area as a potential internal reservoir in which an oxygen concentration could build (Fig. 3-26). The nasal cannula, on the other hand, provides two short prongs, which are inserted into the anterior nares and through which gas flow enters. Because of anatomy of the nasal pharynx, it would appear that those devices which incorporate a curve in the prongs to direct the gas posteriorly would be optimum, since this design would tend to direct gas flow through the turbinates where the gas can be properly humidified. Fig. 3-27, *A*, shows the conventional straight prong, which directs the flow upward toward the opening of the frontal sinuses; thus excessive flows could be irritating. Incorporating a curved prong as well as a flare in the prong's end, as in Fig. 3-27, *B*, may also be advantageous to provide a smoother gas flow, which is spread over a wider area and directed posteriorly.[5] Those cannulas which incorporate these features may have a higher flow capability and, potentially, a higher oxygen concentration delivered.[5]

Aerosol masks, tracheostomy aerosol masks, and endotracheal tube tees were designed originally for the administration of aerosols. However, with the onset of precise oxygen percentage control with high gas flows to the patient, these units have found an increasingly wider use in oxygen administration. They can be fitted to cover the opening to the patient's airway, and then relatively high flow of gas of a precise percentage can be delivered to the nose and mouth, tracheostomy, or endotracheal tube (Fig. 3-28).

Oxygen should be ordered by percentage; optimally, this should be coupled with proper physiologic monitoring of its administration by blood gases, hemoglobin content, arterial oxygen concentration, cardiac output, lactic acid production,

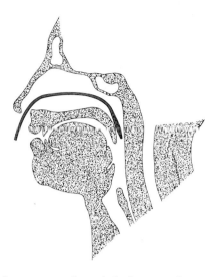

Fig. 3-26. Nasal catheter. Catheter is inserted straight back posteriorly into nasal pharynx so that it comes to rest behind uvula. Purpose is to utilize nasal and oral pharynx as internal reservoir.

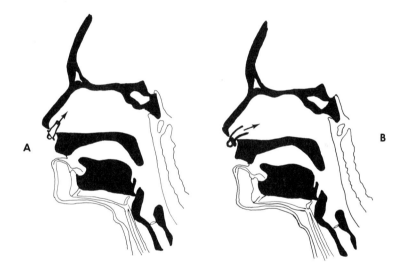

Fig. 3-27. Cannula comparison. The two prongs of nasal cannula are inserted into nares and oxygen is directed into nasal cavity. Anatomy of nasal cavity would indicate that optimal direction of gas flow should be toward posterior portion of cavity (as in **B**) and away from frontal sinuses.

DPG levels, etc.[3,6] The specific oxygen concentration and total gas flow must be properly maintained to ensure proper oxygenation that will keep the arterial oxygen content of the blood as near normal as possible and thereby assure that the cells of the body are actually receiving the necessary amounts of oxygen to maintain their normal function.[6] If the basic devices for oxygen administration mentioned in the earlier part of this chapter are used, then the range of oxygen-percentage delivery should be known (Table 3-1). The respiratory therapist must also acquire the ability to adapt the equipment available to deliver the concentrations necessary

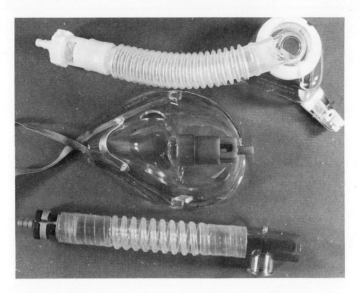

Fig. 3-28. Tracheostomy mask, aerosol mask, and endotracheal tube tee fitted for low-oxygen-percentage delivery.

Table 3-1. Commonly obtainable oxygen concentrations from various oxygen administering devices

Device	Commonly used flows (L/min)	Oxygen concentrations
Simple mask	6 to 10	35 to 55%
Partial-rebreathing mask	6 to 10*	Up to 60%
Nonrebreathing mask	6 to 10*	Up to 95% ± 5%
Nasal catheter	Up to 6 or 8	Up to 50%
Nasal cannula	Up to 6 or 8	Up to 50%

*Flow should be adequate to prevent the reservoir bag from collapsing each breath.

to maintain proper arterial oxygen levels. All the steps just mentioned should be taken so that oxygen, as a pharmacologic agent, can be administered in controlled dosages, as with other medications.

Other medical gases have specific indications for and potential problems associated with their use and should therefore be well understood by personnel involved in their administration. All medical gases are pharmacologic agents, and their use should be monitored carefully, as with any drug.

Whenever oxygen is in use, a "No Smoking" sign must be posted and patients and visitors instructed as to the potential hazards associated with oxygen's use.[7]

TENTS

The value of tent-type environmental enclosures was established in 1920 by Leonard Hill, who invented the first oxygen tent.[1] The oxygen tent's environmental control ability was expanded by Alvin Barach, in 1924, when he added ice and a fan for cooling.[4] Refined versions of tents produced since that time provide environmental control of (1) oxygen concentration, (2) temperature, (3) humidity/aerosol, and (4) filtered gas.

Table 3-2. Minimum oxygen flows needed to provide oxygen levels of up to 50% and carbon dioxide levels below 1% for various tent devices

Device	Minimum oxygen flow (L/min)
Adult console tent	12 to 15
CAM Tent	7 to 12
Croupette Child Tent	10 to 12
Croupette Model D	8 to 10

In many styles of tents, the oxygen percentage attained is a function of the incoming flow, tent canopy volume, and the degree the canopy is sealed or tucked in around the bed. Minimum flows have been selected for various tents, based on the canopy volume (Table 3-2). These flows are designed to maintain the oxygen percentage at maximum (40% to 50%) and carbon dioxide at minimum (below 1%).[3] With an oxygen percentage-control approach of this type, continuous oxygen monitoring is optimum, since entry into a tent for patient care purposes alters the oxygen percentage. A more refined method of oxygen percentage control is use of high-flow (20 to 40 L/min) set percentages into the canopy through some aerosol generator, such as an ultrasonic nebulizer (Fig. 3-29).

All tent canopies should have three "No Smoking" signs on them.[7] One should be located so the patient can read it and two positioned on opposing sides so they are visible externally. A "No Smoking" sign must be placed on the door to the room, and patients and visitors instructed as to the potential hazards involved with oxygen.[7] Electrical appliances are also restricted from being used in an oxygen environment (Fig. 3-30 shows examples).

Temperature control of the environment is necessary to remove the patient's body heat. Temperature controls on small units, such as so-called croup tents, incorporate ice to cool the environment. Flow diagrams for two popular units are

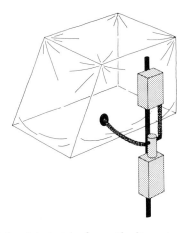

Fig. 3-29. High flow into tent (such as with ultrasonic nebulizer and fan).

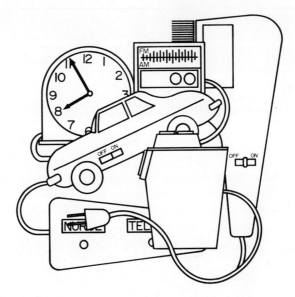

Fig. 3-30. Items *not* to be placed in oxygen-enriched tents include toys, radios, nurse call buttons, electric razors, and other appliances.

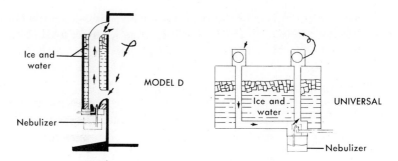

Fig. 3-31. Functional flow diagrams for Air Shields Croupettes.

depicted in Fig. 3-31. A jet nebulizer entrains canopy gas through one tube and exposes the gas and aerosol mixture to the cold wall of that tube, which absorbs heat from the gas.

Other units utilize a refrigeration cycle to cool the environment (Fig. 3-32). The coolant fluid, such as Freon, is compressed into a high-pressure hot gas. The hot gas under pressure passes through condensing coils, which have room air blown over them. The room air removes heat, lowering the coolant temperature below its critical temperature, and the gas changes to the liquid state. The liquid coolant passes into a liquid reservoir and is pushed through a heat exchanger, which cools the liquid below room temperature. The liquid then travels through an expansion valve. At the expansion valve, the high-pressure liquid is allowed to reexpand and convert to the gaseous state. This expansion throughout the cooling coils allows the coolant to absorb heat from the tent environment. The coolant gas passes from

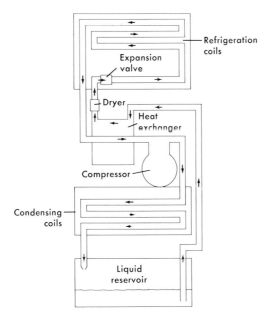

Fig. 3-32. Refrigeration cycle.

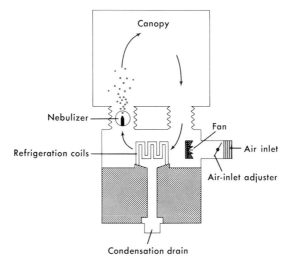

Fig. 3-33. Adult console tent incorporating refrigeration coils for cooling.

the evaporator (cooling) coils through the heat exchanger, where the gas absorbs heat from the liquid coolant traveling to the condensing coils. The gas coolant is drawn to the compressor, and the process is repeated. In a console tent, the refrigeration cycle accomplishes transfer of heat from the tent to the room, resulting in the cooling of the patient's environment (Fig. 3-33). Because the cooling coils are exposed to the patient's environment and may have an aerosol condensation on them, they must be cleaned and decontaminated between patients. An example of this type of tent is the Ohio Environmental tent.

The Child Adult Mist (CAM) Tent made by Mistogen employs the refrigeration cycle to cool water, which is then circulated through a cooling panel in the tent's environment for heat removal (Fig. 3-34). The circulation of the gas within the canopy caused by the nebulizer's gas flow causes contact of the tent's gas with the cooling panel, and heat is absorbed by the cold water.

Most tents with direct exposure of tent gas to refrigeration coils have the capability of cooling the environment to 10° to 12° F below room temperature. Units using ice or having indirect gas contact with the refrigeration coils are generally able to cool the environment only to 6° to 8° F below room temperature or less.

Aerosol is added to the tent by either a pneumatic nebulizer, which is often built into the tent frame (Figs. 3-31 and 3-33), or by an ultrasonic nebulizer (Fig. 3-29). An increased humidity content of the environment results from evaporation

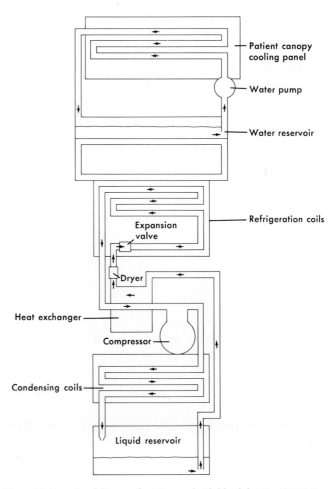

Fig. 3-34. Functional diagram for Mistogen's Child Adult Mist (CAM) Tent.

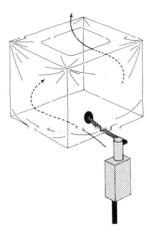

Fig. 3-35. Open-top tent.

of the aerosol within the canopy. A filtered environment is accomplished by either having all gas entering the tent come from a piped source that is free of dust particles or, if ambient air is utilized, by drawing it through a filter as in Fig. 3-33.

Open-top tents (Fig. 3-35) are selected in some instances rather than a refrigerated console primarily when oxygen concentrations above room air are not needed. The open tent allows any heat inside to rise and escape from the top. Since there is no cooling ability other than simple evaporation of aerosol within the tent, high flows (20 to 40 L/min) should be utilized to keep the tent's temperature from rising above ambient temperature.

INCUBATORS

The first incubator was designed by Denuce of Bordeaux, France, in 1857.[4] The first enclosed incubator was designed by Dr. Tarnier and built by Odile Martin, Director of the Paris Zoo, in 1880, for use in Paris maternity hospital.[4] These units' designs were conceived to provide a warm environment for premature infants. Later designs have expanded the capabilities of incubators to provide control of (1) temperature, (2) oxygen concentration, (3) humidity, and (4) an isolated or filtered gas environment. The design of an incubator has the same basic objectives as a tent, but the temperature control is normally for heating a unit rather than cooling it, and the isolation incubator is a more tightly sealed enclosure.

Heating is accomplished by use of heating coils. (Care should be taken not to use a spray disinfectant when cleaning the coils, since they may then produce a toxic gas when heated from any residual cleaning agent left on them.) A fan circulates environmental gas through the coils and over a blow-by humidifier, which is used to keep the air moist.

Most incubators have dilution devices on the incoming gas inlet to limit oxygen-concentration potential to 40%. To accomplish higher percentages, the air entrainment ports are occluded, and, on some units, this is indicated by a visible red flag.

Since the oxygen concentration is difficult to keep constant, particularly with the larger isolation incubators, *hoods* are often used (Fig. 3-36). These are generally

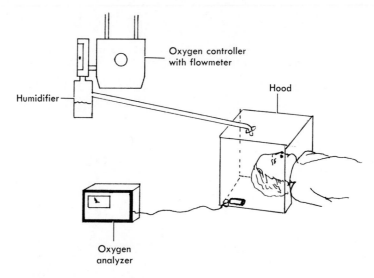

Fig. 3-36. Oxygen hood for infants with humidified preblended oxygen.

small clear plastic enclosures designed to be placed over just the infant's head. Preblended, humidified oxygen is then administered so that the monitored oxygen levels remain relatively constant and the exhaled carbon dioxide is flushed out. This allows for general nursing care of the infant without interfering with the infant's oxygen therapy. It should be noted that the noise levels from incoming gas flows can be loud in these devices and special care should be provided so as to avoid this problem.

REFERENCES

1. MacIntosh, R. R., Mushin, W. W., and Epstein, H. G.: Physics for the anaesthetist, ed. 3, Oxford, England, 1963, Blackwell Scientific Publications, Ltd.
2. Spearman, C. B.: The Bourdon regulator, Respir. Care **20:**750, Aug., 1975.
3. Egan, D. F.: Fundamentals of respiratory therapy, ed. 3, St. Louis, 1977, The C. V. Mosby Co.
4. McPherson, S. P., and Roads, J. S.: History of respiratory therapy. (To be published.)
5. Barach, A.: Personal communication, 1972.
6. Miller, W. F.: Physiological basis for oxygen therapy, Bulletin, Methodist Hospital of Dallas Medical Staff **3:**1, July, 1968.
7. Standard for respiratory therapy, NFPA No. 56B, Boston, 1973, National Fire Protection Association.

4 Humidifiers and nebulizers

Nearly every form of therapeutic intervention employed in respiratory therapy utilizes some form of either humidity or aerosol. In fact, many therapeutic modalities are designed to administer one of the two for specific disorders.

HUMIDITY

Humidity is invisible moisture, that is, *water in the form of individual molecules in its vapor or gaseous state.* These gaseous water molecules (Fig. 4-1) are present in the air we breathe and are all around us. To be even more precise, humidity is actually *vapor.* As defined in Chapter 1, vapor is composed of individual free molecules existing below the critical temperature of that substance (Fig. 4-2). Therefore humidity is not true gaseous water because our environment is at a temperature below the critical temperature of water (374.1° C). For the purposes of this discussion, however, the terms *gas* and *vapor* can be used synonymously.

Humidity may be measured in three different ways. The first method is *absolute humidity,* or the *actual water content of a gas.* The humidity content is recorded in terms of weight per volume, usually in *grams per cubic meter* or *milligrams per liter* (Fig. 4-3). Absolute humidity is usually measured by extracting the water vapor from a known volume of gas and measuring the weight of the water removed.

Since humidity is gaseous vapor, it exerts a pressure; this fact is the basis for the second method of measuring humidity in a gas. As the humidity content or temperature increases, the *partial pressure* of water vapor also increases (Table 4-1). The reason for this increase, as discussed in Chapter 1, is that as the temperature of gaseous molecules increases, their velocity increases. Therefore the molecules now hit objects in their path with greater force, and these collisions are measured as a greater partial pressure.

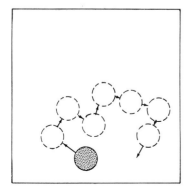

Fig. 4-1. Humidity is water as vapor. Water molecules act as gas, moving in random fashion and exerting pressure.

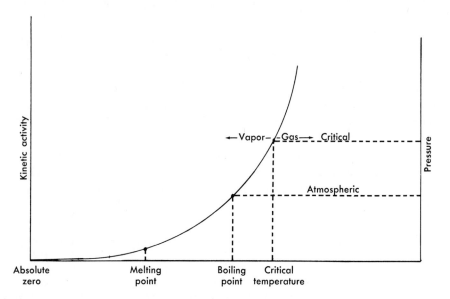

Fig. 4-2. As temperature of molecules rises, their kinetic activity also increases. This is measured as increased pressure. Once sufficient kinetic activity is reached, molecules change their state of matter. Temperatures at which transition of states occur establish both gas melting point and critical temperature. Boiling point represents temperature at which molecular activity equals atmospheric pressure. Below critical temperature, state of free molecules is considered vapor, and above critical temperature, molecules are considered true gas.

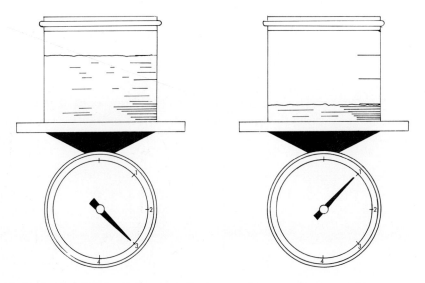

Fig. 4-3. Absolute humidity is actual content of water vapor in gas, usually measured in grams per cubic meter or milligrams per liter. (Modified from Barnes, T. A., and Israel, J. S.: Fundamentals of inhalation therapy principles, Lippincott overhead transparencies, Bowie, Md., 1969, Robert J. Brady Co.)

Table 4-1. Water vapor pressures*

Temperature (°C)	P_{H_2O} (mm Hg)	Temperature (°C)	P_{H_2O} (mm Hg)
20	17.5	29	30.0
21	18.7	30	31.8
22	19.8	31	33.7
23	21.1	32	35.7
24	22.4	33	37.7
25	23.8	34	39.9
26	25.2	35	42.2
27	26.7	36	44.6
28	28.3	37	47.0

*Water vapor pressures increase with a rise in temperature. As the temperature of the water molecules rises, the increased molecular velocity causes them to exert more force. (From Comroe, J. H., Jr.: Physiology of respiration, Chicago, 1965, Year Book Medical Publishers, Inc.)

The third method of measuring water vapor is in terms of relative humidity. *Relative humidity is a percentage expression of the actual water vapor content of a gas as compared to its capacity to carry water at any given temperature.* The capacity of a gas to hold water in its vapor state will increase as the temperature of the gas rises. The capacity of gas to contain water vapor relates to the molecular velocity of the gaseous water molecules (Chapter 1). As the temperature of the individual molecules of water increases, the molecules' velocity exerts a greater force, which pushes other gas molecules aside and joins them in the gas mixture. Therefore the number of water vapor molecules present increases. As a result of the increased force or partial pressure of water vapor, the humidity increases (Fig. 4-4). Thus as temperature increases, it is commonly stated that the *capacity* of a gas to hold water is also increased. If the temperature of the gas is known and either (1) the absolute humidity of the gas or (2) the partial pressure of water vapor of the gas is known, then the relative humidity can be calculated. By referring to the appropriate charts, one can find either the gas vapor pressure or its maximum capacity for holding water. Vapor pressure is actually the maximum pressure that water can exert at a given temperature. The actual maximum capacity of the gas for holding water is measured by total vapor content, or weight per volume at a given temperature. These figures can be substituted into one of the simple formulas listed in the following examples to calculate the percent of relative humidity.

EXAMPLE 1:

$$\text{Given: Absolute humidity} = 18.4 \text{ mg/L}$$

$$\text{Temperature} = 98.6° \text{ F}$$

$$\% \text{ R.H.} = \frac{\text{Content}}{\text{Capacity}} \times 100$$

$$= \frac{18.4 \text{ mg/L}}{43.8 \text{ mg/L}} \times 100$$

$$= 0.42 \times 100$$

$$= 42\%$$

EXAMPLE 2:

Given: Vapor pressure = 19.8 mm Hg

Temperature = 37° C

$$\% \text{ R.H.} = \frac{P_{H_2O}}{P_{Vapor\ H_2O}} \times 100$$

$$= \frac{19.8 \text{ mm Hg}}{47.1 \text{ mm Hg}} \times 100$$

$$= 0.42 \times 100$$

$$= 42\%$$

Humidity therapy

The rationale for uses of humidity in respiratory therapy can be placed in two general categories: (1) supplying enough water vapor to the inspired gas to make it comfortable for the patient and (2) heating the gas to provide 100% relative humidity at body temperature. Normally, the air that people inhale contains some humidity. Since nearly all the gases utilized in respiratory therapy are 100% dry, they must have water vapor added to them before being delivered to patients.

Humidifiers

To accomplish the first type of humidity therapy, simple nonheated humidifying devices are employed. The factors affecting the efficiency of humidifying devices are (1) *time* of contact between gas and water, (2) the *surface area* involved in gas/water contact and (3) the *temperature*. The longer gas and water are in contact with each other, the higher the chance will be of the humidity molecules having sufficient time to displace as many gas-mixture molecules as they can. If these water molecules do attain the greatest quantity possible in the gas mixture at that temperature, then the maximum vapor pressure will be reached. The exposure time and gas/water con-

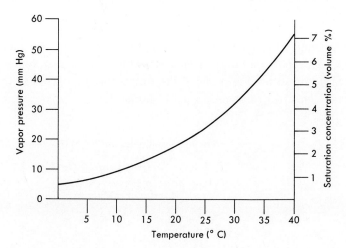

Fig. 4-4. As water vapor pressure increases, water molecules' increased force pushes other gas molecules aside, and water content of gas increases. (From MacIntosh, R. R., Mushin, W. W., and Epstein, H. G.: Physics for the anaesthetist, ed. 3, Oxford, England, 1963, Blackwell Scientific Publications, Ltd.)

tact were optimum if 100% relative humidity was reached at that temperature. If this was not so, then the quantity of water held in the gas at that temperature would not equal the capacity of that gas for holding water vapor. Thus the relative humidity would be below 100% at that temperature. The greater the surface area of the gas-and-water interface, the greater the chance of water molecules pushing their way into the gas mixture. The temperatures of the gas and water are also important. As the temperature increases, the force exerted by the water molecules increases. This increased vapor pressure allows the water molecules to push more gas mixture molecules aside; hence the humidity content will increase.

Simple humidifiers. Simple humidifiers do not employ heat, since they are designed to add only enough humidity to make the gas being administered more comfortable. As the gas enters the patient's airways, the normal humidification mechanism of the nose will supply the balance of moisture not provided by the humidifier. However, if the upper airways are bypassed by a tracheostomy or an endotracheal tube, then the humidity content of the inspired gas must be increased to 100% relative humidity at body temperature. Simple nonheated humidifiers (when working optimally) may provide 100% relative humidity at their operating temperature. However, this amount of moisture supplies only about a third of the total moisture required for the respiratory tract's humidification at body temperature (Fig. 4-5). There are several types of simple nonheated units. The first has been utilized in respiratory therapy for many years and is the *pass-over* or *blow-by* humidifier.[1] This type is the simplest in design (Fig. 4-6). In this unit, the gas merely passes over the water surface and then flows to the patient. The efficiency of this unit is rather low because the time of exposure and the surface area of gas/water contact are reasonably limited. Some examples of blow-by units are those found in a few models of

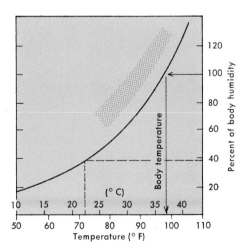

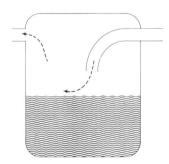

Fig. 4-5. Humidity content graph. At room temperature, 100% relative humidity is only about 37% of total quantity of humidity necessary at body temperature. (Modified from Cushing, I. E., and Miller, W. F.: Nebulization therapy. In Safar, P., editor: Respiratory therapy, Philadelphia, 1965, F. A. Davis Co.)

Fig. 4-6. In blow-by or pass-over humidifier, gas is directed over surface of water and then out of unit.

incubators and some respirators, such as the Emerson Post-Op, although these units generally incorporate the use of a heater.

The second type of simple humidifying device is the *bubble* humidifier[1] (Fig. 4-7). This is probably the most common unit used in respiratory therapy. In this device, gas is conducted below the surface of the water and allowed to bubble back to the top. The time and the surface area contact have been increased over the blow-by humidifier, and therefore its efficiency is also increased (Fig. 4-8). These units are also sometimes called *diffuser* types because several incorporate a device used to break up the gas into smaller bubbles. The smaller the bubbles created, the greater the gas/water surface area, enhancing the efficiency of the unit. Nearly all bubble humidifiers used today by respiratory therapy employ some kind of diffuser device, so, for practical purposes, bubble and diffuser humidifiers can be considered to be the same type.

The third type of simple humidifying device is a *jet* humidifier[1] (Fig. 4-9). It actually produces an aerosol; however, it employs a baffle system whereby these particles are either removed or evaporate before leaving the unit. This type of unit increases both time and gas/water surface area contact over the bubble type (Fig. 4-8).

The fourth type of simple humidifier is the *underwater jet*[1] (Fig. 4-10). It actually

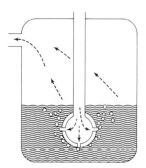

Fig. 4-7. In bubble humidifier, gas is directed below surface of water and bubbles back to top.

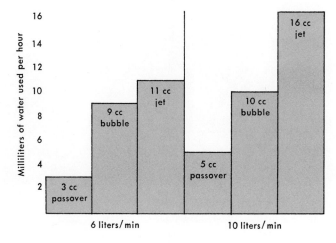

Fig. 4-8. Comparative output of nondisposable humidifiers. (Courtesy Ohio Medical Products, Madison, Wis.)

incorporates the principles of both a bubble and a jet humidifier into one concept. The gas is conducted below the surface of the water to a jet that utilizes Bernoulli's principle, as does the jet humidifier, to produce an aerosol. As gas bubbles containing aerosol float to the surface of the water, the gas/water interface and time of exposure are increased, and the result is improved efficiency of the unit.

Within the past few years, many *disposable*, simple humidifiers have been produced. Nearly all of these are the bubble type. Their engineering provides that their efficiency is sufficient to produce from 80% to 100% relative humidity at operating temperature. All units, to varying degrees, lose their effectiveness as the water level decreases. This occurs because the time of gas/water exposure decreases. To accurately evaluate a humidifier, the clinician should be aware of all the above factors. He should also be able to test the humidifier to ascertain (1) the ability of the unit to deliver 100% relative humidity, (2) the level at which its efficiency drops significantly, and (3) most importantly, whether the unit leaks gas.

Heated humidifiers. The second category of the use of humidity in respiratory

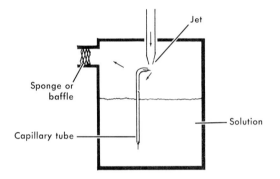

Fig. 4-9. Jet humidifier produces aerosol that is baffled sufficiently so that particles evaporate to form humidity.

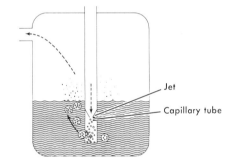

Fig. 4-10. In underwater jet, gas is directed to jet under surface of water where aerosol is produced. Gas containing aerosol bubbles back to surface.

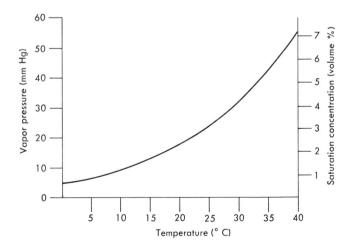

Fig. 4-11. Increased temperature enhances capacity of gas to carry water vapor. (From MacIntosh, R. R., Mushin, W. W., and Epstein, H. G.: Physics for the anaesthetist, ed. 3, Oxford, England, 1963, Blackwell Scientific Publications, Ltd.)

therapy requires control of a third ingredient, *heat*, to increase humidifier efficiency. *100% relative humidity at body temperature* is necessary to humidify the inspired gas when the upper airway has been bypassed. The nose provides an extremely effective humidification mechanism due to the large surface area of the turbinates. When a patient is tracheostomized or intubated, this mechanism is lost, and the humidification must now be supplied by respiratory therapy apparatus. By increasing the gas or the water temperature, the capacity of the gas to carry water vapor increases as it passes through the heated humidifier (Fig. 4-11). Normally, these units can be heated above body temperature, since the gas will cool on its way through the delivery tubing to the patient. As heat is lost through the tubing water, *condensation* will occur. Therefore the tubing must be placed at a downward angle away from the patient, with no low spots, to allow the moisture to drain back into the humidifier (Fig. 4-12). The Bennett Cascade is a heated type of humidifier (Fig. 4-13) and has been employed in respiratory therapy since the 1960s. It is an advanced bubble-type humidifier in which gas travels down a *tower* and passes through a *grid*. From the tower, gas enters a chamber below the grid, and water in the chamber is displaced by the gas. This raises the water level in the Cascade reservoir, allowing some water to enter above the grid through a *port*. Water then forms a film over the grid that becomes a *froth* as gas passes from the chamber through the grid. This design was employed to reduce resistance to gas flow through the unit. A *one-way valve* in the tower acts to retard the drift of humidity back toward the apparatus to which it is attached. A *sensing port* in the tower allows for gas communication with a ventilator inlet, so that the patient's effort can be sensed in the machine. Other units of similar design are now available: (1) the disposable unit produced by Respiratory Care, Inc., (2) the reusable humidifier sold with the Ohio Critical Care and 550 ventilators, (3) the Monaghan 225 ventilator's humidifier, and (4) Searle's disposable unit.

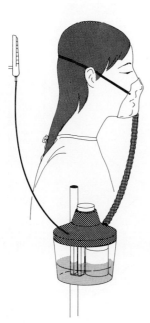

Fig. 4-12. Tubing should be arranged so that low spots are avoided to prevent moisture accumulation and potential blockage.

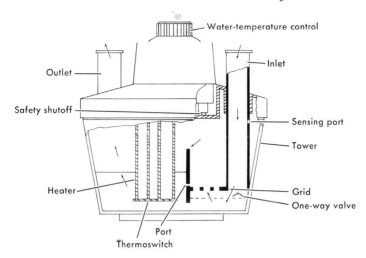

Fig. 4-13. Diagram of Cascade Humidifier. Gas is directed down tower to chamber below grid. Gas displaces water in chamber, which causes rise in water level in remainder of reservoir. Water then enters port above grid forming liquid film on top of grid. Gas passes through grid, froth is formed from hot water, and humidification of gas occurs. (Courtesy Bennett Respiration Products, Inc., Santa Monica, Calif.)

Summary

What humidity is and how it may be measured have been discussed. Humidity can be delivered either at room temperature, to make a gas more comfortable, or at body temperature, to increase the amount of water that it can hold. There are five types of humidifying devices: (1) the blow-by humidifier; (2) the bubble humidifier; (3) the jet humidifier; (4) the underwater jet humidifier; and (5) the heated humidifier.

AEROSOL

Aerosol consists of liquid or solid particles of a substance suspended in a gas (Fig. 4-14). These particles could be cigarette smoke, dust, fog, aerosolized water or medication, etc. If water is used as a basis for comparison, humidity and aerosol can be contrasted. Humidity is water in the gaseous state, whereas this aerosol is water in the liquid state (water droplets suspended in a gas).

Methods of measuring aerosol

Aerosol is measured primarily in two fashions. The first method is the measurement of *particle size* in microns, μ (abbreviation of micrometers, μm) (Fig. 4-15). Particle size is a major factor in determining the depth to which a particle will penetrate the respiratory tract (Fig. 4-16). The particle's *stability* is also determined by its size (Table 4-2). Unfortunately, the different methods of measuring particle size yield inconsistent results.[2] However, with new methods such as the electron micrograph and laser photography, results in the future may prove to be more uniform.

The second method of measuring aerosol is in *total volume output*, mainly in *cubic centimeters per minute or hour*. The basic factors that control output are (1) *particle size* and (2) the *number of particles*. By knowing both of these measurements of aerosol, one can predict where the majority of particles will be deposited and the volume of deposition in the respiratory tract. With this knowledge, the clinician

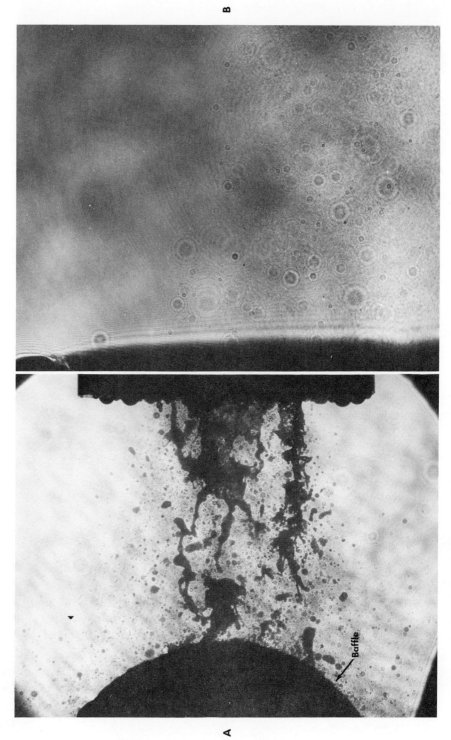

Fig. 4-14. A, Particle baffling. **B,** Hologram of aerosol particles. (Courtesy Respiratory Care, Inc., Arlington Heights, Ill.)

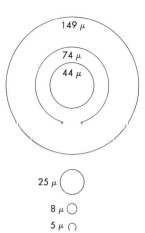

Fig. 4-15. Comparison of particle sizes. (Courtesy Monaghan, Littleton, Colo.)

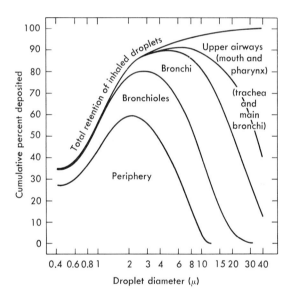

Fig. 4-16. Particle deposition in respiratory tract. The smaller the particle, the deeper into respiratory tract particle will potentially deposit. (From Cushing, I. E., and Miller, W. F.: Nebulization therapy. In Safar, P., editor: Respiratory therapy, Philadelphia, 1965, F. A. Davis Co.)

then has an idea of the actual quantity of aerosol produced and can roughly estimate the quantities deposited. Particle size also has a definite relationship to volume produced. For example, a 40 μ particle contains about a million times more volume than a 0.4 μ particle.[3] The clinician must keep in mind that if the particles must go *deep* into the respiratory tract, then the nebulizer must provide *small particles*.[3,4] This attempt to obtain deeper particle deposition may well lead to a substantial *reduction in volume* output when compared to a nebulizer that produces larger particles. This should not be disconcerting if it is realized that smaller particles traveling to the proper location should provide *optimal local effect* with minimal systemic side effects when the aerosol consists of a pharmacologic agent.[2,3]

Table 4-2. Data on particles issuing from 1 ml liquid according to their diameter*

Particle diameter (μ)†	Brownian movement in 1 second (μ)	Sedimentation rate in still air in 1 second (μ)
10	1.75	6096
5	2.5	1550
2	3.8	400
1	5.9	70
0.1	29.4	1.7
0.05	60.0	0.7

*From Dautrebande, L.: Microaerosols, New York, 1962, Academic Press, Inc.
†The smaller the particle, the lesser the effect gravity has on it (that is, decreased sedimentation rate) and particle is more stable. However, as particles get smaller, molecular bombardment by surrounding gas molecules tends to move them around (increased Brownian movement). This tends to cause particles to hit objects and be deposited.

Factors affecting particle deposition

There are six primary factors that affect the deposition of aerosol particles. The first factor is *gravity*.[5] Its effect on particle deposition is best described in *Stoke's law*.[5] This law states that the rate of sedimentation of the particles nearly equals the density times their diameter squared. Basically, this means that as particles become larger, gravity will have a greater effect on them, and they will settle out of suspension more quickly. Therefore the *larger particles are less stable and will be deposited sooner* than smaller particles.

The *viscosity* of a gas also plays a role related to gravity. A suspension of particles in a gas results from the gas molecules hitting the aerosol particles on various

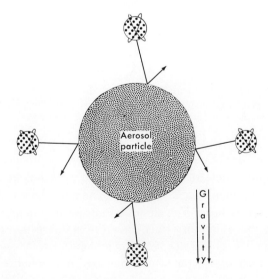

Fig. 4-17. Molecular bombardment from all sides tends to provide equalizing force surrounding aerosol particle, holding it in suspension. Opposing force to this equalization is gravity. The larger the particle and its mass, the greater gravity's effect and the less stable the particle.

sides. On the other hand, the force of gravity is trying to pull the particles out of suspension (Fig. 4-17). Moreover, if the molecules of the carrier gas are small, as with helium, they tend not to stabilize the aerosol particles as well. As the smaller gas molecules hit the aerosol particles from all sides, there is less net force with their impact, so that now gravity, not the collisions, exerts a greater force. For this reason, helium-oxygen mixtures may be poor carriers of aerosol particles.

The second factor relating to aerosol deposition is the *kinetic activity* of the carrying gas molecules.[5] All molecules are continually in motion, colliding with each other and their environment, thus forming the motion called kinetic activity. It is similar to that phenomenon observed by Brown as he examined an agar plate under magnification; he noticed that particles suspended in the liquid medium displayed random motions. These movements observed by Brown were described as "Brownian movement"; they were actually the effect of kinetic activity on the particles. Small therapeutic aerosol particles tend to undergo a phenomenon similar to Brownian movement. The smaller an aerosol particle is, the closer it approaches the size of gas molecules hitting it (Fig. 4-18), and thus the more susceptible its activity is to the force of collision with gas molecules. Small aerosol particles, those below 1 μ in size, are more likely to collide at random and deposit themselves on an object. Before aerosol deposition is significantly enhanced by kinetic activity, the particle's size must be in this submicronic range. A 0.1 μ particle is considered to be most stable, and it is more likely to be inhaled and exhaled without depositing in the airway. Thus the effects of gravity and kinetic activity tend to be cancelled by each other in a particle of this size. Fig. 4-19 graphs the stability of particles.[5] As an aerosol particle's size increases above 0.1 μ, gravity exerts the greater force in affecting its settling.

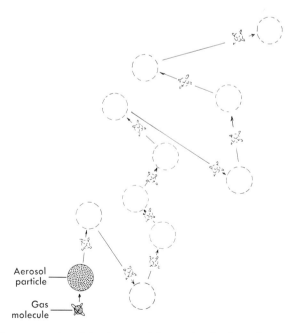

Aerosol particle

Gas molecule

Fig. 4-18. The smaller an aerosol particle, the more influence bombardment by gas molecules has on its path of travel, and the greater the Brownian movement.

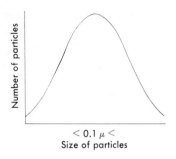

Fig. 4-19. As aerosol particles increase in size above 0.1 μ, gravity plays greater role in removing them from suspension. As particles decrease below 0.1 μ in diameter, kinetic activity (Brownian movement) has greater effect and tends to remove particles from suspension as they collide and become deposited. (From Egan, D. F.: Fundamentals of respiratory therapy, ed. 3, St. Louis, 1977, The C. V. Mosby Co.)

The third factor affecting aerosol deposition is *particle inertia.*[5] The larger the mass of a particle, the more it tends to travel a straight course, even as the gas stream carrying it changes direction. Particles that are to be deposited in the alveoli must make several turns on their way. Thus they must not be markedly affected by inertia. They must be small particles with little mass to successfully reach their destination. The *larger* aerosol particles with their greater mass are less likely to make these turns; they are more apt to be *deposited in the upper respiratory tract* and at each *bifurcation* of the conducting airways.

The fourth factor involved in aerosol placement is the *physical nature of the particle itself.* For example, *hygroscopic* particles such as *propylene glycol* tend to absorb water. This property is responsible for their increase in size in the patient's airway, now causing them to deposit sooner than if they retained their original size. Particles that tend to stick together consolidate to form larger particles and also will deposit sooner in the respiratory tract. This is a factor to be considered when administering solid particles of medication. Another important physical aspect to keep in mind is the type of solutions being aerosolized. *Hypertonic* solutions tend to *absorb water* and their particle size tends to *increase.* *Isotonic* solutions tend to *remain reasonably stable* in particle size, and *hypotonic* solutions tend to *lose* water to the airway and tend to *evaporate.* Thus as their particle size *decreases*, they will travel further down into the respiratory tract than expected from their original mass.

A fifth influence on aerosol deposition is that of *heating* and *humidifying* the carrier gas stream. If aerosol is injected into a warm, humid gas stream, the particles would tend to *grow* due to humidity *coalescence* on the aerosol as the gas cools on the way to the patient. The particles increasing size causes them to deposit much *higher* in the airways. This is an important consideration when administering solutions such as bronchodilators, for which optimal deposition should be deep in the respiratory tract.[3]

The final factor to consider affecting aerosol deposition is the *patient's ventilatory pattern.*[3,5] The clinician should encourage the patient to attain optimum results in aerosol therapy. For maximum aerosol deposition deep in the respiratory tract, the patient should (1) take a *slow, deep breath* (at a flow rate less than 300 ml/sec) and (2) develop a *large tidal volume* (1200 to 1400 cc), including a *breath hold*.[3]

Using aerosols therapeutically

The six factors affecting aerosol deposition in the respiratory tract, then, are enhanced under the conditions previously discussed. In addition, a slower inspiratory flow rate decreases premature particle deposition caused by the effects of inertia. It also provides increased time for gravity of kinetic activity to promote particle deposition. The breath hold provides additional time for the particles to deposit at the optimum levels; *15 seconds allows maximum deposition of particles smaller than 0.5 μ.*[3] Furthermore, the deeper breath provides the patient with (1) a larger volume of gas containing aerosol and (2) an improved and *more uniform distribution* of inspired air. These techniques should be employed especially with the use of *hand nebulizers*, which generate smaller particles. It would help to maximize the local desired effect of aerosols by increasing deposition in the lower respiratory tract. Although a breath hold by the patient with IPPB has not been statistically proved effective in improving aerosol distribution, an attempt should still be made to use low flow rates with large tidal volumes, and the clinician can consider a built-in breath hold with some units.

If the clinician knows the preferred level of aerosol deposition in the airway (Table 4-3), he can select the device best suited for that therapeutic effect. For example, if the objective is to deliver a potent agent such as bronchodilators to the *bronchioles, aerosol particle sizes below* 3 to 5 μ should be attained. Additionally, it has been

Table 4-3. Particle size and site of deposition*

Particle size (μ)	Deposition in respiratory tract
100	Do not enter tract
100 to 5	Trapped in nose
5 to 2	Deposited somewhere proximal to alveoli
2 to 1	Can enter alveoli, with 95% to 100% retention of those down to 1 μ
1 to 0.25	Stable, with minimal settling
0.25	Increasing alveolar deposition

*From Egan, D. F.: Fundamentals of respiratory therapy, ed. 3, St. Louis, 1977, The C. V. Mosby Co.

Table 4-4. Particle size, deposition, and location*

Particle size	Deposition	Location
2 μ†	55%	Periphery
8 μ	30%	Bronchioles
15 μ	40%	Bronchi
↑ 40 μ	100%	Upper airways

*From Miller, W. F.: Fundamental principles of aerosol therapy, Respir. Care 17:295, 1972.
†The 2 μ particles have a low percentage of deposition in upper airway, so small particles should be used to minimize upper airway deposition and systemic side effects when administering potent medications. If mild solutions are administered, larger particles can increase volume deposited at bronchiolar level.

demonstrated that submicronic aerosols (below 1.0 μ) provide maximal topical and minimal systemic effects of such potent agents.[2] Decreased particle size will reduce the amount of upper-airway deposition that is likely to cause systemic side effects. However, if *volume deposition of bland solutions* is the clinician's objective and systemic side effects are of no concern, a particle size of 8 to 20 μ will deposit larger volumes at the bronchiolar level (Table 4-4).

Nebulizers in general

Aerosols are produced in respiratory therapy by devices known as *nebulizers*. Among the many different types of nebulizers employed in respiratory therapy, the most common are the *jet nebulizers*. They utilize *Bernoulli's principle* of lowering the lateral pressure around the jet to draw water up a capillary tube (Chapter 1). When this fluid reaches the gas stream, it is drawn into it and shattered into small particles. Once these particles are produced, they may or may not be baffled (Fig. 4-20). A *baffle* is a means of *reducing the average size of aerosol particles* to be delivered to the patient by *removing larger particles*. Without baffling, larger particles can be delivered by an *atomizer* (Fig. 4-21). Because of the larger particle size produced by atomizers, they are not commonly encountered in respiratory therapy. They do find some use, however, as spray devices used to deposit medication in the pharynx or nasal cavity such as topical anesthetics.

Baffling (Fig. 4-22) can be accomplished with a variety of structures. A *ball* placed in the path of the aerosol, the *surface of the water* in a container, or the *sides of the*

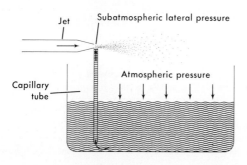

Fig. 4-20. Jet nebulizers utilize Bernoulli's principle to create lateral negative pressure at jet. *Atmospheric* pressure, pushing down on water's surface, forces water up capillary tube. As water leaves capillary tube, it hits gas stream and is broken up into aerosol particles by forward force of gas flow from jet.

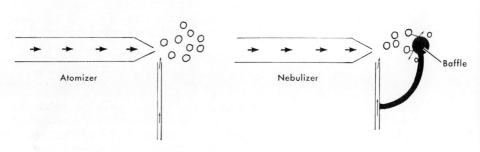

Fig. 4-21. Nebulizer utilizes baffles to produce smaller particle, whereas atomizer does not.

container are all examples of baffles. Actually, any object in the path of the aerosol particles can be a baffle, as can any right-angle bend of the gas flow carrying the aerosol. Baffling results in a loss of the larger particles due to the effects of inertia and gravity (Fig. 4-23), and the smaller particles travel on with the gas stream.

Pneumatic nebulizers. The first medical nebulizer was the *hand-held type* introduced in 1938[6] (Fig. 4-24, *A*). This device incorporates a flexible bulb that, when squeezed, produces gas flow to a jet, which then entrains the medication and produces an aerosol (Fig. 4-24, *B*). Since that time, many devices have been produced with similar design. Once IPPB was employed to a reasonable extent, aerosol nebulizers were incorporated into its circuitry. Driven by a pressurized gas source, they were included as either a *sidestream* nebulizer, in which the aerosol was *injected into the gas stream*, or a *mainstream* nebulizer, where the *main flow of gas* actually passed

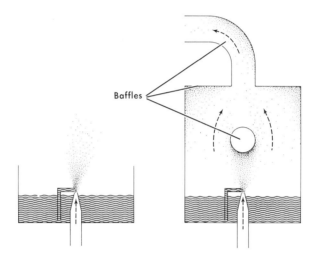

Fig. 4-22. Baffling is provided whenever any object is in path of aerosol flow. (Modified from Cushing, I. E., and Miller, W. F.: Nebulization therapy. In Safar, P., editor: Respiratory therapy, Philadelphia, 1965, F. A. Davis Co.)

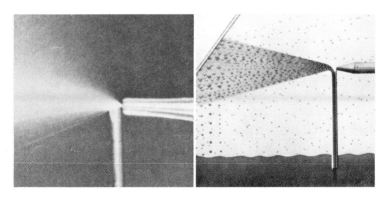

Fig. 4-23. Inertia tends to carry larger particles into baffle, which breaks them up as they strike. (Courtesy Bennett Respiration Products, Inc., Santa Monica, Calif.)

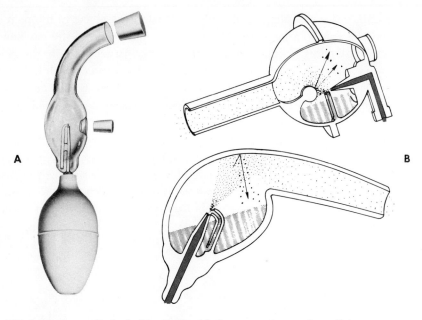

Fig. 4-24. A, The first medical nebulizer. **B,** Hand-bulb compression supplies sufficient pressure to power jet. Lateral negative pressure at jet causes liquid entrainment from capillary tube. (Courtesy Bennett Respiration Products, Inc., Santa Monica, Calif.)

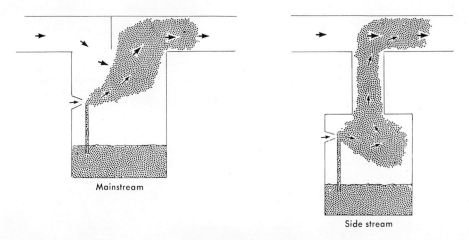

Mainstream

Side stream

Fig. 4-25. Main gas flow passes through mainstream nebulizer and carries aerosol particles with it. Aerosol simply drifts into main gas flow with sidestream nebulizer.

through the aerosol generator (Fig. 4-25). Bennett and Bird produce the most common IPPB units in use today. The Bennett units commonly utilize the Slip/stream nebulizer. This device acts like a mainstream nebulizer in that it utilizes a partition (Fig. 4-26) to direct part of the main flow of gas through the nebulizer vial; here it picks up the aerosol particles created at the pressurized jet site and carries them out. The Bennett Twin is a sidestream nebulizer that encompasses two jets and capillary tubes to produce the aerosol (Fig. 4-27). Only the flow of gas from the jets carry the aerosol particles up to the main stream of gas being delivered to the patient. Based on its construction, a greater number of *large* particles tend to *rain out* in the

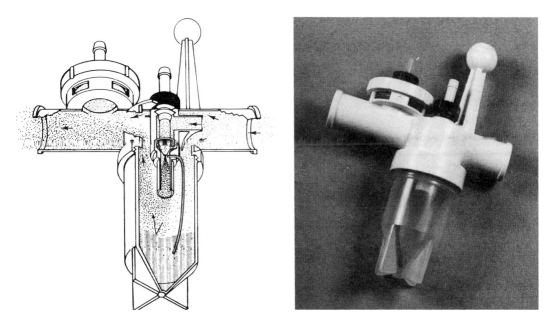

Fig. 4-26. Bennett Slip/stream nebulizer functions as mainstream nebulizer. (Courtesy Bennett Respiration Products, Inc., Santa Monica, Calif.)

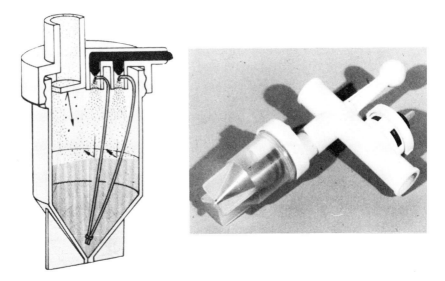

Fig. 4-27. Bennett Twin acts as sidestream nebulizer. (Courtesy Respiration Products, Inc., Santa Monica, Calif.)

Bennett Twin; the aerosol spends more time in the twin (sidestream) unit than in the Slip/stream, and, therefore, the total aerosol output of sidestream nebulizers is most likely lower, but the average particle size is usually smaller. Fig. 4-28 indicates the comparative outputs of the Bennett Twin (sidestream) and the Bennett Slip/stream (mainstream) nebulizers. The Bird Micronebulizer (Fig. 4-29) can be used in either of these ways. As supplied by the company, this nebulizer is often employed as a mainstream device. However, by using the optional Bird Tee (Fig. 4-30), the Micro-

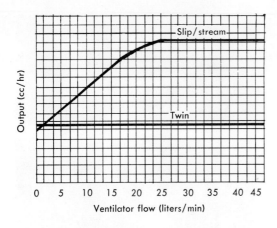

Fig. 4-28. Slip/stream unit has higher aerosol output than Bennett Twin, but Twin has smaller particle size. (Courtesy Bennett Respiration Products, Inc., Santa Monica, Calif.)

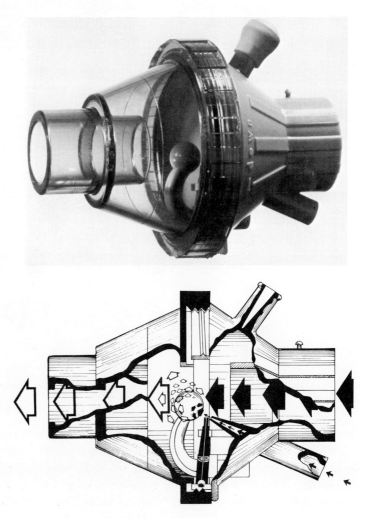

Fig. 4-29. Bird Micronebulizer is normally supplied by manufacturer as a mainstream nebulizer. (Courtesy Bird Corp., Palm Springs, Calif.)

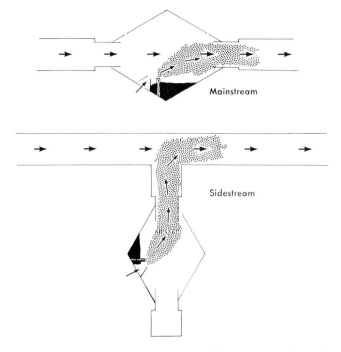

Fig. 4-30. Bird Micronebulizer can be used as mainstream nebulizer. With Bird Tee and nebulizer cap, it can also be utilized as sidestream device to attain smaller particles.

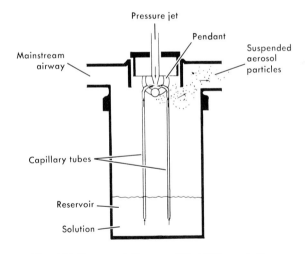

Fig. 4-31. Functional diagram of Bird 500 cc nebulizer.

nebulizer can also be used as a sidestream nebulizer. There are several nebulizers with the newer disposable circuits, most of which can be adapted to either mainstream or sidestream placement.

Some nebulizer units have been developed to deliver aerosol over longer periods of time (Fig. 4-31). The Bird Micronebulizer with its 500 cc reservoir is an example of this type. It incorporates Bernoulli's principle to entrain fluid to the jet. This unit is normally placed in-line with the Bird ventilators. One of the first models of this

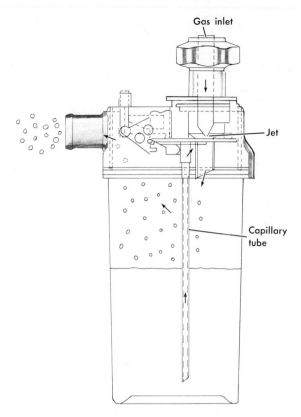

Fig. 4-32. Puritan All Purpose Nebulizer.

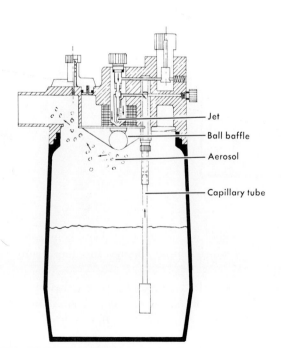

Fig. 4-33. Ohio Deluxe nebulizer. (Modified from Ohio Medical Products, Madison, Wis.)

type of nebulizer was the Puritan All Purpose (Fig. 4-32). It has not only the capacity for nebulizing the large quantities of fluid in the reservoir, but it also has a provision for air entrainment. When operated with oxygen, the settings available are 100%, 70%, and 40% oxygen (Table 4-5). The Ohio Deluxe (Fig. 4-33) may be used with settings of 100%, 60%, and 40% oxygen through its air dilution system. In the delivery of aerosol to patients, *if the total flow from the unit does not meet or exceed the patient's inspiratory flow demands, then the delivered aerosol density and oxygen percentage will drop.* This occurs because the patient also inhales room air through the aerosol delivering device's exhalation ports; the added gas dilutes the aerosol/gas mixture coming from the nebulizer. Therefore a nebulizer should have high enough flow capabilities to meet or exceed the patient's inspiratory flow demands. The nebulizer's total flow output should be adjusted so that aerosol continually drifts out of the exhalation ports, even during the patient's inhalation. Table 4-5 indicates the total flow of the Puritan All Purpose on the various settings. A *normal, peak inspiratory flow rate is about 25 to 30 L/min.* This must be matched or exceeded with total gas flow from the aerosol-creating device to avoid room air dilution.

Both the Puritan All Purpose and the Ohio Deluxe nebulizers can be used with immersion heaters to provide heated aerosols, and both can be used in-line with IPPB apparatus.

After the production of the All Purpose, other units of similar design were introduced. Since then, greater variability of oxygen-percentage control was included on some devices, such as the OEM and Bard-Parker disposable units. There are also some types of nebulizers that employ a device similar to a *Pitot tube* (Chapter 1). This device has the ability to maintain reasonably high amounts of fluid uptake, yet it allows for placement of a baffle close to the jet to attain a small particle size (Fig. 4-34). Nebulizers employing devices similar to this principle are the Aquapak, the Ohio Deluxe, the Micromist, and the Ohio High Output units.

Table 4-5. Gas flow from Puritan All Purpose Nebulizer*

Total unrestricted gas flow from nebulizer (L/min)		Flowmeter setting (L/min)
Diluted to 40% oxygen concentration	Diluted to 70% oxygen concentration	
4	1.6	1
8	3.2	2
12	4.8	3
16	6.4	4
20	8.0	5
24	9.6	6
28	11.2	7
32	12.8	8
36	14.4	9
40	16.0	10
44	17.6	11
48	19.2	12

*Total gas flows from nebulizer should exceed patient's peak inspiratory flow rate (average 25 to 30 L/min) to achieve (1) maximum aerosol density and (2) stable inspired oxygen concentrations. For accurate flow setting, use a pressure-compensated flowmeter. (Courtesy Bennett Respiration Products, Inc., Santa Monica, Calif.)

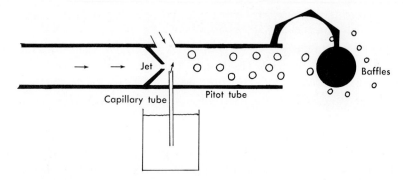

Fig. 4-34. Use of Pitot tube maintains high forward gas pressure. This forward pressure allows for placement of baffle close to jet to attain small particle size without jeopardizing fluid entrainment.

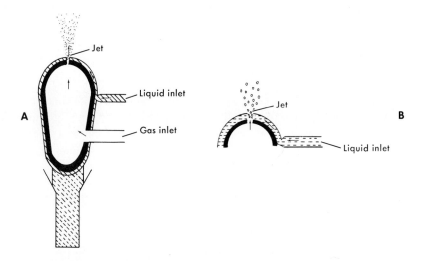

Fig. 4-35. A, Hydro-sphere nebulizer. Source gas enters hollow sphere and travels to small particle size without jeopardizing fluid entrainment. **B,** Small tube carries fluid to outside of hollow sphere, and lateral negative pressure created by jets pulls fluid over sphere into gas stream, producing aerosol. (**A** modified from Litt, M., and Swift, D. E.: Respir. Care **17:**414, 1972.)

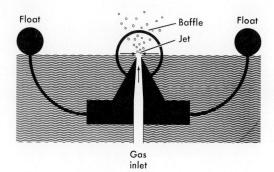

Fig. 4-36. Floating-island nebulizer places jet just below surface of water, and lateral negative pressure entrains water at surface. Depth of jet below surface regulates particle size and affects total aerosol output. The higher the jet is, the smaller the particles are and the lower the particle output is.

Recently a new concept in nebulizers has been developed called the *Hydro-Sphere* or *Babington* nebulizer (Fig. 4-35, *A*).[7] Source gas enters a hollow glass sphere, the outside of which is covered with a thin film of water. At the top are *small slits* or ports in the sphere, which act as jets. A small tube carries fluid to the outside of the sphere; here the lateral negative pressure created by the jets and natural cohesive forces pull fluid over the sphere and into the gas stream, producing an aerosol (Fig. 4-35, *B*). The particle range is reasonably stable, regardless of source gas pressure or gas flow through the slits. The particle size (mass median diameter) is between 3 and 5 μ.[7]

Another change from the standard jet, but still utilizing Bernoulli's principle, is the *floating-island nebulizer*.[1] The most common models are the Win-Liz and a unit produced by Air-Shields. In these devices, the jet is located just below or at the surface of the water. Decreased lateral pressure by the jet draws surface water into the gas stream, producing an aerosol (Fig. 4-36).

Centrifugal nebulizers. Centrifugal nebulizers have been in use for some years, starting with so-called fog-generating devices. A *spinning disk* rotates on a hollow shaft, which acts similarly to an auger, drawing water up the center of the shaft (Fig. 4-37). Once the water reaches the spinning disk, it is thrown outward by *centrifugal force* through the *breaker cones*, and aerosol particles are produced. The Walton and John Bunn units used this principle in the large fog generators these companies produced. Most room-humidifying units used today operate on this principle. Common examples of room humidifiers are made by DeVilbiss and Hankscraft. The nondisposable humidifier unit once used in the Air-Shields 10,000 respirator was also a centrifugal nebulizer.

Ultrasonic nebulizers. During their production within the past decade, ultrasonic nebulizers have gained widespread application in respiratory therapy. The basic principle of ultrasonic nebulization is that *electric current produces sound waves that are utilized to break up water into aerosol* particles. An electric charge is applied

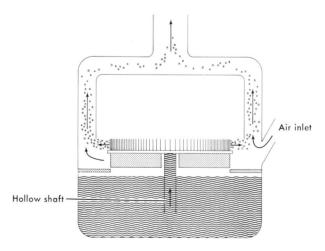

Fig. 4-37. Hollow shaft of centrifugal nebulizer draws water upward. Once water reaches spinning disk, it is thrown outward by centrifugal force through breaker combs, and aerosol is produced. Fan blades on bottom of disk draw air in and blow it out top port, carrying aerosol out of unit.

intermittently (at a high frequency of vibrations) to a substance that has a *piezoelectric* quality, that is, the ability to change shape when a charge is applied to it. This electric current causes vibrations at the same frequency as the electric charge applied to the piezoelectric transducer. These ultrasonic vibrations travel through the water to the surface, where they produce an aerosol (Fig. 4-38).

In the past, ultrasonic nebulizers, such as the 800 series from DeVilbiss, focused these sound waves at a point slightly above the surface of the liquid to be aerosolized (Fig. 4-41, *A*). The Mistogen models 142 and 143 and the previously produced DeVilbiss 900 series utilize flat transducers, which create straight, unfocused sound waves (Fig. 4-39, *B*). The DeVilbiss 35 and 65 series use flat transducers that are shielded by a bonded stainless steel plate (Fig. 4-39, *C*). A glass covering is used on the Monaghan 650 and 670 models.

There are two general output ranges for commonly used ultrasonic aerosol gen-

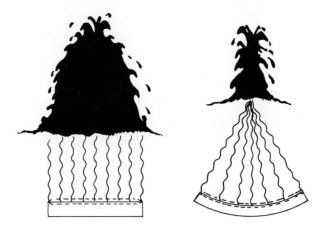

Fig. 4-38. Electric energy supplied to piezoelectric transducer produces sound waves. When sound waves hit water's surface, aerosol is produced.

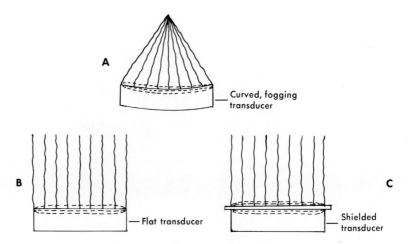

A — Curved, fogging transducer

B — Flat transducer

C — Shielded transducer

Fig. 4-39. Piezoelectric transducer configurations. (Modified from The DeVilbiss Co., Somerset, Pa.)

erators, 0 to 3 ml/min and 0 to 6 ml/min. The DeVilbiss 900 and 35 series, Mistogen's 142 and 143 units, and Monaghan's models 650 and 670 all fall into the 0 to 3 ml/min category. The 0 to 6 ml/min output units include the DeVilbiss 800 and 65 series, Mistogen's EN-145 model, and Monaghan's model 675.

The ultrasonic transducer is often placed in a *coupling chamber* filled with water (Fig. 4-40). The water (1) helps absorb the mechanical heat produced and (2) acts as a transfer medium for the sound waves to the nebulizer chamber. The frequency of the electric energy supplied to the transducer is usually around 1.35 megacycles.

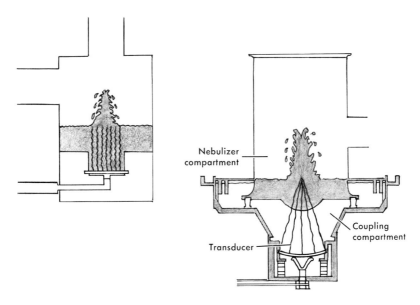

Fig. 4-40. Focusing sound waves usually breaks up aerosol to greater degree; it increases output but requires controlled water level. This is usually accomplished with some type of automatic-feeding system. Flat transducer units usually have lower output, but they do not require specific water level. Transducer is placed in coupling chamber filled with water. Water within it helps absorb mechanical heat and acts as transfer medium for sound waves to nebulizer chamber. (Modified from The DeVilbiss Co., Somerset, Pa.)

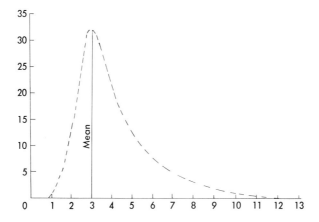

Fig. 4-41. Particle-size dispersement of ultrasonic nebulizer. (Courtesy Monaghan, Littleton, Colo.)

When this frequency is matched with a transducer that can react optimally to it, a vibration is produced at that same frequency. It is this *frequency* that *determines the particle size* when water is broken up at its surface. The *amplitude* or strength of the sound waves *dictates aerosol output* by altering the number of particles produced. Most ultrasonics have been constructed so that their range of particle size falls between 1 and 10 μ with a *mean particle size* of about 3 μ (Fig. 4-41), although some investigators have found units that produce particles with a mass median diameter of around 6 μ.[8]

Aerosol for humidification

Aerosol is often used to simply provide humidity. The evaporation of aerosol particles forms humidity that may provide sufficient moisture to humidify a gas to 100% of body temperature. This would usually require a heated aerosol (Fig. 4-42)

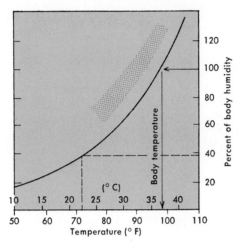

Fig. 4-42. Aerosol needed to supply humidity sufficient to meet body's requirements is indicated by dotted area. (Courtesy Ohio Medical Products, Madison, Wis.)

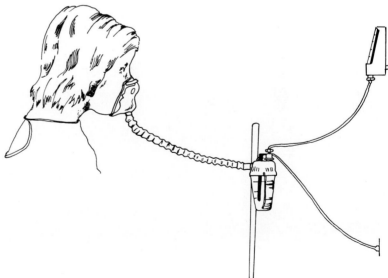

Fig. 4-43. Device for delivering heated aerosol in use.

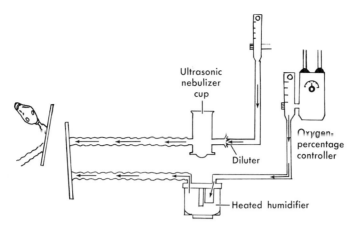

Fig. 4-44. Simple dilution device can be utilized for low resistance systems such as ultrasonic nebulizer. With higher-resistance systems, controller must be used to provide stable oxygen concentration. Flow must meet patient's peak inspiratory flow rate.

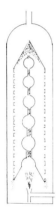

Fig. 4-45. Filtration of particles. (Modified from Dautrebande, L.: Microaerosols, New York, 1962, Academic Press, Inc.)

or, perhaps, ultrasonic nebulization. The utilization of aerosol as a means of humidification is not optimum if simple humidification is the only goal, since microorganisms may be provided a carrier by the particulate matter to transport them into the respiratory tract. Heated *humidification* devices that produce *100% relative humidity* without aerosol, at body temperature, have a reasonably small chance of causing a pulmonary infection. Aerosol nebulizers should be used when liquid volume or medication deposition is required, realizing, however, the potentials of pulmonary infection and the medication's side effects. Fig. 4-44 demonstrates methods of administering both aerosol and humidity with set oxygen concentrations; however, sufficient flows must be supplied to meet the patient's peak inspiratory-flow requirements.

Looking ahead

In the future, there seems to be good potential for more sophisticated nebulizers. For example, jet nebulizers with more sophisticated baffling systems could incorporate such principles as the *Pitot tube* and *particle filtration* (Fig. 4-45) to control precisely the range of particles administered. As materials have become more sophisticated, ultrasonic nebulizer transducers may some day be designed to produce different particle size ranges simply by a knob's adjustment. All of these improvements should provide more efficient and effective therapeutic aerosols for respiratory therapy.

REFERENCES

1. McPherson, S. P.: Humidity and aerosol, Ohio Items and Topics, Aug., 1970.
2. Dautrebande, L.: Microaerosols, New York, 1962, Academic Press, Inc.
3. Miller, W. F.: Fundamental principles of aerosol therapy, Respir. Care 17:295, 1972.
4. Miller, W. F.: Aerosol therapy in acute and chronic respiratory disease, Arch. Med. 131:148, 1973.
5. Egan, D. F.: Fundamentals of respiratory therapy, ed. 3, St. Louis, 1977, The C. V. Mosby Co.
6. McPherson, S. P., and Roads, J. S.: History of respiratory therapy. (To be published.)
7. Litt, S. D.: The Babington nebulizer, a new principle for generation of therapeutic aerosols, Respir. Care 17:414, 1972.
8. Goddard, R. F., et al.: Output characteristics and clinical efficiency of ultrasonic nebulizers, J. Asthma Res. 5:355, 1968.

5 Oxygen-controlling devices and analyzing devices

OXYGEN-CONTROLLING DEVICES

In recent years, increased attention has been placed on the devices utilized for the control of oxygen percentage. These devices can be categorized into four distinct types of units. *Oxygen adders*, the first type, are devices in which oxygen and air are mixed by simple oxygen addition. The second type is the *entrainment device*, which employs Bernoulli's principle to maintain a stable oxygen concentration. The third type is a *precision metering device*, in which two types of restrictions can be altered to change the flow of oxygen and air, therefore controlling the oxygen percentage. The fourth type, *oxygen controllers*, incorporate precision metering devices plus add mechanisms to equilibrate the air and oxygen pressure sources to maintain a stable concentration.

Oxygen adders

Oxygen adders are normally employed with apparatus in which the gas to be administered is first drawn through some system. Most commonly, these units are found in association with certain ventilators in which a piston, bellows, or Venturi of the machine draws in gas from the room. By *adding oxygen in the proximity of the intake*, increased oxygen percentages can be delivered (Fig. 5-1). By inserting a *reservoir system* on the air-intake side and adding oxygen between the intake reser-

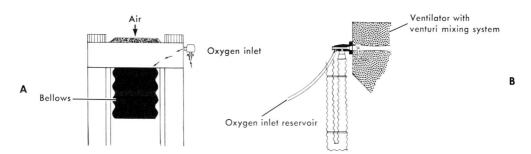

Fig. 5-1. **A**, Example of oxygen addition system. On this ventilator (Air Shields Model ICV-10), bellows falls during expiratory phase and refills with filtered room air and oxygen is added, increasing oxygen concentration inside bellows. **B**, Example of oxygen addition system (Bennett oxygen adder for TV/PV and PR series ventilators) utilizing reservoir system. Venturi entrains oxygen-enriched gases from open-ended reservoir tube during ventilator's inspiratory cycle.

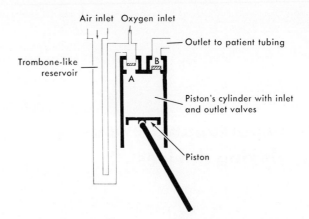

Fig. 5-2. Example of oxygen adder (Emerson 3PV ventilator oxygen system) utilizing reservoir. As piston moves downward, inlet valve, *A*, opens (outlet valve, *B*, closes) and oxygen-enriched gases fill piston's cylinder. During ventilator's inspiratory phase, piston moves upward, closing valve *A* and opening valve *B*. During this phase, oxygen is entering reservoir tube and mixing with ambient air.

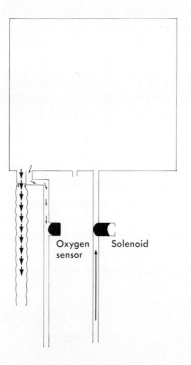

Fig. 5-3. Mixing chamber oxygen adder.

voir and machine, more stable oxygen percentages can be delivered (Fig. 5-2). The reservoir allows for mixing or blending of air or oxygen; therefore gas is drawn into the system, and the mixture remains reasonably stable in oxygen percentage. A more sophisticated type of adder incorporates an oxygen analyzer that monitors the oxygen concentration within the mixing chamber or within an environment (Fig. 5-3). When the sensor detects an oxygen concentration approximately 2% below the desired (set) level, a solenoid valve opens and allows oxygen to enter the system. Oxygen continues to be added until the sensor detects a concentration approximately 2% above the desired level; at this point the solenoid valve is automatically closed. Examples of these devices have been marketed by Bio Marine Industries (BMI), Inc., Bourns, Inc. (Life Systems), Sinclair Scientific, Inc., and the IMI Division of Becton, Dickson, and Company.

Entrainment devices

The second type of oxygen control units are *entrainment devices*. These utilize *Bernoulli's principle* to cause a low lateral pressure, which, in turn, causes air entrainment. By altering the *jet size* (Fig. 5-4) or the *entrainment-port size* (Table 5-1), the oxygen percentage can be maintained at a specific level.[1] Examples of these devices are the so-called Venturi masks. The name is not entirely accurate, since none actually contain a Venturi tube. Units such as the Ventimask, OEM's Mix-Omask, Inspiron's Accur-OX Mask, and Scott Diluters use different jet sizes to attain different oxygen concentrations while maintaining a set-size entrainment port for each device. The *smaller* the *jet size*, the *lower* the *lateral pressure*, the *higher* the *air entrainment*, the *lower* the *oxygen concentration*, and the *higher* the *total flow* from the unit will be (Table 5-1). Other units, such as Hudson's Multi Vent Mask, use a principle similar to Dr. Barach's original Mix Mask,[2] which is produced by OEM. In these units, the entrainment port size is altered and the jet size remains constant to attain different oxygen concentrations.[1] This same principle is incorporated in most nebulizers that have percentage-control provisions.

Some devices, such as the Ohio Diluter, which normally comes supplied with the Ohio 100 Mask, employ a *Pitot tube*–like device (Fig. 5-5).[1] The Pitot tube affords

Table 5-1. Entrainment ratios for commonly used oxygen concentrations

Oxygen percentage	Ratio air : oxygen	Total parts*
100	0:1	1
70	0.6:1	1.6
60	1:1	2
50	1.7:1	2.7
40	3:1	4
35	5:1	6
28	10:1	11
24	20:1	21

*Total parts × Oxygen flow = Total flow

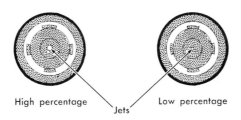

High percentage   Jets   Low percentage

Fig. 5-4. Entrainment devices' jet size. (Modified from Barnes, T. A., and Israel, J. S.: Fundamentals of inhalation therapy principles, Lippincott overhead transparencies, Bowie, Md., 1969, Robert J. Brady Co.)

a greater ability to operate efficiently in the presence of resistance in the form of *back pressure* placed on it.[1] Units of this design have improved application in systems in which mild resistance may be a factor. *All entrainment devices become inaccurate with resistance placed downstream,* since this reduces the lateral, negative pressure after the jet and, therefore, the air entrainment. The result is an *increased*

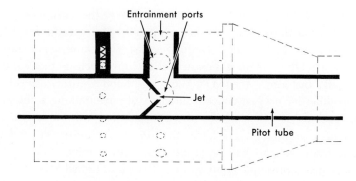

Fig. 5-5. Ohio Diluter with Pitot tube–like system.

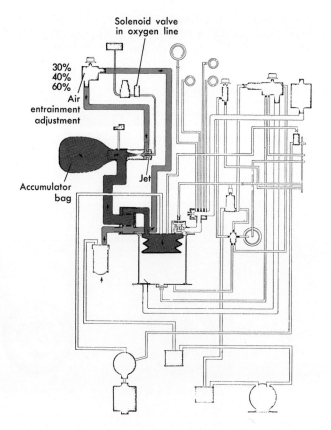

Fig. 5-6. MA-1 oxygen system on early units. (Courtesy Bennett Respiration Products, Inc., Santa Monica, Calif.)

delivered oxygen percentage and a *decreased total gas flow*. Those units incorporating a Pitot tube have a greater ability to accommodate back pressure.

Ventilators often employ oxygen-powered Venturis that entrain air and therefore lower the oxygen concentration to something below source-gas percentage in their delivery of gas to the patient's system.[2] The Venturi primarily increases the total flow capabilities of the unit and is *not designed to specifically control oxygen percentage.* As pressure rises in the patient's circuit, the percentage of oxygen delivered by these units will increase. The greater the patient's airway resistance or the worse the patient's compliance, the higher the delivered oxygen percentage will be.

Other ventilators employ more sophisticated entrainment devices in their oxygen-control systems. The system of the older-model Bennett MA-1 (Fig. 5-6) *altered the entrainment port size* of a Venturi device that supplied an *accumulator bag.* A *solenoid* in the system opened and closed oxygen flow to the jet of the device. As the bag filled, a microswitch shut the solenoid, stopping gas flow to the jet. As the bag collapsed, another switch opened the solenoid. The oxygen-driven Venturi-type percentage unit in the Ohio 560 has a different method of supplying premixed oxygen for filling a reservoir bag. Instead of adjusting entrainment ports, a needle valve–like device adjusts a flow of oxygen to be entrained by the *Venturi mechanism* (Fig. 5-7). For higher oxygen concentrations, the oxygen percentage dial, which functions like a needle valve, is opened more to allow more oxygen to flow into the unit's entrainment area. Thus the oxygen powered jet entrains increasingly higher portions of oxygen as the dial is turned to greater percentages. Finally, on the 100% setting, no more room air is drawn in because the oxygen flow from the control is sufficient to supply the entire entrainment demands of the jet. The lowest oxygen concentration obtainable from this system is approximately 30%. When the control is set below this value, the Venturi oxygen system is *off.*

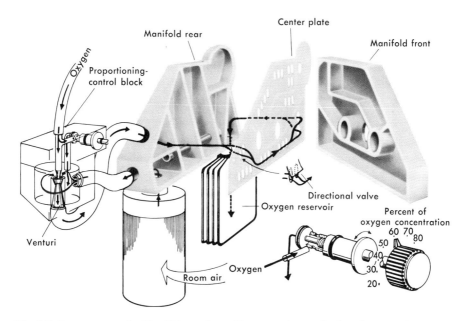

Fig. 5-7. Oxygen system for Ohio 560 ventilator. (Courtesy Ohio Medical Products, Madison, Wis.)

Precision metering devices

The third type of unit is the *precision metering device.* The most common example of a precision metering device consists of *two flowmeters* using needle valves, one for oxygen and one for air, supplying a single reservoir or delivery system. By altering their respective flows, different blends of oxygen and air can be acquired; thus oxygen percentages can be controlled (Fig. 5-8). Fig. 5-9 demonstrates the formulas that can be employed in calculating the approximate oxygen percentage, oxygen, air, or total flow for these systems. The Engstrom 150, 200, and 300 series ventilators incorporate a similar system with their *rotometers* or flowmeters and an *air dosage valve.* The rotometers *adjust the flow of oxygen* into the patient's system, while the dosage valve *adjusts the amount of room air* pulled in during the bag refill phase of the ventilator's cycle (Fig. 5-10). By altering either or both flows, the oxygen percentage can be changed. The Bird Parallel Inspiratory Flow Mixing

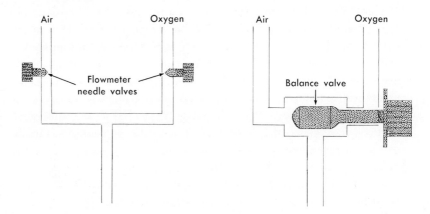

Fig. 5-8. Precision metering devices. In both of these types, air and oxygen should have matching inlet pressures. Balance valve type is single control which, when turned, opens one side as it proportionately closes other side.

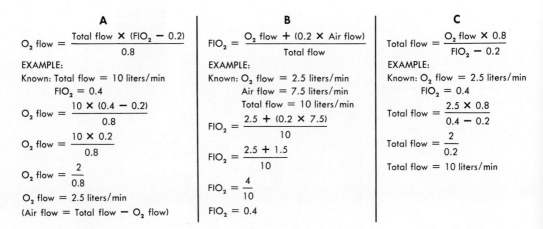

A

$$O_2 \text{ flow} = \frac{\text{Total flow} \times (\text{FIO}_2 - 0.2)}{0.8}$$

EXAMPLE:
Known: Total flow = 10 liters/min
$\text{FIO}_2 = 0.4$

$$O_2 \text{ flow} = \frac{10 \times (0.4 - 0.2)}{0.8}$$

$$O_2 \text{ flow} = \frac{10 \times 0.2}{0.8}$$

$$O_2 \text{ flow} = \frac{2}{0.8}$$

O_2 flow = 2.5 liters/min
(Air flow = Total flow − O_2 flow)

B

$$\text{FIO}_2 = \frac{O_2 \text{ flow} + (0.2 \times \text{Air flow})}{\text{Total flow}}$$

EXAMPLE:
Known: O_2 flow = 2.5 liters/min
Air flow = 7.5 liters/min
Total flow = 10 liters/min

$$\text{FIO}_2 = \frac{2.5 + (0.2 \times 7.5)}{10}$$

$$\text{FIO}_2 = \frac{2.5 + 1.5}{10}$$

$$\text{FIO}_2 = \frac{4}{10}$$

$\text{FIO}_2 = 0.4$

C

$$\text{Total flow} = \frac{O_2 \text{ flow} \times 0.8}{\text{FIO}_2 - 0.2}$$

EXAMPLE:
Known: O_2 flow = 2.5 liters/min
$\text{FIO}_2 = 0.4$

$$\text{Total flow} = \frac{2.5 \times 0.8}{0.4 - 0.2}$$

$$\text{Total flow} = \frac{2}{0.2}$$

Total flow = 10 liters/min

Fig. 5-9. Examples of formulas approximating **A,** oxygen flow needed if fraction of inspired oxygen (FIO_2) and total flow are known, **B,** FIO_2, when known flows of oxygen and air are used, and **C,** total flow being used when oxygen flow and mixed FIO_2 are known.

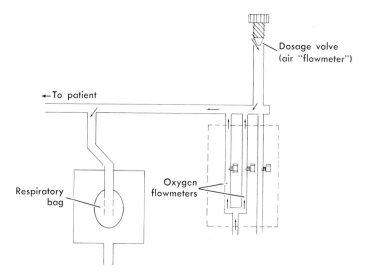

Fig. 5-10. Oxygen mixing system used for Engström 300 series ventilators. When respiratory bag is filling, air and oxygen are mixed from dosage valve and oxygen flowmeters, respectively.

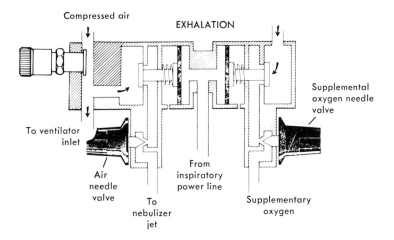

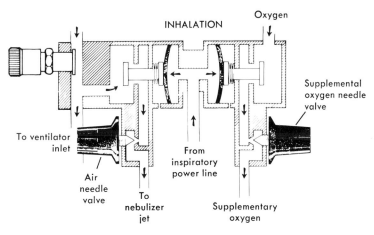

Fig. 5-11. Bird Parallel Inspiratory Flow Mixing Cartridge for use with Bird Respirators. (Modified from Bird Corp., Palm Springs, Calif.)

Cartridge has a design that *interrupts the flows of gases* on specific portions of the ventilatory cycle. By using the air and oxygen *needle valves*, it adjusts the flow of oxygen and air into the respiratory circuit on inspiratory phase of ventilation (Fig. 5-11), thus tending to control oxygen concentrations.

Oxygen controllers

The fourth type of controlling device is an *oxygen controller*. It incorporates both a *precision metering device* as well as the addition of a *unit to maintain stable inlet pressures*, so that slight line pressure changes do not alter the oxygen percentage delivered. One of the first devices of this type was the new version of the MA-1 oxygen control system (Fig. 5-12). This controller both brought oxygen into the system and then *reduced its pressure* to a maximum of 1.85 to 2.1 cm H_2O in the *accumulator*.[3] The feedback line maintained air and oxygen at the same pressures when the bellows dropped and drew the two gases through the oxygen percent valve (precision metering device). By *altering the opening through which air and oxygen pass*, different oxygen concentrations could be acquired. As an example, when the oxygen percentage valve control is turned so that it partially occludes the air intake port

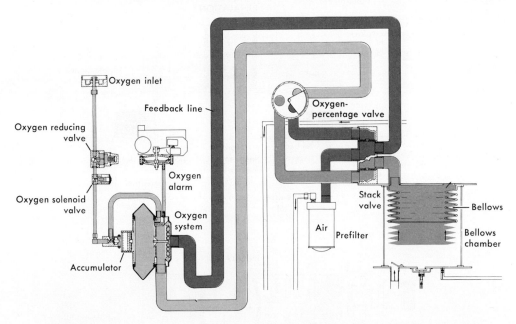

Fig. 5-12. MA-1 oxygen percentage system for newer models. (Courtesy Bennett Respiration Products, Inc., Santa Monica, Calif.)

Fig. 5-13. A, Functional schematic of Bird Oxygen Blender. Compressed air and oxygen enter and their respective pressures are equalized so that gas of higher pressure is reduced to match that of lower-pressure gas. Mixer control (precision metering device) controls amount of each gas reaching outlet. **B,** Functional schematic of Bennett Model AO-I Air-Oxygen Mixer. Compressed air and oxygen pressures are matched by their respective first- and second-stage regulators. Amount of each gas reaching outlets is determined by mixture control (precision metering device). Note that air pressure is referenced to both oxygen regulators to facilitate pressure equalization. (**A** courtesy Bird Corp., Palm Springs, Calif.; **B** courtesy Bennett Respiration Products, Inc., Santa Monica, Calif.)

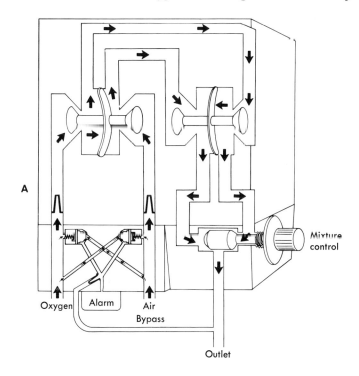

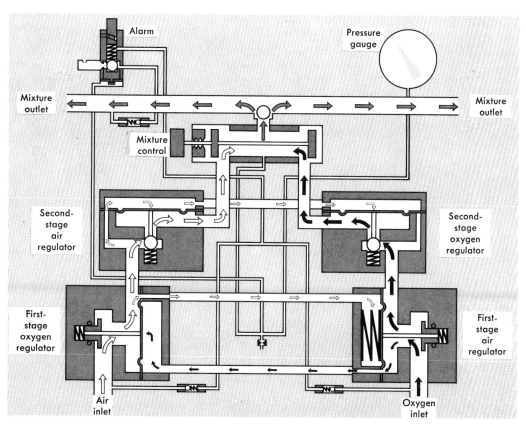

Fig. 5-13. For legend see opposite page.

while *proportionately* opening the oxygen port, an increased oxygen percentage into the bellows can be acquired and vice versa.

Oxygen controllers, such as the Bird Oxygen Blender (Fig. 5-13, *A*) and the Bennett Air-Oxygen Mixer (Fig. 5-13, *B*), provide controlled oxygen mixtures in a fashion similar to that of the MA-1 system just described, except that they operate at higher inlet and outlet pressures. That is, instead of reducing 50 psig oxygen pressure to match ambient air pressure, these units take *compressed* oxygen and air, usually near 50 psig each, and by using reducing valves (regulators), match the two pressures. These gases then move to the area of the mixture control (precision metering device) and flow through to a common outlet or outlets. Because the pressure gradient across the mixture control is the same for both gases now, the amount of each allowed out the outlet is governed by the mixture control's opening for each gas. Again, as in the MA-1 system, turning the knob to set the oxygen concentration opens one side (air or oxygen) and it *proportionately* closes the other side (air or oxygen).

Other units operating on similar principles are the Precision Air-Oxygen Controller by Bendix, the Air-Oxygen Proportioner by Ohio, and the MR-I Controller by Veriflo.

These oxygen controllers have several advantages. They can *potentially deliver 40 to 50 psig,* and most ventilators or respirators can be placed on the 100% setting and deliver a set oxygen percentage. Special points of consideration are that (1) the *Bird Mark 7 and 8's 100% setting* provides a *constant or square-wave flow pattern* at a reduced maximum flow and (2) the Bennett *PR-2 terminal flow control entrains air* into the patient system. If the terminal flow control on the PR-2 is utilized, the set oxygen percentage will consequently be lowered. In addition, *HAFOE* (High Air Flow with Oxygen Enrichment)[2] can be expanded with the use of oxygen controllers to provide high flows of preset gas mixtures in high-resistance systems (Fig. 5-14). Another application of controllers shows that ventilators that do not have oxygen systems built in can have a reservoir tube placed on their intake and, with high enough flows from the oxygen controller, preset oxygen concentrations can be delivered. The Bourns LS 104-150 infant ventilator can be modified in this fashion

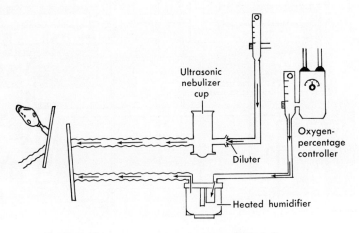

Fig. 5-14. Using preset oxygen percentage for high flow usage.

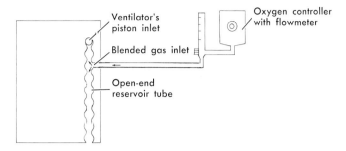

Fig. 5-15. Bourns Infant Ventilator with reservoir and oxygen percentage controller.

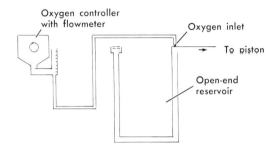

Fig. 5-16. Emerson Post-Op 3-PV volume ventilator's oxygen system with oxygen percentage controller and flowmeter.

(Fig. 5-15).[4] The Emerson 3-PV volume ventilator can be used in this way as well, except that an oxygen reservoir is already present. Flow from a controller can be run directly into the oxygen intake of the ventilator at a rate high enough to ensure that the only gases from the controller flushing the reservoir enter the piston's chamber (Fig. 5-16).

OXYGEN ANALYZERS

There are five types of oxygen analyzers in common use: (1) the *physical analyzer* utilizes the Pauling principle, (2) the *electrical analyzer* works on the principle of thermal conductivity, (3) the *chemical analyzer* uses chemical absorbers for the gases being measured, (4) the *electrochemical analyzers* (encompassing the polarographic and galvanic types) use oxygen to generate electric current, and (5) the *mass spectrometer* separates gases because of their ionic mass.

Physical analyzers

Physical analyzers work on a principle described by Pauling, Wood, and Sturidivant.[5] Oxygen possesses the specific characteristic of *paramagnetic susceptibility.* When introduced into a magnetic field, *oxygen tends to alter the design of the magnetic force* (Fig. 5-17). Being paramagnetic, oxygen locates itself in the strongest portion of a nonhomogeneous magnetic field; a diamagnetic gas (such as nitrogen) is attracted to the weaker portion. The Beckman D-2 oxygen analyzer is a common example of a unit using the physical paramagnetic property of oxygen (Fig. 5-18). A *glass dumbbell* filled with nitrogen is suspended on a *twisted quartz fiber.* The magnets normally hold the dumbbell in a specific position. Once oxygen is added to the mag-

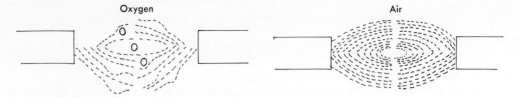

Fig. 5-17. Pauling's (Paramagnetic) principle.

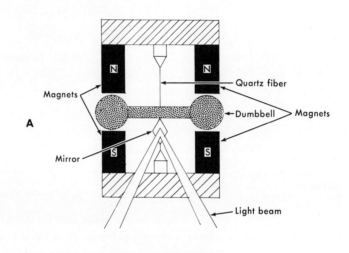

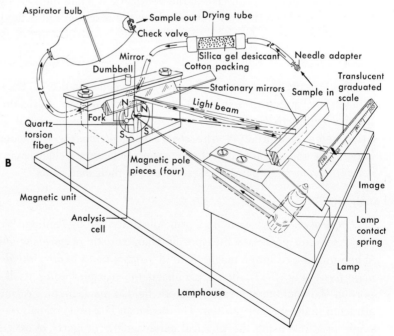

Fig. 5-18. A, Physical (Pauling) analyzer. **B,** Beckman D-2. (**A** modified from Wilson, R. S., and Laver, M. B.: Anesthesiology **37:**112, 1972; **B** courtesy Beckman Instruments, Inc., Irvine, Calif.)

netic field, the alteration in the magnetic field allows the dumbbell to rotate slightly. A *mirror* is attached to the dumbbell and reflects a *light focused on it to a translucent scale* that is calibrated in both mm Hg partial pressure and oxygen percentage. Any rotation of the dumbbell is reflected as a change in oxygen partial pressure or concentration on the scale. The Beckman's reading *does require adjustment for different altitudes* and, even though it is recalibrated at 21%, the accuracy progressively deteriorates at higher percentages when used at higher altitudes. This is because as the dumbbell tends to rotate, it relinquishes some portion of the torque on the quartz fiber, normally present at sea level. Therefore at higher altitudes the torque of the fiber is less and the dumbbell does not rotate as much as it would at sea level when oxygen is introduced. The Beckman uses *blue silica gel* as a *drying agent* to absorb moisture from the sample and prevent corrosion of the internal chamber. Once the silica gel has turned pink, it should be changed to prevent alterations in reading as well as corrosion of the dumbbell chamber itself due to water vapor in the gas sample. The Beckman reading relates to the *quantity of oxygen molecules* present in the magnetic field and, therefore, more closely measures the *partial pressure* of oxygen rather than the oxygen percentage.

Electrical analyzers

Electrical analyzers utilize the principle of *thermal conductivity* and a *wheatstone bridge to compare the resistance to current flow through two wires* (Fig. 5-19).[2] One is a *reference wire* and is exposed to room air. The other wire, which is a *sampling wire*, is in the gas sample chamber. The larger the mass is of the molecules exposed to the wires, the more heat that is removed and the cooler the wire will be. As the wire is cooled, more electric current can flow through it. This *change in current flow* is proportional to the cooling (thermal conductivity) and is compared to the reference wire. The difference *is read out on a meter as oxygen percentage.* Oxygen, having a higher mass than nitrogen, the major component of ambient air surrounding the reference wire, *tends to cool the wire more,* thereby *allowing more current to*

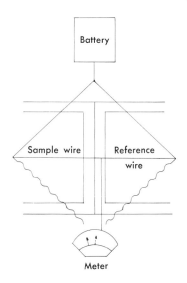

Fig. 5-19. Wheatstone bridge of electrical analyzer.

flow through it. Therefore, as higher oxygen concentrations are introduced in the sampling chamber, the higher current flow reads out as a higher percentage on the meter face. Other gases of high mass, such as carbon dioxide, will alter the accuracy of the analyzer, and the reading will be erroneously high. Examples of this type of unit are the Mira and OEM units. These units also use *silica gel;* here it acts as a *ballast* to provide uniform humidity input into the unit. As in the physical analyzer, the electric analyzer is also subject to the *quantity of molecules* hitting the wires; therefore their reading most closely relates to *partial pressure* rather than to actual percentage.

Chemical analyzers

The third type of oxygen analyzer, and probably the most precise, is the *chemical analyzer.* The most common unit is the Scholander (Fig. 5-20). A sample is drawn into the chamber and measured *volumetrically by mercury displacement.* Then a *carbon dioxide absorber* is allowed to enter the chamber, and carbon dioxide is chemically extracted. The volume change is recorded, and then an *oxygen absorber* is added. Again, the volume change is noted. By *calculating* (Fig. 5-21) *the difference in volumes,* actual volumetric percentage can be attained. This unit gives a *true oxy-*

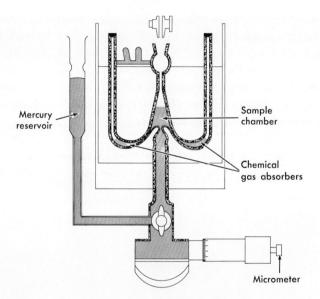

Mercury reservoir

Sample chamber

Chemical gas absorbers

Micrometer

Fig. 5-20. Example of chemical analyzer.

$$CO_2\% = \frac{\text{First reading} - \text{Second reading}}{\text{First reading}}$$

$$O_2\% = \frac{\text{First reading} - \text{Third reading}}{\text{First reading}}$$

$$N_2\% = \frac{\text{Third reading}}{\text{First reading}}$$

Fig. 5-21. Chemical analyzer formulas. Initial reading on micrometer provides total sample gas volume. After carbon dioxide absorber is added, second reading indicates sample volume with oxygen and carbon dioxide removed. Third sample reading is taken after oxygen absorber is added and both oxygen and carbon dioxide are removed.

gen percentage reading. The measurements of the others are influenced the most by partial pressure, since their response is related to the actual number of oxygen molecules present and not to what part of the total volume they represent in the mixture.

Electrochemical analyzers

The fourth type of oxygen analyzer is the *electrochemical,* which is subcategorized into (1) the *galvanic fuel cell* and (2) the *polarographic electrode.* The galvanic fuel cell[5] incorporates a semipermeable membrane, often Teflon, which isolates the gas sample from a *hydroxide bath.* In the bath are located a *gold* and usually a *lead electrode* (Fig. 5-22). As oxygen enters the hydroxide bath, it combines with water to form *hydroxyl ions* by absorbing electrons from the negative gold electrode. By virtue of simple diffusion, the hydroxyl ions travel to the lead electrode, where they decompose to form *lead oxide, water, and electrons.* The *electron current is measured on a meter as oxygen percentage.* Therefore, the higher the *quantity of oxygen molecules* entering the unit, the higher the oxygen percentage displayed. Examples of these would be units produced by Teledyne Analytical Instruments, Hudson, and Biomarine Industries.

The second type of electrochemical analyzer is the *polarographic (Clark) elec-*

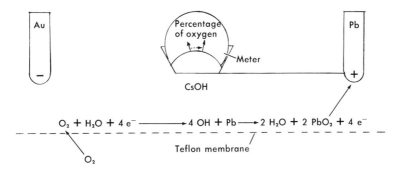

Fig. 5-22. Example of galvanic fuel cell for gaseous oxygen analysis.

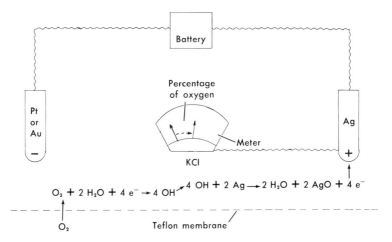

Fig. 5-23. Example of polarographic (Clark-type) electrode for gaseous oxygen measurement.

trode. Its structure is similar to the galvanic cell except that it utilizes a *battery to polarize the electrodes* (Fig. 5-23).[5] The result is an *improved response time,* since the hydroxide ions are actually attracted by the difference in electrical charge of the electrode.[5] The reaction formula is basically similar but occurs much faster. These electrodes tend to be spent or used up much more quickly as a result of their improved sensitivity. Examples of polarographic units would be those by IMI Division of Becton, Dickson and Company, the 406 and 407 models from Instrumentation Laboratory, Inc., the 200, 400 and 600 models by Ohio Medical Products, and the IBC Multipurpose Differential Oxygen Analyzer from International Biophysics Corporation.

To compare the polarographic and galvanic analyzers, the polarographic electrode uses batteries to polarize the electrode and has a quicker response time. On the other hand, the electrodes do not last as long. The galvanic cell does not utilize batteries to polarize the electrodes. As a result, the *response time is slower,* but the *electrodes last longer.* Whenever batteries are found in a galvanic analyzer, it is understood that they power the unit's various alarm systems. Both the polarographic and the galvanic analyzers are sensitive to the *quantity of oxygen molecules* diffusing across their membranes and, therefore, their readings are most closely related to *partial pressure* rather than actual oxygen concentration. Both are *affected by water* collected on their sensors, *altitude,* and *marked increases in system pressure* (such as with higher levels of PEEP or CPAP).

Mass spectrometry

Mass spectrometry is based on the ability of gases to be *ionized and separated* due to the *molecular mass of their ions* (Fig. 5-24).[5] A small sample of the gas to be analyzed is drawn from the sampling area by a vacuum pump. A small portion of this sample passes into the *ionization chamber* consisting of a *heated filament,* which produces a *bombarding electron beam.* The beam converts the gas molecules to positive ions by causing the molecules to lose electrons. The ions are drawn into the

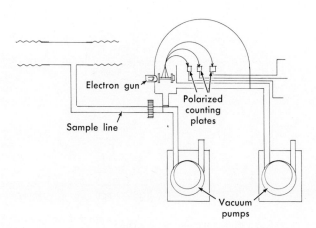

Fig. 5-24. Mass spectrometer. (Modified from Wilson, R. S., and Laver, M. B.: Anesthesiology **37:** 112, 1972.)

analysis chamber due to the *diffusion pump*. Within the analysis chamber is a magnetic field that causes the molecules to be deflected downward. The larger the ions, the farther inertia will carry them before they hit the *collecting plate* within the negative portion of the magnetic field. As an example, oxygen ions have a larger mass than nitrogen ions and will therefore hit farther on the plate. The plate collectors *count the numbers of ions* hitting them and therefore determine the *relative percentage* of the total sample.

Mass spectrometers are generally stable and accurate and can measure the true percentage of molecules in a sample.[5]

REFERENCES

1. McPherson, S. P.: Editorial: Oxygen percentage devices, Respir. Care **19:**658, 1974.
2. Egan, D. F,: Fundamentals of respiratory therapy, ed. 3, St. Louis, 1977, The C. V. Mosby Co.
3. Service and repair instructions, Bennett Model MA-1 Respiration Unit, Form 3190A (MA 11-1-74).
4. Spearman, C. B.: Control of inspired oxygen concentration and addition of PEEP or CPAP with the Bourns Pediatric Ventilator, Respir. Care **18:**405, 1973.
5. Wilson, R. S., and Laver, M. B.: Oxygen analysis: advances in methodology, Anesthesiology **37:**112, 1972.

6 Airways and manual resuscitators

There are numerous apparatus employed in respiratory therapy to either establish or maintain an airway for ventilation of the patient in acute care situations. Those to be described first are types of equipment utilized for airway maintenance.

AIRWAYS

Nasopharyngeal airways are inserted into the nose and aimed posteriorly. Once the device is in place, its terminal portion is located so that it can provide a clear path for gas flow into the pharyngeal area[1,2] (Fig. 6-1, *B*). *Oropharyngeal airways* are usually inserted into the mouth from the side and, once inserted, are twisted into position so that they project down into the inferior oropharynx (Fig. 6-1, *A*).

Proper size of airways, whether they are nasopharyngeal or oropharyngeal airways, is extremely important. If they are too long, they may potentially push the epiglottis down posteriorly, occluding the larynx, reducing effective ventilation and promoting gastric insufflation. If the oropharyngeal airway is too small, it may tend to push the tongue anteriorly, producing rather than preventing pharyngeal obstruction.

Oropharyngeal airways come in several varieties to provide various features to clinical use. Generally, the designs (as typified in Fig. 6-2) provide an *I-beam support* for rigidity, which prevents the patient's teeth clamping closed (such as the Berman type), thus occluding the airway, or have a *hollow passageway* through which pharyngeal suctioning can be performed[2] (such as the Rosser, Guedel, Connel, Waters, and Cath-Guide Guedel types). The Safar and Rosser tubes (or S-tubes) have an outward projection for mouth-to-tube–like ventilation. However, the adequacy of their use for this type of ventilation has been questioned, and other disadvantages are listed elsewhere.[3]

The *esophageal obturator* was designed for quick airway maintenance in emergency situations.[1] The closed-end tube (Fig. 6-3) is inserted *into the esophagus*, and the cuff is inflated to seal the tube in place. The incoming gases pass through an inlet into the face mask and out many small ports in the tube in the area of the pharynx and continue on into the larynx.[4]

Endotracheal tubes of various designs are employed for quick insertion into the trachea by way of the larynx in emergency situations to provide a *sealed airway* for improved ventilation and to *prevent aspiration of vomitus* into the respiratory tract.[1,2,4]

Initially, endotracheal tubes were structured from metal, such as the one used by

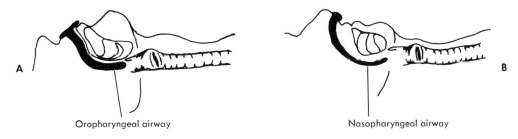

Oropharyngeal airway

Nasopharyngeal airway

Fig. 6-1. Oropharyngeal and nasopharyngeal airways in relationship to proper anatomic placement

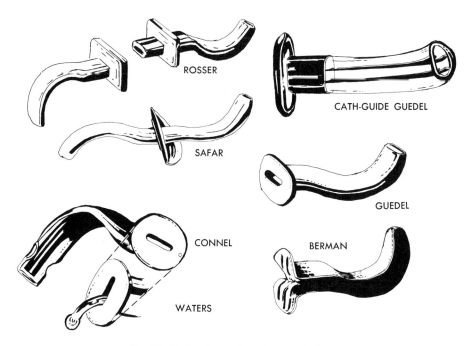

ROSSER

CATH-GUIDE GUEDEL

SAFAR

GUEDEL

CONNEL

BERMAN

WATERS

Fig. 6-2. Various types of oropharyngeal airways.

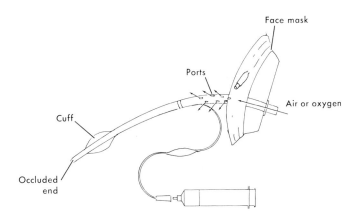

Face mask

Ports

Air or oxygen

Cuff

Occluded end

Fig. 6-3. Esophageal obturator is inserted into esophagus and cuff is inflated. Mask makes seal against face, and air or oxygen entering through ports cannot enter esophagus due to inflated cuff, so it enters larynx.

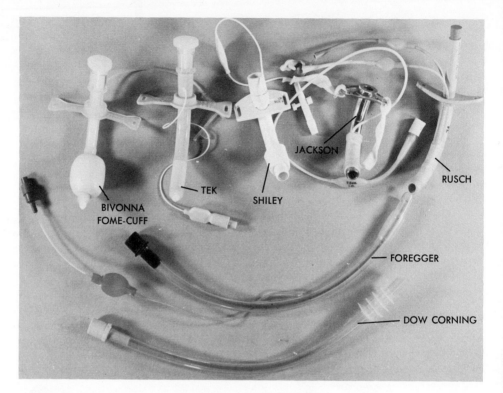

Fig. 6-4. Various types of tubes.

Smellie in 1763 to perform the first intubation.[6] Metal tubes first gave way to ones made of rubber and then to various types of plastic tubes. Initially, tubes were not cuffed; later a rubber *replaceable cuff* was added to the tube if desired by the physician. Problems associated with the use of replaceable cuffs on tubes were (1) the nonuniform expansion, (2) the lack of cuff strength, and (3) the acutely dangerous situation that could develop if the cuff were to *slip over the end* of the endotracheal tube.[5] The result of a cuff migrating off the end of a tube was the effective sealing of the airway, through which inspiratory pressures were excessive, and the seal made exhalation impossible.[1]

The most common type of tube currently available incorporates a cuff built onto the tube itself, which eliminates the problem of the cuff slipping off. Examples of commonly available tubes are shown in Fig. 6-4.

Types of cuffs

Since cuffs of *low residual volume and high pressure* (Fig. 6-5) tend to cause sufficient pressure on the respiratory tract mucosa of the trachea to stop capillary blood flow, maneuvers such as the *minimal leak* technique[1,11] are employed. In this technique a slight leak during inhalation is allowed around the cuff for those patients on long-term mechanically supported ventilation. *Periodic deflation*[7] of the cuff every hour for 5 minutes has also been utilized, although the adequacy of this technique has been questioned.[8] These methods have been devised to try to minimize the potential of tracheal wall dilation and mucosal necrosis with long-term use of cuffed tubes.[9]

Reducing the potential of *necrosis* also prompted the development of other types of cuff designs with *high residual volume* and *low pressure* (Fig. 6-5). These cuffs are larger than high-pressure cuffs and are actively deflated for insertion, then partially inflated with enough air to obtain a seal against the tracheal wall. Low-volume, high-pressure cuffs have been shown to exert pressures from *40 to over 200 mm Hg*, and high-volume, low-pressure cuffs may exert less than 25 mm Hg pressure.[9-11] Examples of tubes incorporating the newer low-pressure designs are the Soft-Cuf by Forreger and the Soft-Seal by Portex. Shiley also makes a tube with a cuff that has a relatively large residual volume. This cuff is cylindrical in shape, made of comparatively rigid material, and is said to inflate evenly.[1,12]

The tubes produced by Lanz Medical Products Corporation and Extracorporeal Medical Specialties, Inc., which utilize a *McGinnis* pressure-regulating balloon,[13] were devised to maintain a low pressure against the tracheal wall (Fig. 6-6). The elasticity of the *external pressure-regulating valve and control balloon* is the factor limiting the pressure developed in the tube's cuff to 20 to 25 mm Hg.[14] The control balloon, however, must never be allowed to be inflated to the size of the *outer cover*, or the 25 mm Hg pressure will be exceeded rapidly.

Shiley Laboratories, Inc., produces a tracheostomy tube utilizing a low-pressure cuff with a pressure-regulating valve (Fig. 6-7). A spring-loaded relief valve is set to

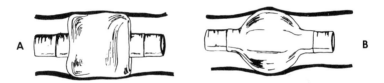

Fig. 6-5. Diagram comparing shapes of **A**, high-residual-volume, low-pressure cuff and **B**, low-residual-volume, high-pressure cuff.

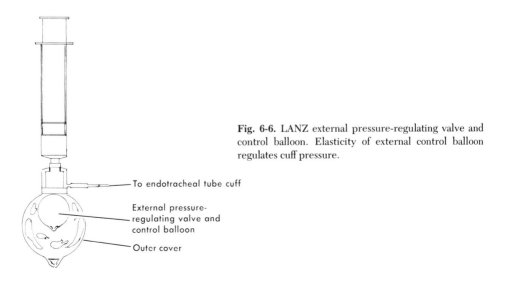

Fig. 6-6. LANZ external pressure-regulating valve and control balloon. Elasticity of external control balloon regulates cuff pressure.

To endotracheal tube cuff

External pressure-regulating valve and control balloon

Outer cover

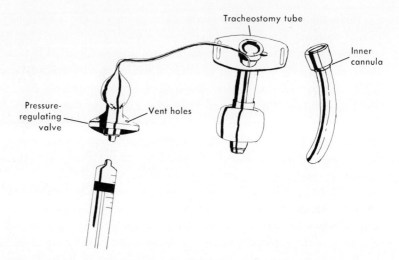

Fig. 6-7. Shiley's tracheostomy tube with pressure-regulated valve for its low-pressure cuff. Shiley tracheostomy tubes can be used with inner cannulas.

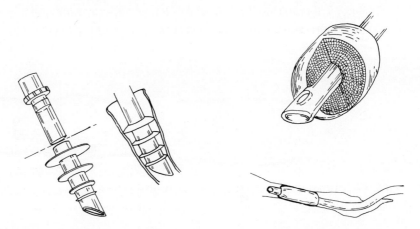

Fig. 6-8. Dow Corning tube with ring seals.   **Fig. 6-9.** Kamen-Wilkinson Fome Cuff.

vent excess air *during active cuff inflation* so as to maintain a pressure of approximately 25 mm Hg within the cuff. Once the filling syringe is removed from the filling port of the valve, however, this vent system is bypassed, and pressure fluctuations above 25 mm Hg can occur.

With these same concerns in mind, a tube of *silicone* was devised by Dow Corning with *flexible silicone rings of decreasing diameters* to form a seal (Fig. 6-8). The tube is inserted and *pulled back slightly*, which aims the rings inferiorly, sealing the trachea and attempting to minimize pressure on the tracheal mucosa. However, pressure developed by the rings can be as high as 55 to 100 mm Hg.[14]

Recently, the *Fome Cuff* was introduced by Kamen and associates,[15] in which the cuff (Fig. 6-9) is filled with a *soft, spongy foam.* The cuff is deflated, flattening the foam for insertion, and then it is allowed to attempt to resume the *normal shape of the foam,* providing an effective seal against the tracheal wall. These cuffs also exert a low pressure against the tracheal wall of about 20 mm Hg pressure[16] when properly used.

Intubation and tracheostomy tubes

The *endotracheal tube* must be *long enough* to pass the cuff through and *past the cords*, but not so long as to allow any danger of the tube being misplaced or *migrating into the right* mainstem bronchus (Fig. 6-10, *A*).[1] Were this to happen, the result would be *hyperinflation* of the right and *no* ventilation of the left (Fig. 6-10, *B*). The average distance from the teeth to the carina in adults is *27 cm*[17]; therefore a tube cut to that length accommodates nearly all adults and reduces the danger of migrating into the right mainstem bronchus.[17] Once the tube is inserted, both *auscultation* of the chest as well as *radiography* (some tubes have *radiopaque markings* along their length) can indicate the proper placement of the tube. Once in place, the tube should be *firmly secured* to maintain its proper location.

Endotracheal tubes can be inserted either nasally or, more commonly in adults, orally. It usually requires 2 cm of extra tube or an average of *29 cm total* length to insert a tube nasally.[17]

Tracheostomy tubes have followed cuff designs similar to those found on most endotracheal tubes. Those units which have *removable cuffs* such as the *Jackson silver tubes* (Fig. 6-11) have found decreasing use in respiratory care because of the potential of the cuffs slipping off the end of the tube and occluding the airway, as described with endotracheal tubes (Fig. 6-12). The availability of the newer low-pressure cuffs have also contributed to the Jackson's disuse.

Since tracheostomy tubes tend to be left in place during certain long-term situations, attempts were made through design innovations to *prevent secretion accumulation* in the tube. Some units utilize an *inner cannula* that can be *removed* and cleaned periodically, as do the Jackson and Shiley units. Materials such as silicone have also been tried in an attempt to reduce the sticking of secretions to the inner surface.

The *fenestrated tracheostomy tube* is a device that can be useful for assessing the patient's ability to be extubated and to allow the patient to verbalize when the tube is occluded and the cuff deflated[1,18] (Fig. 6-13). This tube utilizes an opening in its posterior portion above the cuff. An inner cannula must be used when a seal is desired. When the inner cannula is removed, the cuff is deflated, and the normal inlet

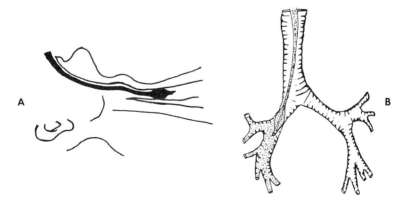

Fig. 6-10. Proper tube placement is with cuff's position between vocal cords and carina, **A.** If tube is placed too low, it may migrate into right bronchus, and no ventilation of left lung will occur, **B.**

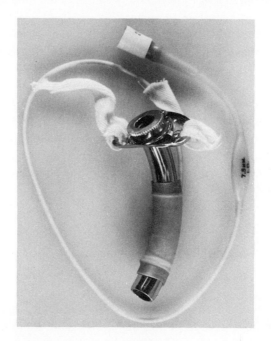

Fig. 6-11. Jackson silver tracheostomy tube with removable cuff.

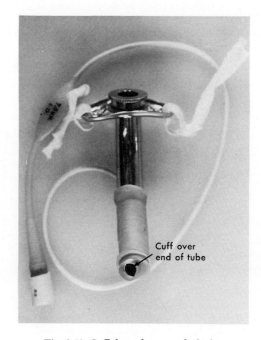

Fig. 6-12. Cuff slipped over end of tube.

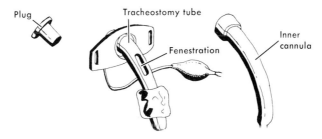

Fig. 6-13. Example of fenestrated tracheostomy tube with removable inner cannula and plug. (Modified from Shiley Laboratories, Inc., Irvine, Calif.)

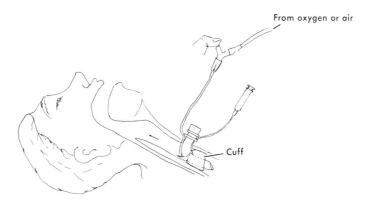

Fig. 6-14. Pitt Speaking Tracheostomy Tube. Small tube open above cuff allows for low flow (2 to 4 L/min of oxygen or air) to pass through vocal cords for vocalization. Intermittent control can be occluded by patient or clinician. (Modified from Safar, P., and Grenvik, A.: Crit. Care Med. 3:23, 1975.)

is occluded, the patient can inhale and exhale through the fenestration and around the tube. Shiley produces a disposable fenestrated tube supplied with a plug and removable inner cannula.

Another type of tube that can be used to allow tracheostomized patients to talk is the *Pitt Speaking Tracheostomy Tube*[18] (Fig. 6-14). A small tube with an opening above the tube's cuff is connected to a source of 4 to 6 liters of air or oxygen and a Y connector for intermittent control. When the open port on the Y is occluded, gases flow out the small tube and out through the patient's larynx and upper airway, allowing for vocalization. The cuff must be inflated during this procedure.

RESUSCITATORS

Resuscitators can be divided into two general categories: *manual* resuscitators and *gas-powered* resuscitators.

Manual resuscitators using self-inflating bags can be subdivided by the design characteristics of their valves. The first valve of this type is the *disk* type. The earliest of these units was the early model *AMBU* unit.[19] It incorporated a *spring-loaded* disk that moved on a *shaft* in the patient valve (Fig. 6-15). On the outlet side of the disk was the spring that held the disk valve to the right, allowing communication of the patient outlet with the exhalation port. Compression of the bag forced the disk forward, occluding the exhalation port and directing gas flow into the patient. On

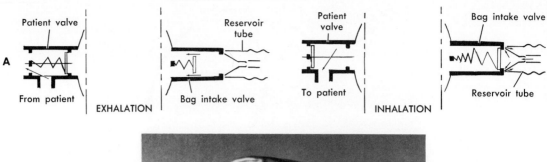

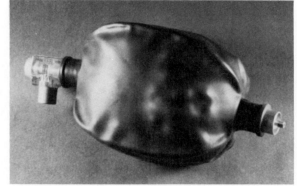

Fig. 6-15. **A,** Model of early AMBU Resuscitator's valve. **B,** AMBU Resuscitator bag and valve.

releasing the bag, changes in pressure and the spring simply push the disk back toward the bag, allowing the patient to exhale into the room. The *bag intake valve* for the resuscitator was also a simple spring and disk valve that allowed the bag to fill by drawing in room air and oxygen. The negative pressure that was caused internally by the bag expanding, as it attempted to resume its normal shape, drew gas in through the valve. Oxygen entered a *nipple* on the bag into the cone at the spring/disk valve of the bag intake valve (tailpiece). When the bag was not drawing gas in during refill, the oxygen was simply flushed out the cone and went into the room. During refill of the bag, oxygen in the cone and area around it was drawn into the bag. The addition of a *reservoir tube at the tailpiece* for the accumulation of oxygen when the bag was not refilling allowed the unit to deliver nearly 100% oxygen to the patient. Another reservoir tube attachment is described elsewhere.[20]

Some important considerations for the early AMBU resuscitators include the following. (1) The self-inflating characteristic was accomplished by an insert of *foam rubber*, which with time would deteriorate and flake as well as make cleaning of the unit difficult. (2) Oxygen flows of greater than 10 to 15 L/min connected directly to the bag intake valve can force that valve's disk to open, the bag to pressurize, and the patient's valve to jam in an *open* position (closing the exhalation port) and cause excessive pressures within the patient's airway.

The AMBU units currently produced are of a different design and will be covered later in this chapter.

Another disk-type unit is the *Ohio Hope* (Fig. 6-16). The Hope valve was similar in design to the original AMBU except the shaft, disk, and spring are *connected* to the exhalation outlet; that is, when the exhalation valve is removed, the disk valve assembly comes with it. The gas *inlet* valve for the bag itself is a *leaf valve* and is

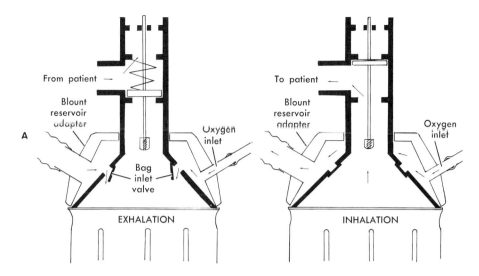

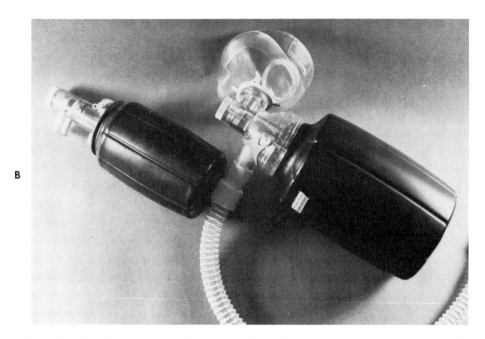

Fig. 6-16. A, Ohio Hope Resuscitator's valve with Blount Oxygen Reservoir Adapter. **B,** Hope Pediatric and Adult (with oxygen adapter) resuscitators.

located in the neck of the valve body. The disk valve works principally the same as the AMBU valve. Oxygen is added into the valve neck and mixed with the air drawn in during bag refill. A sleeve produced by Blount fits around the neck of the Hope and provides a *reservoir volume* for oxygen accumulation, with delivery of up to 100% oxygen[21] (Fig. 6-16).

Earlier models of the Hope did not have ports on the oxygen inlet, and excessive flows tended to inflate the bag and hold the bag valve at the inspiratory position. This was modified by placing the holes in the inlet to reduce the buildup of pressure.

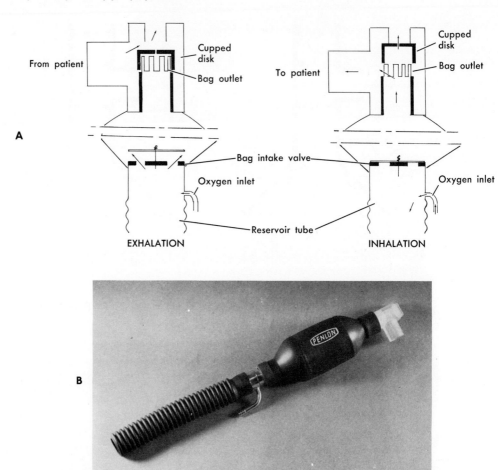

A

EXHALATION   INHALATION

Fig. 6-17. A, Penlon Infant Resuscitator's valve. **B,** Penlon resuscitator bag, valve, and oxygen reservoir.

The Hope resuscitators can be obtained with or without a magnetic pressure relief valve preset to open when a pressure of 40 cm H_2O is within the valve.[19] Since the relief port itself is relatively small, pressures above 40 cm H_2O can be exerted at the patient connection with rapid compression of the bag. In other words, the valve is *flow dependent*. The adult bag contains 2 liters when full, and a pediatric model uses a bag containing 730 cc.[19]

The *Penlon Infant Resuscitator* has a *cupped-disk valve* (Fig. 6-17). Instead of employing a spring to seat the valve when flow from the bag stops, the valve uses only changes in pressure within the bag to move the valve. During bag compression, the gas flow from the bag pushes a cupped disk away from the bag outlet port and against the exhalation port. With the *exhalation valve* occluded, gas is directed to the patient. A *small hole* in the cupped disk serves to provide a *leak* to reduce the peak pressure delivery potential. Like the pressure relief on the Hope units, this system is flow dependent; that is, the higher the flow from the bag, the higher the generated pressure will be in the valve, in spite of the leak. On exhalation, the subatmospheric pressure generated within the bag causes the cupped valve to close the *bag outlet,*

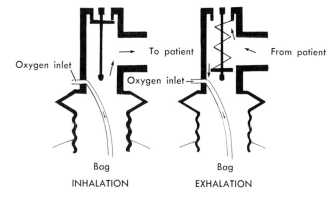

Fig. 6-18. Air Viva Resuscitator's valve.

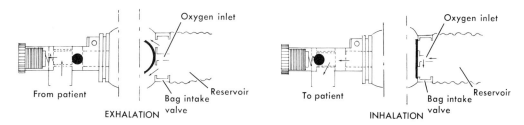

Fig. 6-19. Valves for Ohio's Hope II prototype resuscitator.

and exhalation occurs out of the exhalation port. Both an *oxygen inlet* and a *reservoir volume* allow the administration of up to 100% oxygen.

Since the oxygen inlet is angled so that the forward force of the oxygen does not influence the bag intake valve directly, even high flows into the open-end reservoir tube will not interfere with the resuscitator's normal function. This device is primarily designed for neonates[19] and should not need oxygen flows of more than 5 to 8 L/min under usual circumstances.

The *Air Viva* also employs a *spring-disk* principle similar to the AMBU and Hope units (Fig. 6-18). As gas travels from the bag during compression, a disk is pushed against a spring and exhalation valve and gas travels to the patient. On exhalation, the spring and pressure changes in the bag return the disk toward the bag. The bag fills with oxygen from the oxygen inlet, room air from the exhalation port, and some exhaled gases. The continuous flow of oxygen flushes the bag to reduce carbon dioxide levels in the bag and increase oxygen content. Even fairly low flow rates of oxygen into the bag (above 5 L/min) can stick or jam the disk against the exhalation valve.[22] This could then create excessive pressures within the patient's airways; therefore high flows should be avoided. Oxygen concentrations of 50% to 80% with flows of 5 to 15 L/min have been reported.[22]

The prototype of *Ohio's Hope II* utilizes a *spring and ball,* rather than a spring and disk, but works fundamentally the same. As the bag is compressed, gas pushes the ball against the spring, compressing it, and gas travels to the patient. Once gas flow from the bag compression has stopped, the spring seats the ball on the bag outlet, and the patient's gases exit through the exhalation ports (Fig. 6-19). The *reservoir*

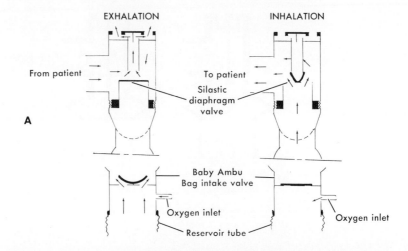

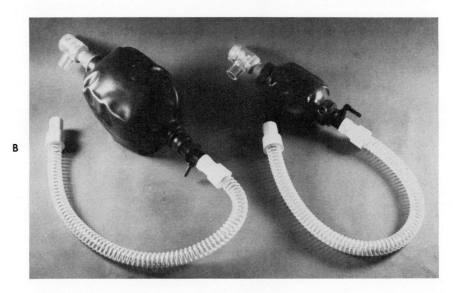

Fig. 6-20. A, New AMBU Resuscitator's E-2 valve and Baby AMBU Bag's intake valve. **B,** Adult and baby AMBU resuscitators with oxygen reservoir system.

on the bag inlet allows for oxygen accumulation and for the potential of 100% oxygen delivery. The angle of the oxygen inlet opening allows for high (over 20 L/min) oxygen flows to be used *without* interruption of normal function.

The second general type of resuscitator valve incorporates a *diaphragm.* The current AMBU (E-2) valve (Fig. 6-20) allows a Silastic diaphragm to be pushed upward, *occluding the exhaust port* when the flow of gas from the bag being compressed enters the valve, directing gas to the patient. Once flow from the bag stops, the diaphragm is moved away from the exhalation port by the patient's exhaled gas and by the subatmospheric pressure of the bag re-expanding. The E-2 valve has been used for both adult and pediatric models.[19] The *bag intake valve* for the Baby AMBU is shown in Fig. 6-20. A simple one-way leaf valve opens when the bag is refilling (exhalation) and closes with the positive pressure from bag compression (inhalation).

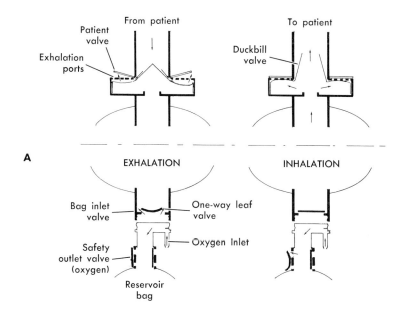

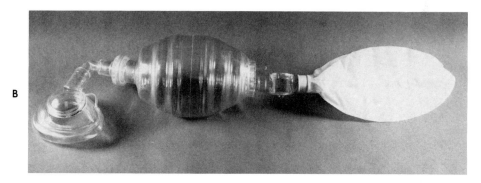

Fig. 6-21. **A,** Valves for Laerdal Resusci Folding Bag II (RFB-II) for adults with oxygen reservoir bag system. **B,** Adult Laerdal Resusci Folding Bag II with oxygen reservoir system.

During bag refill, oxygen and/or air from the bag intake valve and reservoir move through the valve. As with the Penlon unit, the angle of the oxygen inlet allows for high flows of oxygen to fill the open-end reservoir, allowing for up to 100% oxygen delivery and no malfunctioning of the E-2 valve.

Recently, this same bag intake valve from the Baby AMBU has been used with the adult model with good results.[23,24] Its function is similar to an adaptation used for the early model AMBU.[20]

When gas flow from the bag enters the valve of the *Laerdal Resusci Folding Bag II* (RFB II), the force pushes the *diaphragm* up against the exhalation ports, occluding them (Fig. 6-21). This gas flow then opens a *duckbill valve*, allowing gas to go to the patient. Once flow from the bag has ceased, exhaled gas from the patient pushes the diaphragm back and gas flows out the exhalation ports. The bag inlet is a simple *leaf valve* with a *reservoir* attached for it to attain up to 100% oxygen.[19]

The *Laerdal Infant Resuscitator* has recently been reported[25] to be a safe, multi-

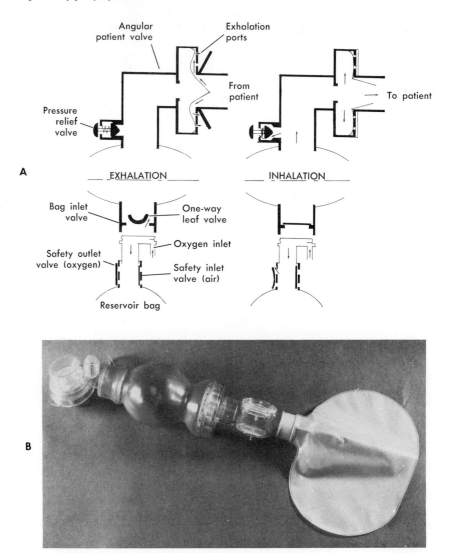

Fig. 6-22. A, Valves for Laerdal Infant Resuscitator with oxygen reservoir system. **B,** Laerdal Infant Resuscitator with oxygen reservoir system.

purpose device. The unit incorporates the *Laerdal Valve III—Angular* (Figs. 6-22 and 6-23). The diaphragm and duckbill valves function in a similar fashion to the RFB II adult model. When the bag is compressed, gas pressure swells the diaphragm and occludes the exhalation ports, directing gases through the open duckbill valve and to the patient. During exhalation, the subatmospheric pressure of the bag refilling and the slight positive pressure of the patient's exhaled gases move the duckbill valve closed and the diaphragm away from the exhalation ports, allowing the patient's gases to exit. A pressure relief is set to open at about 35 cm H_2O but can easily be occluded with the index finger of the hand compressing the small bag, so that pressures of over 100 cm H_2O can be obtained if needed.[25] The bag size is 240 ml, and tidal volumes of up to 200 ml can be delivered.[25]

As shown in Fig. 6-23, this unit can be adapted for use with continuous positive

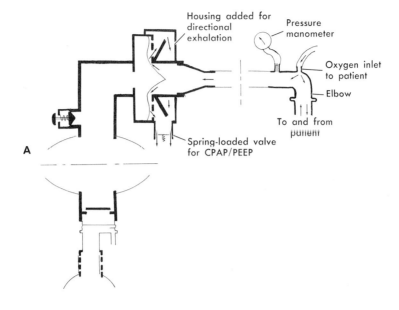

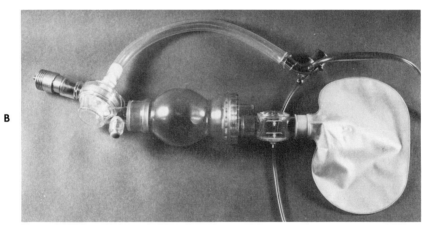

Fig. 6-23. A, Laerdal Infant Resuscitator with system added for using continuous positive airway pressure (CPAP) and intermittent bag inflations. **B,** Infant Resuscitator modified for use with CPAP.

airway pressure (CPAP) or positive end expiratory pressure (PEEP) combined with intermittent bag inflations.[25] A continuous flow of oxygen enters at an *elbow* connection for spontaneous patient breathing. That gas plus any exhaled gases flow out the exhalation port where a device, such as the spring-loaded relief valve shown, creates a positive pressure in the system and the patient's airway. That pressure is monitored by an aneroid manometer connected to the elbow. When the bag is compressed, the exhalation port is occluded, and gases enter the patient as usual. During exhalation, the patient's gases mix with the oxygen source and exit through the sping-loaded valve, and pressure in the system is not allowed to drop to atmospheric level. Since the bag's intake valve is separated from the patient connection, its refilling does not interfere with the CPAP or PEEP level.[25]

An optional reservoir assembly with a valve system is available for both the adult

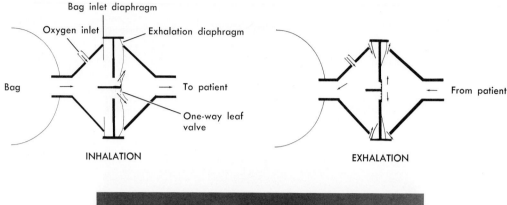

INHALATION   EXHALATION

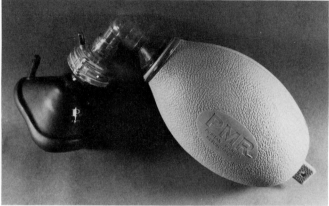

Fig. 6-24. Puritan Manual Resuscitator's (PMR) valves.

and infant Laerdal resuscitator bags and is shown in Figs. 6-21 and 6-22. The bag inlet valve for both the RFB II adult bag and the Infant Resuscitator are functionally identical. The reservoir assembly has two one-way leaf valves: (1) an *inlet* valve and (2) an *outlet* valve. Oxygen entering from its inlet in the bag inlet valve travels into the reservoir assembly if the resuscitator bag is not in its refilling stage. If the reservoir assembly is full, the excess oxygen flows through the outlet one-way valve. The inlet one-way valve serves as a safety inlet to the resuscitator in case the oxygen flow is inadequate or absent. Utilization of this reservoir system allows for high oxygen concentrations of up to 100% to be delivered with either the RFB II or the Laerdal Infant Resuscitator.[19,25]

The *Puritan Manual Resuscitator* (PMR) (Fig. 6-24) uses *two diaphragms* and a *leaf valve* incorporated into the main valve to direct both outgoing gas flow from the bag and incoming gas flow from the inlet for its refill. As gas flow from the bag compression enters the valve, its force causes (1) the *bag diaphragm inlet valve* to occlude the bag refill ports and (2) the *exhalation valve diaphragm* to occlude the patient exhalation ports. The gas flow from the bag then opens the one-way leaf valve to travel to the patient. On exhalation, the patient's exhaled gas pushes the exhalation diaphragm back, and patient gases flow out the exhalation ports. The subatmospheric pressure generated in the bag, once it is released, causes the back diaphragm to move away from the exhalation port and air is drawn in. *Oxygen is added* at the bag

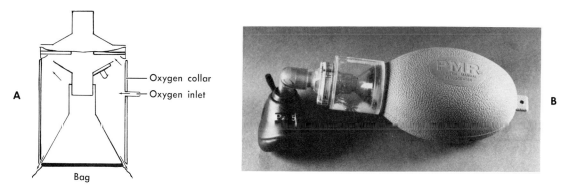

Fig. 6-25. A, PMR valve with oxygen collar for reservoir added. **B,** PMR modified with oxygen reservoir collar.

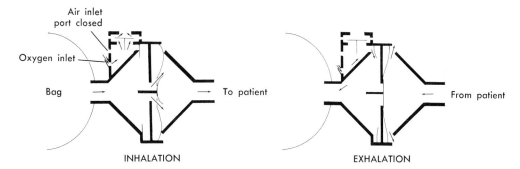

Fig. 6-26. High Oxygen PMR valves with oxygen in use. Air inlet port is closed, and only oxygen flow rate fills bag.

refill ports and is drawn in with room air. Fig. 6-25 shows a handmade collar that fits around the PMR valve, providing some reservoir area for oxygen accumulation. An oxygen inlet is attached to the collar. Although this attachment is not currently available commercially, clinical and laboratory data show delivered oxygen concentrations of nearly 100% when incoming flows are above 15 L/min[26] compared to nearly 70% without the collar,[19] using slow bag refill in both cases.

When using the standard PMR valve as shown in Fig. 6-24, high oxygen flows above 15 L/min will *not jam* the valve although some *resistance* to exhalation can occur.

Recently another model, the *High Oxygen PMR* (Figs. 6-26 and 6-27), has become available. This unit incorporates a spring-loaded valve that closes the air intake port to the bag when oxygen is connected. The bag's refill is therefore dependent on the oxygen flow rate, and delivered oxygen concentrations exceed the 95% level.[19] Because this unit is flow dependent when an oxygen tube is connected, high flow rates should be used. An adaptation of the valve shown in Fig. 6-28 has also been devised. The spring-loaded device is removed and a 24-inch reservoir tube added to its seat. Flows of oxygen from 20 to 22 L/min have provided 100% oxygen delivered during clinical and laboratory trials. The bag is not solely dependent on the oxygen flow rate for its filling, only its oxygen concentrations.

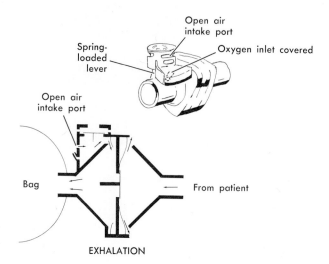

Fig. 6-27. High Oxygen PMR in air mode. (**A,** Bag filling with air. **B,** Spring-loaded lever, which covers oxygen inlet in this mode.)

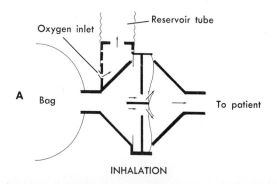

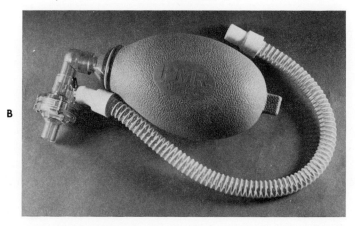

Fig. 6-28. A, Modified High Oxygen PMR. Spring-loaded lever (shown in Fig. 6-27) has been removed and 24-inch reservoir tube added. **B,** Modified High Oxygen PMR showing oxygen reservoir tube added.

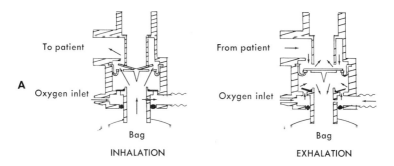

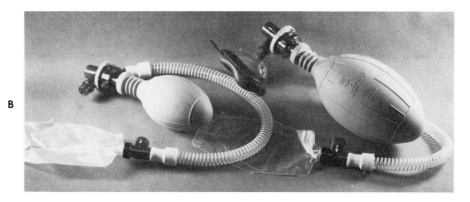

Fig. 6-29. A, AIRbird Resuscitator's valve. **B,** Infant and adult models of AIRbird Resuscitator with oxygen reservoir systems attached.

The AIRbird (Fig. 6-29) also employs *diaphragm and leaf valves.* On bag compression, the gas flow opens the *center* leaf valve of the top diaphragm. The leaf occludes the exhalation port, and gas travels past the leaf to the patient. On exhalation, the leaf *reseats,* and gases flow out the exhalation valve. The negative pressure generated in the bag as it is released causes gas to enter past the bottom leaf. An adapter, available for attachment onto that portion of the valve which enclosed the bottom, allows for a tube and/or bag *reservoir* to develop high oxygen concentrations up to 95%.[19] Using high oxygen flow rates will not compromise the AIRbird's valve operation.

All the self-inflating manual resuscitator units just mentioned can be used with supplemental oxygen[19] and can achieve from 60% to 100% delivered oxygen when the following criteria are considered:

1. *The highest acceptable oxygen flow rate should be utilized.* "Acceptable" means that flow rate which will not cause sticking or jamming of the valving mechanisms.

2. *A reservoir for oxygen collection should be utilized where available.*

3. *The longest possible bag refill must be utilized.* Clinical and laboratory experience has shown that even resuscitators such as the adult Hope and the original PMR units without a reservoir system can achieve oxygen concentrations above 60% when 3 to 4 seconds are allowed for refill and oxygen flows of 10 to 18 L/min are used.

Table 6-1 summarizes some characteristics of the manual resuscitators presented.

Table 6-1. Summary of self-inflating manual resuscitators' characteristics

Resuscitator	Type of patient valve	Type of bag inlet valve	Approximate volume of full bag	Maximum suggested oxygen flow rates
AMBU (early models)	Spring disk	Spring disk	2000 ml	Less than 10 to 15 L/min to avoid valve jamming
Hope	Spring disk	One-way leaf valve	Adult, 2000 ml; pediatric, 730 ml	Less than 15 L/min to avoid valve sticking or chattering
Penlon	Cupped disk	Spring disk		High oxygen flow rates will not affect proper function
Air Viva	Spring disk		2000 ml	5 L/min may cause chattering, 10 to 15 L/min jamming of valve
Hope II (prototype)	Spring ball	One-way leaf valve	2000 ml	High oxygen flows will not affect proper function
AMBU E-2	Diaphragm	One-way leaf valve	Adult, 1800 ml; Baby, 500 ml	High flows may be used when unit is equipped with valve shown in Fig. 6-20 without affecting proper function
Laerdal RFB II	Diaphragm and duck bill	One-way leaf valve	2000 ml	High oxygen flows will not affect proper function
Laerdal infant resuscitator	Diaphragm and duck bill	One-way leaf valve	240 ml	High oxygen flows will not affect proper function
PMR	Diaphragm and leaf valve	Diaphragm	2000 ml	Oxygen flows up to 20 L/min will not affect proper function; flows from 20 to 50 L/min may cause some resistance to patient's exhalation
High oxygen PMR	Diaphragm and leaf valve	Diaphragm and one-way leaf valve (air) or oxygen inlet	2000 ml	High oxygen flows will not affect proper function; low oxygen flows less than 12 L/min decrease bag refill and available breathing rates (high or low oxygen flows will not affect operation on modified unit, see Fig. 6-28)
AIRbird	Diaphragm and leaf valve	One-way leaf valve	Adult, 2000 ml; Pediatric, 500 ml	High oxygen flows will not affect proper function

Gas-powered resuscitators are usually *pressure-limited* units that may also be used as *demand valves*. Pressure-limited resuscitators work in a manner similar to reducing valves (Fig. 6-30) in that they *reduce* incoming (usually 50 psig) oxygen to a preset level. The *advantage* of using this type of unit is that the obtainable *100% oxygen* concentration is important in a hypoxic patient with a respiratory arrest. A notable *disadvantage* would include decreasing the effectiveness of volume delivery when *ventilatory pressure needs* sometimes *increase above the pressure capabilities of the unit*. A possible *hazard* would be that, in some units, if the *primary diaphragm were to rupture, 50 psig source* gas would be exposed to the patient's airway.

The device shown in Fig. 6-30 can be used as a pressure-limited resuscitator or as a demand valve. Oxygen enters the unit at 50 psig, normally, and travels to the

Type of oxygen reservoir	Maximum oxygen percentage expected with optimum conditions	Type of pressure relief	Spontaneous breathing opens valve for oxygen (inhalator)
Tube or bag with inlet one-way valve such as Laerdal's reservoir assembly	Up to 100%	None	No
Sleeve with tube or bag	Up to 100%	Optional magnetic ball set to open at 40 cm H_2O	No
Tube	Up to 100%	Leak in cupped disk	No
None	Up to 80%	Spring ball set to open near 40 cm H_2O bag pressure	No
"Elephant" bore tube	Up to 100%	None on prototype	No
Tube or bag with inlet one-way valve such as Laerdal's reservoir assembly	Up to 100%	None	Yes
Tube or oxygen reservoir assembly	Up to 100%	None	Yes
Tube or oxygen reservoir assembly	Up to 100%	Spring-loaded valve set to open near 35 cm H_2O bag pressure	Yes
None commercially available	70% to 90%	None	Yes
None (tube on modified unit; see Fig. 6-28)	Above 95%	None	Yes
Tube or tube with bag and safety one-way valve inlet	Above 90% or 95%	None	Yes

top of the *main diaphragm.* The oxygen also passes through a restriction to a *pressure-equalization passage.* This passage leads to (1) another restriction, occluded by a lever on exhalation, and (2) to the bottom of the main diaphragm. The gas pressure supplied to the bottom of the main diaphragm by way of the pressure-equalization passage holds the main diaphragm up, and gas exposed to the top of the main diaphragm is unable to pass. This allows the patient's exhaled gas to push the exhalation valve assembly up and exhale out the ports.

Inhalation can be *initiated by* (1) the *manual control button* being depressed, or (2) the *patient* generating negative pressure, which is transmitted to (1) the *exhalation leaf diaphragm,* (2) *sensing passage,* and (3) the *sensing diaphragm.* In both cases, the sensing diaphragm and lever move *down,* opening the restriction from the

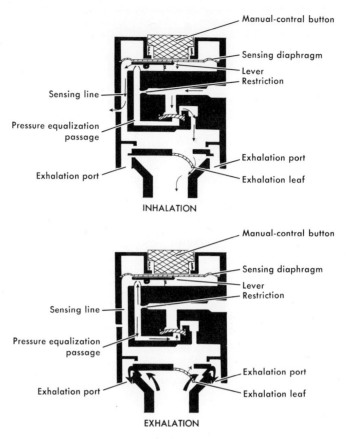

Fig. 6-30. Demand valve pressure resuscitator. (Modified from oxygen demand valve by Robertshaw Controls Co., Anaheim, Calif.)

pressure-equalization passage, which empties, decreasing the pressure on the bottom of the main diaphragm. The 50 psig exposed to the top of the main diaphragm pushes the diaphragm down, and gas flows to the patient. When pressure has developed sufficiently against the sensing diaphragm to compress the spring upward, the lever closes the pressure-equalization chamber, the main diaphragm moves up to stop flow, and exhalation occurs.

REFERENCES

1. Shapiro, B. A., Harrison, R. A., and Trout, C. A.: Clinical application of respiratory care, Chicago, 1975, Year Book Medical Publishers, Inc.
2. Dorsch, J. A., and Dorsch, S. E.: Understanding anesthesia equipment: construction, care, and complications, Baltimore, 1975, The Williams & Wilkins Co.
3. Standards for cardiopulmonary resuscitation and emergency cardiac care, J.A.M.A. (suppl.) **227**:833, 1974.
4. Greenbaum, J. M., et al.: Esophageal obstruction during oxygen administration, Chest **65**:188, 1974.
5. Egan, D. F.: Fundamentals of respiratory therapy, ed. 3, St. Louis, 1977, The C. V. Mosby Co.
6. McPherson, S. P., and Roads, J. S.: History of respiratory therapy. (To be published.)
7. Demers, R. R., and Saklad, M.: A procedure for periodic deflation of endotracheal cuffs of patients on controlled ventilation, Respir. Care **16**:119, 1971.
8. Bryant, L. R. et al.: Reappraisal of tracheal injury from cuffed tracheostomy tubes, J.A.M.A. **215**:625, 1971.
9. Selecky, P. A.: Tracheostomy: a review of present day indications, complications, and care, Heart Lung **3**:272, 1974.
10. Ching, N. P. H., and Nealon, T. F., Jr.: Clinical experience with new low-pressure high-volume tracheostomy cuffs, N.Y. State J. Med. **74**:2379, 1974.

11. Wen-Hsien Wu et al: Pressure dynamics of endotracheal and tracheostomy cuffs, Crit. Care Med. 1:197, 1973.

12. Hardy, K. L., et al.: A new tracheostomy tube, Ann. Thorac. Surg. 10:58, 1970.

13. McGinnis, G. E., et al.: An engineering analysis of intratracheal cuffs, Anesth. Analg. 53:557, 1974.

14. Carroll, R. G.: Evaluation of tracheal tube cuff designs, Crit. Care Med. 1:45, 1973.

15. Kamen, J. M., et al.: A new low-pressure cuff for endotracheal tubes, Anesthesiology 34:182, 1971.

16. Lederman, D. S., et al.: A comparison of foam and air-filled endotracheal tube cuffs, Anesth. Analg. 53:521, 1974.

17. Dripps, R. D., Eckenoff, J. E., and Vandam, L. D.: Introduction to anesthesia, ed. 4, Philadelphia, 1972, W. B. Saunders Co.

18. Safar, P., and Grenvik, A.: Speaking cuffed tracheostomy tube, Crit. Care Med. 3:23, 1975.

19. Product information supplied by the manufacturers of these devices.

20. Saklad, M., and Gulati, R.: Adaptation of Ambu Respirator for high oxygen concentration, Anesthesiology 24:877, 1963.

21. Ziecheck, H. D., Nurick, H., and Fadale, V.: A method for increased inspired oxygen concentration with the Hope Resuscitator, Respir. Care 18:409, 1973.

22. Steinback, R. B., and Carden, E.: 1973 assessment of eight adult resuscitator bags, Respir. Care 20:69, 1975.

23. Cilnyk, P.: Adult AMBU modified for better oxygenation, Respir. Care 20:1024, 1975.

24. Spearman, C. B.: Unpublished clinical and laboratory data from Tucson Medical Center, Tucson, Arizona, 1973 and 1975.

25. Breivik, H.: A safe multipurpose pediatric ventilation bag, Crit. Care Med. 4:32, 1976.

26. McPherson, S. P., and Spearman, C. B.: Unpublished clinical and laboratory data from Tucson Medical Center, Tucson, Arizona, 1972 through 1975.

7 Bedside pulmonary function and monitoring devices

Most modern hospitals today provide some means of measuring pulmonary function. Respiratory therapy departments often provide such services, which may involve relatively simple spirometric measurements at the patient's bedside primarily dealing with single-breath tests or the complex studies requiring an elaborate laboratory. This chapter will deal with devices that can be used primarily on a mobile basis, generally to collect the following data at the bedside:

1. Tidal volume (TV)
2. Respiratory frequency or rate (f)
3. Minute volume ($\dot{V}$)
4. Vital capacity (VC), nonforced or timed (static)
5. Forced vital capacity (FVC)
6. Forced expiratory volume times (FEV_t)
7. Forced expiratory volume timed to forced vital capacity ratio expressed as a percent ($FEV_t/FVC\%$)
8. Forced expiratory flow (FEF)
9. Peak expiratory flow (PEF)

Respiratory therapists should be well acquainted with these and other pulmonary function parameters, which are presented elsewhere.[1-4]

VOLUME-COLLECTING DEVICES

Often called *spirometers*,[4] volume-collecting devices generally utilize a bell, bellows, moving piston, or the like for volume displacement. The most common of these is a series of *water-sealed* spirometers by Warren E. Collins, Inc.

Fig. 7-1 diagrams a water-sealed spirometer after a popular Collins model. A *bell* is sealed by water from the atmosphere. Tubing with *one-way valves* and a container with *carbon dioxide absorber* connect the inside of the bell to the patient in a rebreathing fashion. The bell is suspended by a chain and pulley mechanism, which also connects to a pen for recording the bell movements on a *spirograph*. As the patient inhales from the bell, it moves downward, causing the pen to rise proportionately. Gases exhaled into the bell cause the reverse to occur. The size of the bell basically determines how much volume is displaced for each corresponding distance the bell (and pen) must move. That is, a 9-liter bell will move 1 mm when 20.93

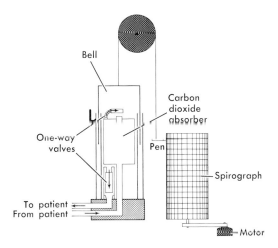

Fig. 7-1. Collins Water-Seal Spirometer. (Modified from Warren E. Collins, Inc., Braintree, Mass.)

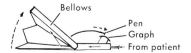

Fig. 7-2. Vitalor Wedge Spirometer.

cc of gas are displaced. This bell factor then can be used after a ventilatory maneuver is recorded as a vertical movement of the bell by the pen and spirograph.

As shown in Fig. 7-1, a *motor* can be connected to the spirograph. The motor turns the graph paper at a selectable, constant speed (in mm/min) providing horizontal markings by the pen. The horizontal movement is the time axis, and the vertical movement is the volume axis of the graph. From this graph provided by the Collins spirometer, a variety of values can be calculated.[4,5]

Although water-sealed units are generally less mobile than other types to be discussed, smaller units with 7-, 9-, and even 13.5-liter bells have been mounted on carts for bedside use. Their degree of accuracy and dependability remain advantages for water-sealed spirometers.

Another type of volume collection pulmonary function device uses an *expandable bellows.* Again, a graph for displaying volume and time is utilized. An early model of this type is the Vitalor (McKesson), still available from Air Shields (Fig. 7-2). As a volume of gas enters this *wedge spirometer*, the bellows expands, moving upward. The amount of this movement is recorded by the pen on a graph calibrated in volume (liters). A motor provides the horizontal markings by the pen for a time axis. Another wedge unit, the Vitalograph by Vitalograph Medical Instrumentation, functions in a similar fashion. A computerized pulmonary function system based around a large surface area wedge spirometer is the Compactest from Med Science.

Other expandable bellows units not in a wedge shape have been produced by Air Shields and Jones Medical Instrumentation. They are diagrammed in Fig. 7-3. By a pulley or lever arrangement, these units indicate the volume displacement of the bellows on a graph. Their recording-paper speeds provide a time axis to the graph.

More recently produced are the *dry rolling-seal* spirometers such as the 800

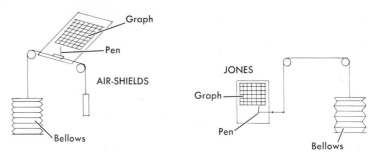

Fig. 7-3. Early Jones and Air-Shields Pulmonary Function Units.

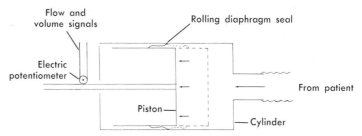

Fig. 7-4. Dry rolling spirometer. (Modified from Ohio Medical Products, Madison, Wis.)

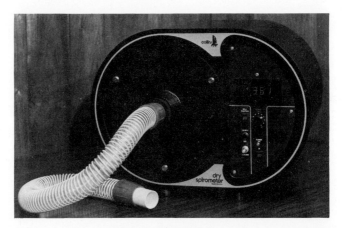

Fig. 7-5. Collins Dry Spirometer with digital display. (Courtesy Warren E. Collins, Inc., Braintree, Mass.)

series spirometers from Ohio Medical Products. Fig. 7-4 diagrams this type of device. Gas enters from the patient and displaces a *piston*. The piston is sealed to its *cylinder* by a rolling diaphragm-like seal. An electric *potentiometer* for detecting the piston's movements can provide electric signals for recording data on a graph or a scope (not shown). The piston generally has a large surface area to keep mechanical resistance to movement minimal.[4,5] Another dry spirometer is the unit from Warren E. Collins pictured in Fig. 7-5.

The *Bennett Monitoring Spirometer* (Fig. 7-6) is also a bellows unit. It is primarily used for monitoring exhaled tidal volumes from a patient receiving supportive mechanical ventilation.[5] The bellows is housed in a calibrated, transparent bell. Exhaled

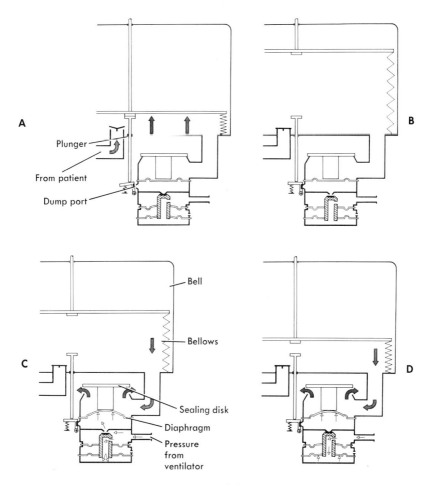

Fig. 7-6. Bennett Monitoring Spirometer. **A,** Start of exhalation. **B,** Exhalation end. **C,** Start of inhalation. **D,** During inhalation. (Courtesy Bennett Respiration Products, Inc., Santa Monica, Calif.)

gases enter the bellows, *A*, causing it to rise away from a *plunger*, *B*. When inhalation occurs, *C* and *D*, positive pressure from the ventilator enters the unit, pushes on a *diaphragm*, and raises a *sealing disk* off its seat. This opens the bellows to atmospheric air and it falls, emptying its previously collected volume. When the bellows reaches bottom, it depresses the plunger and opens a *dump port*, and pressure from the ventilator is released. This allows the sealing disk to fall, closing the bellow's communication to atmospheric air, and the unit is ready to receive another exhaled volume of gas.

FLOW-SENSING DEVICES

Probably the most common device used at the bedside to measure tidal volume, minute volume and nonforced vital capacity is the *Wright Respirometer* (Fig. 7-7). *Rotating vanes* spin with gas flow and, through a series of *gears*, indicate that movement on a *dial* calibrated in liters. *Slots* are used to direct the gas flow through the unit. High flow rates (above 300 L/min) can cause damage to the unit, and low flows (below 3 L/min) can produce inaccurate readings. Inertia can play a significant role

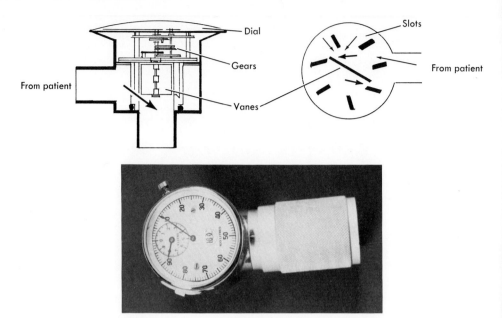

Fig. 7-7. Wright Respirometer. (Modified from operating instructions, Wright Respirometer, Harris Calorific, Cleveland, Ohio.)

in these units' accuracy, and they are delicate. Their portability lends itself to their popularity.

The *Dräger Volumeter* (Fig. 7-8) works in a similar fashion but uses rotating *cogs* rather than vanes. Again, the cogs rotate with gas flow, and a dial indicates the volume of gases passing through the units. The Volumeter also has a built-in timer that stops the collecting of values on the dial at the end of a minute when used. This provides a convenient way to collect minute expired volumes. Again, inertia plays a significant role in the Dräger's accuracy.

The *Wright Peak Flow Meter* (Fig. 7-9) also operates by a flow of gas against a *vane*. As gas flow hits the vane, it moves farther around to expose more ports through which gas escapes. The indicator attached to the vane has a *spring stop* or brake to keep it at the *peak* flow point until mechanically released. This unit is calibrated in liters per minute peak expiratory flow.

The *Emerson Spirometer* is actually a modified gas meter, similar to the type of unit used by gas companies for houses. Internally, it works on a refined method of diaphragm displacement by admitting gas volume within two chambers (Fig. 7-10).

Two *valves*, coordinated by a *gear* and *levers*, control the flow of gas into one of the two diaphragm chambers. When the right valve is open to receive incoming gas, the left is closed. Gas enters a line and flows to the bottom diaphragm chamber. This flow pushes the gas on the other side of the diaphragm out the exhaust port and rotates the gear. As the gear rotates, the right valve closes and the left one opens. The same process occurs in the top diaphragm chamber. This process continually repeats from right to left, and the gear movement is utilized to reflect volume on a meter.

Thermal units use another principle to detect gas flow. These incorporate tem-

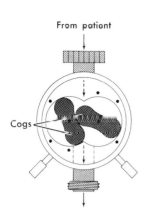

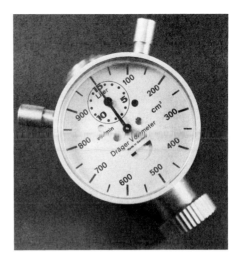

Fig. 7-8. Dräger Volumeter.

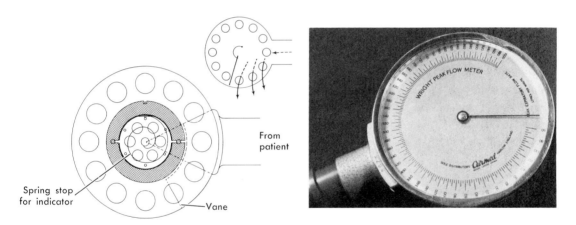

Fig. 7-9. Wright Peak Flow Meter.

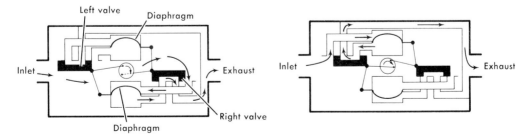

Fig. 7-10. Emerson Gas Meter. (Modified from How things work, vol. 1, New York, 1967, Simon & Schuster, Inc.)

perature-dependent, resistant elements such as a thermistor bead or heated wire.[6] As gases pass through these devices, they cool the heated element, changing its resistance. Flow cooling the thermistor bead causes an *increase* in resistance, whereas flow cooling the heated wire causes a *decrease* in resistance. The *change* in electric current needed to maintain the temperature of the bead or wire is proportional to gas flow.

The Monaghan Pulmonary Function Analyzer models M-402 and M-403 and the Monaghan M-700 Ventilation Monitor utilize a heated thermistor bead in their flow sensors (Fig. 7-11). The pulmonary function units provide values for FVC, PEF, FEV_1, and maximum voluntary ventilation (MVV), and the M-700 monitors TV, $\dot{V}$, and f with adjustable alarms for high and low TV and f. The M-700 can be used for monitoring either mechanically ventilated or spontaneously breathing patients[7,8] and finds valuable use for ventilator weaning circuits as well.[9]

Cavitron's Donti PA-74 Pulmonary Performance Analyzer and RM-73 Respiratory Monitor devices utilize a heated wire transducer (Fig. 7-12) for flow detection. The PA-74 provides a digital display of FVC, FEV_1, FEV_3, MVV, and PEF. The RM-73 monitors TV, $\dot{V}$, and f with alarm capabilities. Like the Monaghan M-700, the Donti RM-73 can also be used during mechanical ventilation or spontaneous breathing as well as the weaning process from the former.[10]

Electrical resistance-dependent devices can be affected by a variety of conditions such as ambient temperature change, different altitudes, and varying gas densities (such as different exhaled oxygen concentrations) and should be calibrated to compensate for these conditions.

Pressure differential devices have been used for flow detection for some years but have only recently become popular for bedside studies and monitoring. The most frequently used of this type is the *Fleisch Pneumotach* (Fig. 7-13). This device consists of a tube with a flow-resistive element, a *capillary mesh*, to produce a slight pressure drop as flow passes through the device. A *pressure differential transducer* monitors the pressure before the mesh (P_1) and after (P_2) so that its *diaphragm* reflects the difference in pressure. Here an electric signal proportional to the pressure difference (and therefore flow—see Chapter 1) is produced. Flow should be as laminar as possible, and screens inside *cones* as well as the capillary mesh itself tend to provide this pattern of gas movement. A *heater* can be used to raise the temperature so that saturated exhaled gases will not condense water vapor in the capillary mesh.

The Fleisch Pneumotach can be used to continuously monitor patients on mechanical ventilators for providing data for flow, volume, and breathing rates, and can be combined with sophisticated analyzing equipment in the respiratory care unit.[11]

This device is also used for a computerized mobile pulmonary function system by Bennett. The Remac system can be used for measuring and displaying a variety of data from single-breath tests done through the pneumotach.[5] Combining a nitrogen analyzing system with the Remac computer and pneumotach system's residual volume (RV), residual volume:total lung capacity ratio (RV:TLC), closing volume (CV), closing capacity (CC), and nitrogen differences (ΔN_2) can be computed from a single exhalation.[5] Flow-volume curves or loops can also be acquired.[5] Another computerized mobile unit, the Medistor from Terra Technology Corporation, also uses the Fleisch Pneumotach as its primary measuring device.[5]

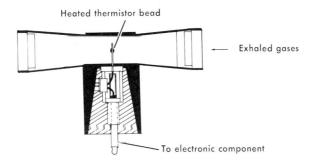

Fig. 7-11. Thermistor bead flow transducer such as used with Monaghan Pulmonary Function and Ventilation Monitors. (Modified from Sutton, F. D., Nett, L. M., and Petty, T. L.: Respir. Care **19**:196, 1974.)

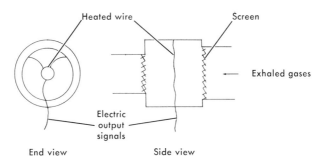

Fig. 7-12. Heater wire flow transducer such as used for Cavitron's pulmonary performance and respiratory monitors (Donti models).

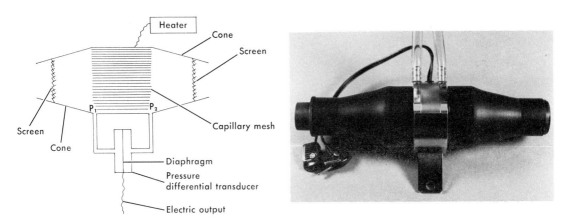

Fig. 7-13. Fleisch Pneumotach. Capillary mesh is heated to avoid condensate from exhaled gases. Pressure differential transducer produces electric signal proportional to flow.

The Bourns LS-75 Ventilation Monitor uses a relatively new flow measuring principle, *vortex shedding*[5,6] (Fig. 7-14). Precisely sized struts are placed into a narrow tube so that a known turbulence occurs, creating vortices or waves as the flow tumbles over the strut. The size of the tube and the size of the strut cause each of these vortices to be 1 cc in volume when flows of from 5 to 250 L/min transgress the device. An *ultrasonic transducer* produces sound waves that are picked up by the

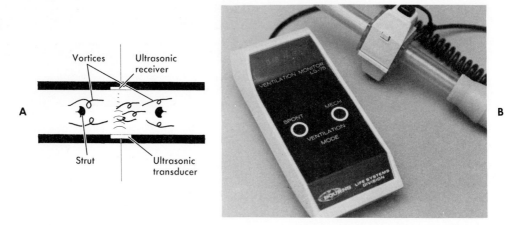

Fig. 7-14. A, Functional diagram of vortex shedding-ultrasonic flow transducer. **B,** Bourns LS-75. (**A** modified from Bourns, Inc., Riverside, Calif.)

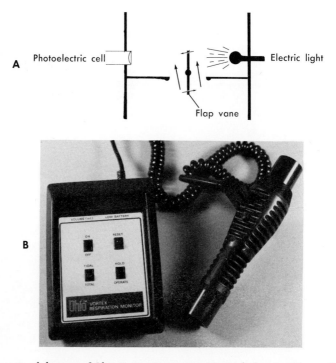

Fig. 7-15. A, Functional diagram of Ohio Vortex Respiration Monitor's flow transducer. **B,** Ohio Vortex Respiration Monitor.

receiver and produce an electric impulse. Each vortex of air interferes with the sound pickup of the receiver and creates a *beat* or known change in current that is proportional to flow. There are no moving parts.

A counting and calculating unit provides computation and digital display of TV, f, and $\dot{V}$ collected by the LS-75. The device is powered by a rechargeable battery system. Vital capacity can be measured with the unit, and, although high flow rates cannot cause damage, flows above 250 L/min will not give accurate readings. Gas composition, temperature, and humidity will not appreciably affect the vortex principle.[5]

The Ohio Vortex Respiration Monitor incorporates a small *flap vane* that flips back and forth with flow through the unit (Fig. 7-15). The vane's oscillation frequency is linearly proportional to each 10 cc passing it. Each time the flap moves, a light beam from a photoelectric cell is broken. The higher the gas flow, the more the flap moves. Increased numbers of photoelectric cell beam breakages are indicated as increased gas volume passes through the unit. The device can display TV breath to breath or accumulated breaths digitally within a flow range of 10 to 150 L/min.[5] High flows can damage the vane, and condensate from exhaled gases or aerosol may stop the unit's functioning.

REFERENCES

1. Comroe, J. H., et al.: The lung: clinical physiology and pulmonary function tests, ed. 2, Chicago, 1962, Year Book Medical Publishers, Inc.
2. Miller, W. F., Paez, P. N., and Johnson, W. C.: Respiratory function testing. In Race, G. J., editor: Laboratory medicine, New York, 1973, Harper & Row, Publishers, Inc.
3. Pulmonary terms and symbols: a report of the American College of Chest Physicians—American Thoracic Society Joint Committee on Pulmonary Nomenclature, Chest 67:583, 1975.
4. Ruppel, G.: Manual of pulmonary function testing, St. Louis, 1975, The C. V. Mosby Co.
5. Product information supplied by manufacturer of these products.
6. McShane, J. L., and Geil, F. G.: Measuring flow, Research/Development, p. 30, Feb., 1975.
7. Sutton, F. D., Nett, L. M., and Petty, T. L.: A new ventilation monitor for the intensive respiratory care unit, Respir. Care 19:196, 1974.
8. Petty, T. L.: Intensive and rehabilitative respiratory care, ed. 2, Philadelphia, 1974, Lea & Febiger.
9. McPherson, S. P., et al.: A circuit that combines ventilator weaning methods using continuous flow ventilation (CFV), Respir. Care 20:261, 1975.
10. Carney, R. T.: Monitoring during IMV, Respir. Therapy 5:37, Sept.-Oct., 1975.
11. Osborn, J. J.: Monitoring respiratory function, Crit. Care Med. 2:217, 1974.

8 Introduction to ventilators

CLASSIFICATION OF VENTILATORS

Classification of ventilators should be structured so as to provide a systematic description of ventilator designs that will be universally applicable to ventilators currently available, as well as to those to come in the future. A design classification should be simple enough to be thoroughly comprehended by clinicians, so that the understanding they acquire will provide information that will be useful at the bedside. The system must also be comprehensive enough to provide sufficient functional details of the ventilators.

The first point for consideration in a theoretical classification of ventilators to be used here is the *type of force*, measured as *pressure*, that the units apply to the body to effect ventilation. Normally, the force utilized to move gases is the energy of the inspiratory ventilatory muscles.[1] By contraction, they enlarge the volume of the chest and create a subatmospheric intrathoracic pressure. This causes the *atmospheric-to-subatmospheric pressure gradient* necessary to move gas into the chest. Exhalation, then, occurs passively because of the elastic recoil of the lung.[1]

To accomplish this same ventilatory activity with mechanical apparatus requires generation of an inspiratory force (or pressure) to supply the active phase of the ventilatory cycle (inhalation) that the ventilatory muscles normally provide. This force generated by ventilators could be of three types. First, a *negative extrathoracic pressure* would cause the atmospheric pressure exposed to the airway to inflate the lungs (Fig. 8-1). The force generated causes a pressure gradient of atmospheric to subatmospheric, which expands the chest and moves gas into the lungs. Examples of this type of unit would be the *iron lung and cuirass*, which generate a negative extrathoracic pressure.[1] This type of ventilation has also been used for neonatal ventilation with a modified isolation incubator.[2]

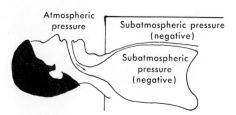

Fig. 8-1. Principle of applying subatmospheric pressure around chest wall to produce drop in pressure in airway and flow into chest.

The second method of generating inspiratory force by ventilators would be to create a *positive intrapulmonary pressure* in the presence of atmospheric extra-thoracic pressures (Fig. 8-2). This force of above-atmospheric pressure applied to the airways is reflected to a degree in the lungs by expansion of the chest and lungs. There are many common examples of this type of device, such as volume and pressure-limited ventilators.

The third mechanism of providing ventilatory force would be a combination of the first two forces just described. A modest *negative extrathoracic pressure and a positive intrathoracic pressure* would provide force necessary to move gas into the lungs (Fig. 8-3). The reason for attempting this combination could be potentially to maintain more normal intrathoracic pressures, which are important in both preserving normal hemodynamics while also providing improved ventilatory ability. This system would combine some of the potential good points of both methods. As will be discussed later in the chapter, negative pressure units, especially the

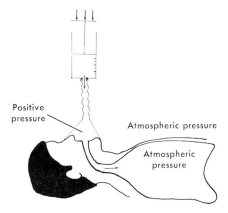

Fig. 8-2. Principle of positive pressure applied at airway to provide pressure gradient and, therefore, gas flow into chest.

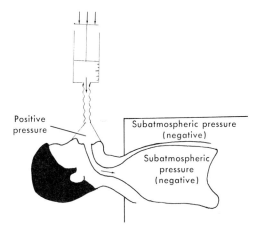

Fig. 8-3. Combination of negative extrathoracic pressure *and* positive airway pressure to establish gas flow into chest.

cuirass type, frequently have difficulty in ventilating abnormal respiratory systems. There are no ventilators of this type currently in use with the exception of the previously produced Engstrom 150, which could potentially provide both a positive inspiratory pressure system and, with its cuirass attachment, could provide negative inspiratory pressure around the thorax on the same patient. Unfortunately, this system also possesses the majority of common problems associated with both positive- and negative-pressure ventilators, which probably negates its potential benefits in most instances. A constant negative pressure around the chest wall with inspiratory positive pressure from a ventilator has been reported in neonatal care.[2]

Based on the classification just given, the major divisions of ventilators would be as follows:

1. Negative-pressure ventilators (iron lung and cuirass)
2. Positive-pressure ventilators (pressure-limited, volume-limited, etc.)
3. Positive/negative pressure ventilators (theoretical)

Once the force sufficient for inhalation has been generated by a ventilator, a *cycling mechanism* for each phase of the ventilation provides the additional ventilatory characteristics.[3] First, since inhalation is generally the focal point, how this is initiated or *what cycles the ventilator into the inspiratory phase* will be examined. The inspiratory phase can begin by (1) *patient cycling*, in which the patient generates a gas flow or slight negative pressure by starting to inhale, (2) *manual cycling* by the patient or by an operator who activates the inspiratory phase, and (3) *time cycling* into inhalation by a timing mechanism. Some ventilatory apparatus provide for all three alternatives.

If the *patient* cycles the unit into the inspiratory phase, the machine is called an *assistor*, since it triggers the ventilator on and assists the patient's own ventilatory endeavor. If *time* cycles the unit into the inspiratory phase, the unit is designated as a *controller*, since that parameter determines the initiation of inspiration. If the patient can assist and the machine can back him up (if his breathing rate drops or stops altogether), the unit is designated as an assistor/controller. Again, it is possible for a machine to be all three. It is (1) an assistor when it is patient-cycled and there is no timed back-up rate, (2) a controller when it is time-cycled and no assist mechanism is provided, or (3) an assistor/controller when the timed rate backs up the patient's rate.[4]

Each of the three divisions of negative, positive, and positive/negative ventilators could have any or all of the cycling subdivisions as follows:

Begin inhalation (cycle)
    Patient-cycled (assist)
    Time-cycled (control)
    Patient/time cycled (assist/control)
    Manual-cycled

Once inhalation has begun, the next cycling mechanism is the ending of inhalation or the cycling of the ventilator into the expiratory phase. Although it is not totally correct, to avoid confusion it may be better to consider the end of inhalation as a limit and to see *what event or mechanism limits the extent to which inhalation occurs.*[3]

If ventilation pressure can be preset at a specific level to limit or end inspiratory phase, the unit would be considered to be *pressure limited*. Some units can preset the volume of gas to be delivered and are therefore *volume limited*. Time, as well, can end the patient's inhalation to provide a *time limit*. A device that could terminate inhalation when a preset or minimum flow was reached would be called *flow limited*. Other units provide a manual override device to lengthen inhalation, and this part of the ventilatory cycle must be ended manually by the patient or by the machine's operator. These units would be classified as *manually limited*.

Therefore all three divisions of the type of force generated by a ventilator could have any or all of these limiting mechanisms available to end inhalation. Usually, a unit is designed to be primarily one specific type, such as a volume-limited ventilator, but it may possess the other mechanisms as additional features. Classification would be as follows:

End inhalation (limit)
  Pressure limit
  Volume limit
  Time limit
  Flow limit
  Manual limit

As mentioned previously concerning the ending of the inspiratory phase, *limit* may not be totally correct terminology, but its inappropriateness in specific instances is generally more of an engineering concern rather than a clinical one.[3] To give a practical example, the Bennett MA-1 and Ohio 560 ventilators can be compared. Both units are primarily volume-limited (or cycled) units. Both, however, do possess a pressure-limiting mechanism. If a predetermined pressure is reached *prior to* the volume delivery pressure, the ventilator limits the extent of inhalation (pressure limit occurs). In the MA-1, the bellows immediately drops to the bottom, starting exhalation, and, thus, cycles the unit into the expiratory phase. In the 560, however, the pressure is not allowed to go higher than is set because of a pressure-release mechanism, and the machine will not cycle into the expiratory phase until the bellows reaches its *full excursion* and expels all the volume it contained. So, to be precise, the MA-1 in this situation is both pressure limited and pressure cycled, whereas the 560 is pressure limited but volume cycled.

The next consideration concerning ventilators' design is that of *drive mechanism* and its design. A clear understanding of these features provides insight into the delivery characteristics of flow and pressure curves as well as I:E ratios.

Two general categories could be devised for the drive mechanisms of ventilators; they are *electric* and *pneumatic*. Under each of these classifications will be subcategories relating more to ventilator specifics. Finally, after these subcategories, the circuitry design of the *power circuit* will be discussed. If the gas supply powering the ventilator goes to the patient, the unit will be considered as having a *single circuit* (Fig. 8-4).[1] If the source gas powering the ventilator compresses another mechanism, such as a bag or bellows that in turn sends gas to the patient, the unit will be classified as having a *double circuit* (Fig. 8-5).[1]

The first category of drive mechanisms to be discussed is the *pneumatic* type. Usually, the unit is powered by one of two types of devices. The ventilator utilizes either a *Venturi* mechanism or *fluidic* components in its power system. Either one

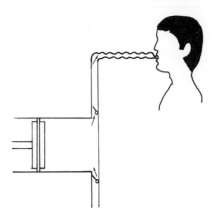

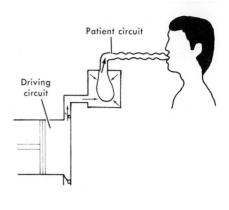

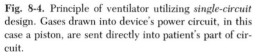

Fig. 8-4. Principle of ventilator utilizing *single-circuit* design. Gases drawn into device's power circuit, in this case a piston, are sent directly into patient's part of circuit.

Fig. 8-5. Principle of ventilator utilizing *double-circuit* design. Here driving (or power) circuits' gases are used only to compress bag (or bellows) containing separate gases, which are sent to patient through patient circuit.

functionally accomplishes the same basic delivery of gas to the patient system, although fluidics have a greater potential for control module use. Either fluidics or refined pneumatics (including Venturis) can be structured into a single- or double-circuit unit.

Electric-drive mechanisms are the second category and can also be split into two subcategories. The first category would be comprised of electric-powered motors that drive small *air compressors*. These are usually *piston* or *rotary* compressors, and the gas pressure produced is used to power a unit within the ventilator (double circuit), although single-circuit units could be structured as well. The remaining subcategory is that of electric, motor-driven *pistons*. They are either *linear* or *rotary* in their movement and can be either single or double circuit (Fig. 8-6).

In summary, a classification scheme concerning *drive* mechanisms for ventilators could be constructed as follows:

I. Pneumatic
    A. Refined pneumatics
        1. Single circuit
        2. Double circuit
    B. Fluidic
        1. Single circuit
        2. Double circuit
II. Electric
    A. Compressor (piston or rotary blower)
        1. Single circuit
        2. Double circuit
    B. Piston
        1. Rotary
            a. Single circuit
            b. Double circuit
        2. Linear
            a. Single circuit
            b. Double circuit

Analysis of the *power-circuit* (pneumatic driving force) design indicates the type of flow and pressure characteristics the ventilator will possess.

Pneumatic units employing a *Venturi or fluidic drive* will generally have a *downward-tapering flow pattern* as their basic waveform, which will cause an *upward-tapering pressure pattern*. The reason for this performance characteristic is that, generally, the fluidic or Venturi unit can, at best, exert pressure *only slightly higher than peak ventilatory pressures*. Therefore, when inhalation is initiated, the pressure gradient allowing gas delivery to the patient is at its peak. The fluidic or Venturi-drive component is delivering its peak pressure against a zero pressure gradient downstream, and at a maximum pressure gradient, the *flow* will be *maximum* as well. As gas continues to enter the ventilator's tubing circuit and the patient during inhalation, the pressure in this system rises. As the system pressure rises and approaches the fluidic or Venturi-drive pressures, the pressure gradient continues to decrease and is accompanied by a *decreasing flow*. As an example, if the fluidic or Venturi drive supplied a pressure of 20 cm H_2O pressure to 0 cm H_2O (ambient) pressure at the patient's airway, the resulting drop in pressure gradient (up to 100%, ultimately) would produce a corresponding drop in flow (Fig. 8-7). As the flow into the circuit gradually decreases, the result is a progressively slower incline to peak pressure (Fig. 8-7).

Pneumatic ventilators that utilize a *high pressure*, such as 15 to 50 psig directly, to supply gas to the circuit produce a *constant-flow, square-wave pattern* (Fig. 8-8).[3] Since the pressure supplying the peak ventilation pressure is *significantly higher*, the pressure gradient throughout inhalation is not sufficiently altered. For example, if the peak ventilation pressure were 20 cm H_2O and if the power source were

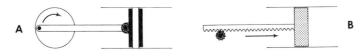

Fig. 8-6. Rotary-drive, **A,** and linear-drive, **B,** piston drive mechanisms for ventilators.

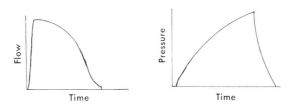

Fig. 8-7. Flow and pressure curves for low-pressure-drive respirator.

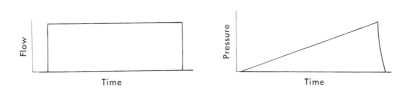

Fig. 8-8. Flow and pressure curves for ventilator using high-driving-pressure pneumatic drive.

50 psig (3500 cm H_2O pressure), the change in pressure gradient producing flow into the circuit would only be from 3500 cm H_2O pressure to 3480 cm H_2O from beginning to end inhalation, respectively. The pressure gradient dropped only slightly, which would produce an undetectable change in flow. The result would be a constant flow produced by the ventilator. With a constant flow into the circuit, the pressure curve would climb in a relatively *linear fashion* to peak pressure (Fig. 8-8).

Direct-drive (single-circuit) *piston* ventilators can be powered in three ways to have a *linear* drive: (1) direct cogs, (2) a spring-loaded piston, or (3) a piston powered by 50 psig (Fig. 8-9). The result would be (1) a *constant flow* due to the constant (linear) speed of the piston, and (2) a *square-wave flow curve* would be produced (Fig. 8-10),[1,3] as shown for the pneumatic units, where the system was supplied with high-pressure gas. As a result of constant flow into the circuit, a relatively *linearly increasing pressure curve* would occur (Fig. 8-10).

Rotary-driven pistons move in an accelerating then decelerating fashion. Fig. 8-11 illustrates a complete forward cycle of such a unit. The *rotary wheel* moves at a constant speed. However, the *piston* is connected to the outer edge of the

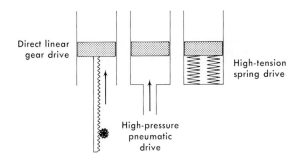

Fig. 8-9. Potential system for providing linear drive piston in ventilators.

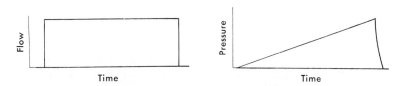

Fig. 8-10. Flow and pressure curves for linear-driven piston.

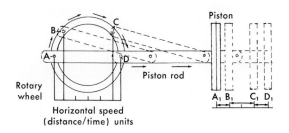

Fig. 8-11. Diagram of rotary-driven piston's movement.

wheel by the *piston rod* in such a way that its movements are not constant. As the wheel turns, the piston rod moves a greater distance vertically than horizontally (points *A* to *B*). Therefore the piston's actual forward (horizontal) movement is relatively short (A_1 to B_1). As the connection point of the piston rod to the wheel moves along the top of the wheel during its rotation (points *B* to *C*), the horizontal speed (distance per time) of the piston rod and piston (B_1 to C_1) increase. That is, the piston's forward motion is faster during this phase. From points *C* to *D* and C_1 to D_1, the piston's movement slows again similar to its speed from points *A* to *B* and A_1 to B_1 previously, and for the same reason, the piston rod's movement is primarily vertical rather than horizontal. This gradually increasing and gradually decreasing piston speed produces a corresponding gas flow pattern from the piston referred to as a *sine-wave*–like curve (Fig. 8-12).[1,3]

Indirect-drive (double-circuit) piston units acquire a different flow pattern than their basic drive flow curve would indicate because this flow is exerted on a bag[3] or bellows (Fig. 8-13). The flow of gas from the drive mechanism into the chamber that houses the bag (or bellows) starts to compress the bag containing the gas used to ventilate the patient. As the bag is compressed, the pressure inside it increases, and a pressure gradient is established for gas flow to the patient system. As more gas enters the chamber, a higher pressure is exerted against the bag. This higher pressure causes the pressure gradient to increase. Even though patient-circuit pressure increases also, the pressure on the bag increases proportionally *higher*. The result is a progressively increasing flow pattern (Fig. 8-14). A pressure pattern

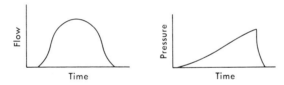

Fig. 8-12. Flow and pressure curves created by rotary-driven piston positive-pressure ventilator.

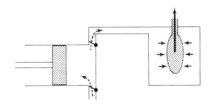

Fig. 8-13. Simple diagram of piston-driven double-circuit system.

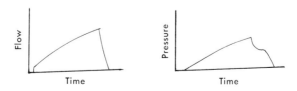

Fig. 8-14. Double-circuit rotary-driven flow and pressure curves.

similar to the flow pattern is created initially by the *accelerating* flow. Once the bag has collapsed, the bag volume is held briefly in the patient system, and circuit pressures start to equilibrate. The result is a *drop* in circuit pressure during the volume hold, causing a notch in the pressure curve (Fig. 8-14).

Bellows ventilators produce flow curves of one of two basic types, depending on the *amount* of pressure compressing the bellows. If the pressure supplied to the bellows chamber is close to the peak circuit or ventilation pressure, then the flow will *taper* until the volume has been delivered, and then it will drop to zero (Fig. 8-15, *A*). As an example, if the peak pressure supplied to the bellows was 140 cm H_2O pressure and system pressure reached 70 cm H_2O, the pressure gradient for gas flow would drop from 140 cm H_2O pressure at beginning inhalation. This 50% drop in pressure gradient would also cause a drop in flow (Fig. 8-15, *B*).[3] If a significant volume were delivered to cause the system pressure to be equal to the bellows' chamber supply pressure, then the flow would have tapered to zero, since no pressure gradient would exist to cause gas flow (Fig. 8-15, *A*). However, under clinical conditions, circuit pressure rarely approaches those levels, so the flow curve drops to zero only when the volume has been delivered. The pressure curve reflects a gradually deteriorating increased tapering pattern caused by the progressively tapering flow (Fig. 8-15, *B*).

Two situations can occur that cause alterations in the flow curve attained. First, with a *low-resistance and high-compliance system*, the pressure gradient is not altered significantly during inhalation, and the flow curve delivered is a constant-flow square wave (Fig. 8-16). Clinically, this would occur only on patients with normal airways and lungs, for whom a reasonably low volume was utilized and low peak system pressures developed.

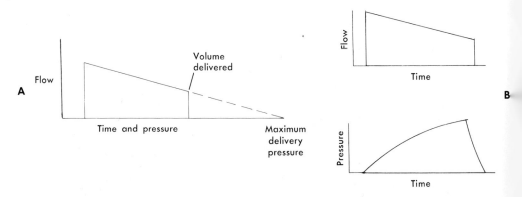

Fig. 8-15. A, Primary flow curve for low-pressure-drive bellows ventilator system. **B,** Flow and pressure curves for low-pressure-drive bellows ventilator system.

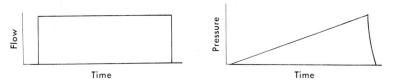

Fig. 8-16. Flow and pressure curves for bellows ventilator against low-resistance high-compliance system.

The second situation that would produce an altered flow pattern would be a situation in which a patient with *high resistance* and *high compliance* was being ventilated. This event would be similar to placing a marked restriction on the ventilator circuit's outflow tract and ventilating a large container or a room (Fig. 8-17). As gas from the bellows reaches the restriction, its *critical velocity* is reached, and the resulting turbulence creates back pressure upstream from the restriction. In relation to the pressure downstream from the restriction, this increased pressure causes an additional and increasing pressure gradient for gas to flow past the restriction and into the patient (or circuit). As additional gas from the ventilator reaches the restriction, an increasing pressure develops. The result is that an *increasing pressure gradient* develops across the restriction, and an *increasing* flow occurs (Fig. 8-18). This could occur clinically with an improperly sized endotracheal tube that is too small to accommodate the flows and volumes generated or in patients with severe airway resistance.

Ventilators that supply *high-pressure* gas (such as 50 psig) to collapse their *bellows* produce a constant-flow, square wave with a linearly increasing pressure curve (Fig. 8-19).[3] The only situation in which this pattern is altered is with the high-resistance, high-compliance systems described above. The resulting flow and pressure curves are similar to those in Fig. 8-18.

Both a *controlled rate* and *inspiratory-time-to-expiratory-time ratio* (I:E) are accomplished by four basic procedures. First, rate can be controlled either by adjusting a *transmission-type gearing mechanism* or by *changing motor speed*. In

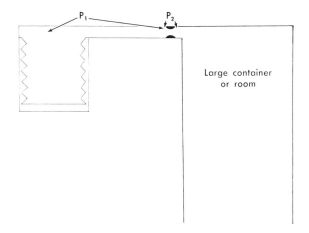

Fig. 8-17. Low-pressure-drive bellows ventilator against high-resistance and high-compliance system.

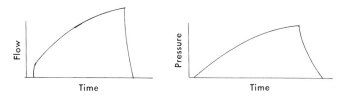

Fig. 8-18. Flow and pressure curves for low-pressure-drive bellows ventilator against high-resistance and high-compliance system.

this fashion, rate is controlled *directly,* and the I:E ratio is fixed at a certain value, such as 1:1 or 1:2. Second, with the rate set on a rate control, I:E can be controlled by *altering the inspiratory time component* of the ventilator's cycle. *Flow and volume* are the important ingredients in controlling inspiratory time (Fig. 8-20, *A*). Since flow is *volume per unit of time,* it controls the time it will take to deliver a certain volume. In essence, the *higher* the flow is at a set volume, the *shorter* the inspiratory time will be. Control of inspiratory time can then be accomplished with the *rate* set in one of two ways. *Flow* and *tidal volume* controls can be used to control inspiratory time. Decreasing the tidal volume or increasing gas flow will *decrease* inspiratory time and *increase* the I:E ratio. *Increasing* the tidal volume or *decreasing* gas flow will *increase* the inspiratory time and *decrease* the I:E ratio (Fig. 8-21). An example of this type of ventilator's control would be the Bennett MA-1.

Third, *inspiratory time and expiratory time* can be controlled separately to acquire rate and desired I:E ratio. With this approach, alterations in either inspiratory time or expiratory time require a proportional change in the other control if a set rate is to be maintained (Fig. 8-20, *B*). This technique can be accomplished with an inspiratory and an expiratory timer (Fig. 8-22), such as in the Emerson 3PV. Inspiratory time can also be controlled directly with a *timer* or *flow transducer* that can control flow to maintain a *set* I:E ratio.

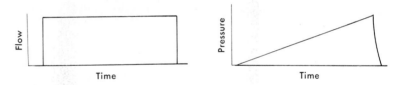

Fig. 8-19. Flow and pressure curves for bellows ventilator driven by high-pressure (such as 50 psig) source.

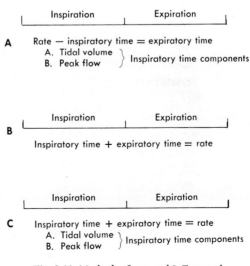

Fig. 8-20. Methods of rate and I:E control.

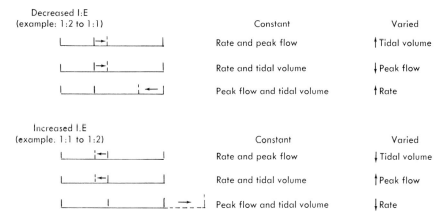

Fig. 8 21. I : E and rate changes with changes in tidal volume, peak flow, and rate.

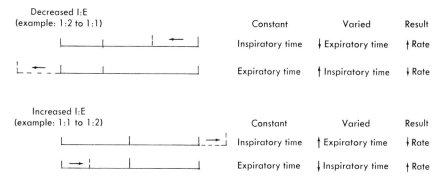

Fig. 8-22. I : E and rate changes with changes in inspiratory or expiratory time.

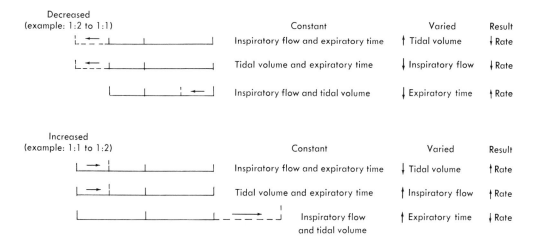

Fig. 8-23. I : E ratio and rate changes with flow, tidal volume, and expiratory time.

Fourth, *tidal volume and flow controls* can be employed to establish *inspiratory time* just as described, and a timer can be utilized to control *expiratory time;* rate can be acquired from the adjustment of the two (inspiratory and expiratory) times (Figs. 8-20, *C,* and 8-23). An example of this type of control mechanism is found on the Ohio 560 Respirator.

It should also be noted that any time a patient is able to trigger the machine causing it to assist, the I:E ratio is always *decreased* from the set controlled value. This decrease is caused by the resulting decrease in *expiratory* time (Fig. 8-24).

NEGATIVE-PRESSURE VENTILATORS

There are basically two types of negative-pressure ventilators employed in respiratory therapy: (1) the *body tank respirator* (commonly called the *iron lung*) (Fig. 8-25), and (2) the *cuirass,* which is a *chest shell piece.*

The first *iron lung* to have widespread use was invented by Drinker and Shaw in 1928 and produced commercially by J. H. Emerson Company.[5] It consists of

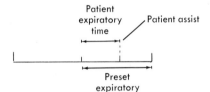

Fig. 8-24. I:E ratio change with patient assist.

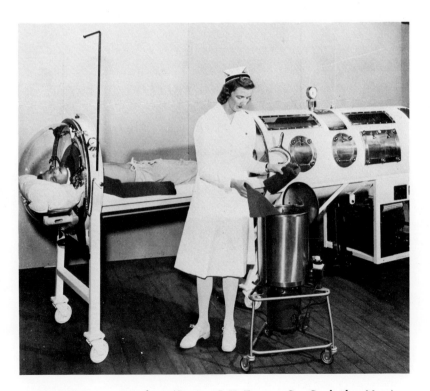

Fig. 8-25. Emerson iron lung. (Courtesy J. H. Emerson Co., Cambridge, Mass.)

an *airtight cylinder* that encloses the patient up to his neck. A seal is formed with foam rubber around the neck so that there is no leak. The cylinder made isolation of the patient's body unavoidable, and even ports on the side made it difficult to provide adequate patient care. In addition, the units had no assist mode, nor was there any means of regulating I:E ratios or respiratory flow rates. The units were reasonably effective on patients who had relatively normal airways, such as polio victims, but they inadequately ventilated patients with significant respiratory disorders. Also, negative pressure exerted on the abdomen often caused *abdominal pooling* of blood, called *tank shock*.[1] Because the abdominal wall is flaccid and, thus, extremely subject to the negative pressure,[1] abdominal pooling of blood can occur, decreasing venous return and cardiac output. These units were difficult or impossible to sterilize and were often noisy as well. Tracheostomy or intubation of the patient was usually *not necessary* for long-term ventilation because maintaining an airway was not a crucial problem affecting volume delivery. This aspect reduced the chance of incurring pulmonary infection or other problems associated with artificial airways. Iron lungs were also rugged and dependable with little maintenance or down time, and were easy to operate by personnel. The newer Isolette negative-pressure ventilator for newborns works basically like an iron lung[2] (Fig. 8-26).

Because of the problems that existed with the body respirator, Drinker and Collins combined in 1939 to produce a *cuirass* or *shell unit* in hopes that they would eliminate the abdominal pooling.[5] Basically, the unit consisted of a rigid shell that came in varying sizes. It confined the thorax so that subatmospheric pressure could be exerted within the shell and *only* around the chest (Fig. 8-27). An electric pump, similar in design to a vacuum cleaner, was used to generate the negative extrathoracic pressure. Maximum pressure was less than that attainable with an iron

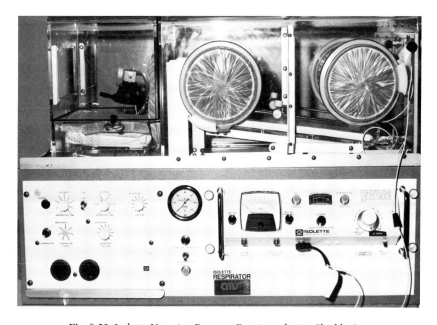

Fig. 8-26. Isolette Negative-Pressure Respirator by Air Shields, Inc.

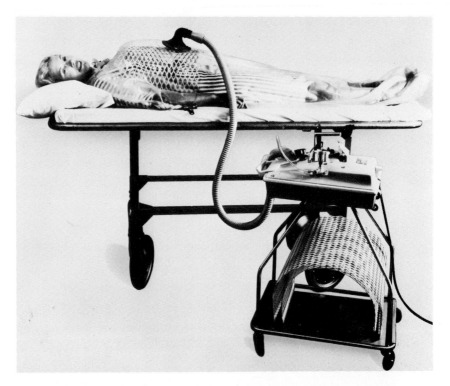

Fig. 8-27. Emerson Cuirass. (Courtesy J. H. Emerson Co., Cambridge, Mass.)

lung and was dependent on the tightness of the fit of the shell. Cuirass-type units also fell into disuse for some of the same reasons as did body-tank respirators: (1) they were excessively noisy, (2) providing patient care was still hampered, although improved over the body respirator type, (3) regulation of I:E ratios was difficult and there was no consideration for the regulation of inspiratory flow rates, (4) the seal around the chest was difficult to achieve, which oftentimes made the unit periodically undependable, and (5) the negative pressure was not as great as in the iron lung, so it was impossible to totally ventilate a patient who had no respiratory drive.[1] These units, however, were used to augment patients with weakened respiratory muscles to ventilate adequately through the night. Because the negative pressure was primarily extrathoracic only, these devices provided for an increased venous return compared to the tank units. In addition, the modification of adding a *flow sensor* at the patient's nose for a triggering mechanism during an assist mode provided easier synchronization of the ventilator and the patient than could be achieved with the iron lung type.[1]

POSITIVE-PRESSURE VENTILATORS

The subclassification of positive-pressure ventilators becomes much larger than the one just described for negative-pressure ventilators. Chapters 11 and 12 deal with time-flow units and volume-limited ventilators. Two common pressure-limited units will be discussed in Chapters 9 and 10. The remainder of this chapter will deal with those simple pressure-limited and manually-limited devices that are not included in the other chapters but find common use in respiratory care.

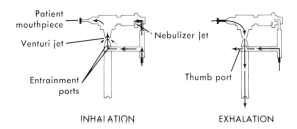

Fig. 8-28. Functional diagram of Ohio Hand-E-Vent. (Modified from Ohio Medical Products, Madison, Wis.)

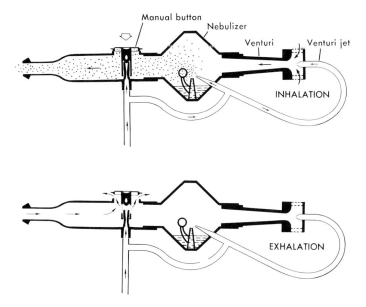

Fig. 8-29. Functional diagram of Bird Asthmastik. (Courtesy Bird Corp., Palm Springs, Calif.)

The first to be discussed are the *manually limited* devices. The *Hand-E-Vent* (Fig. 8-28), produced by Ohio Medical Products, is a device in which gas flow from a compressor can be directed to both (1) the *jet* of the Venturi and (2) the *nebulizer* to supply patient gas and aerosolized medication.[6] Normally, during the expiratory phase with the *thumb port* released, the gas from the compressor simply passes through a channel to the main body of the unit and empties into the room. Once the user's thumb *occludes* this port, gas can go to only (1) the jet of the Venturi and (2) the nebulizer, thus beginning inhalation, which lasts until the thumb is removed. This unit is somewhat more advanced than the hand-held nebulizer, and it is designed for use with patients who require *some* assistance in active hyperinflation of their lungs.

The Bird *Asthmastik* works on the same principle (Fig. 8-29). Again, by occluding the port with a finger on the *manual button*, gas is directed to both the *jet* of the Venturi and the *jet* of the nebulizer. Inhalation lasts until the finger is removed.

Another group of units has been devised using *fluidics* to deliver a flow of gas with medication to the patient, and do not require the manual dexterity needed to coordinate the effort of the hand-held ventilator with the patient's inhalation.

The principle of operation for fluidic, pressure-limited respirators employs what is known as the *Coanda effect* (Fig. 8-30).[7] This phenomenon is caused when *an air stream passes by a wall and turbulent gas flow causes an attachment* of the stream *to the wall*.[7] This wall attachment then forms the basis for a fluidic element. In essence, the turbulence produced by the gas tends to cause a phenomenon similar to Bernoulli's effect, in that the pocket of turbulence forms an *air foil*, similar to what occurs with an airplane wing.[7] As gas travels faster over a pocket of

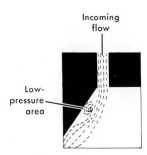

Fig. 8-30. Coanda effect. Low-pressure bubble is created next to wall, and gas stream tends to adhere to that wall. (Modified from Smith, R. K.: Respir. Therapy 3:29, May-June, 1973.)

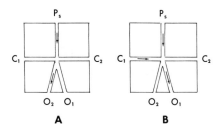

Fig. 8-31. Example of fluidic flip-flop component. Outflow remains at O_2, **A**, until input signal (pressure) is applied at C_1, **B**, which causes outflow to flip to O_1.

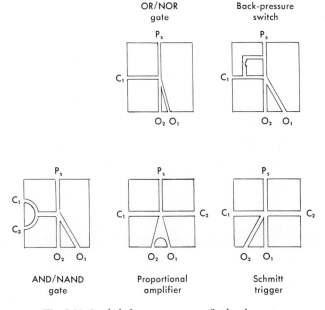

Fig. 8-32. Symbols for some common fluidic elements.

turbulent air, the increased forward molecular velocity of the gas causes a *decreased* lateral pressure by the pocket; the surrounding gas molecules not in the stream then possess a *higher* pressure, thus holding the stream against the wall. Fig. 8-31 is a schematic of a simple *flip-flop* unit, which is the basic design for the *fluidic-breathing assistors* being described in this section. The source gas is applied to port P_s. Once gas supply enters at P_s, it *arbitrarily* picks an *outflow tract* (O_2 and O_1). It will remain in that position unless encouraged to go the other way by an *input pressure* (at C_1 or C_2) being supplied. For example, if the output O_2 is arbitrarily selected, A, the gas flow would remain there until sufficient positive pressure is exerted at C_1 to *push it over* to O_1, B. Flow will then remain at O_1 until there is an input force at C_2 to cause gas to flow out O_2, A. Fig. 8-32 provides symbols of various fluidic components. For the OR/NOR gate, the *back-pressure switch* and the AND/NAND gate output flow will always be at O_2 when control inputs are absent. A pressure must be present at C_1 of the OR/NOR gate for it to switch its output to O_1. (OR/NOR gates generally have several input choices, any one of which can be used.) The back-pressure switch allows some gas from P_s to escape *out* C_1. When C_1 is *occluded*, pressure is applied, causing gas to switch to ouput O_1. The AND/NAND gate requires that *both* C_1 and C_3 must have inputs to switch output from O_2 to O_1. The *proportional amplifier* can have flow out both O_2 and O_1. When a greater pressure is applied at C_1 than at C_2, then O_1 will have the higher output, and vice versa. The Schmitt trigger is actually several proportional devices together and is used to provide a device for sensing minute pressure changes between C_1 and C_2 to cause outputs at O_1 and O_2. Fig. 8-33 provides a diagram of the inhalation-exhalation phase of a fluidic breathing device that would be *pressure* limited. During inhalation gas leaves the outflow tract to the patient. As pressure builds up in the patient circuitry, pressurized gas comes back to a *feedback channel* through a feedback orifice, and this orifice acts as a pressure-limit adjustment. Once enough gas leaks back through the orifice, due to pressure increasing in the patient system, the gas stream will be forced over the left side (exhalation). In this instance, the left side is the exhaust side so that the

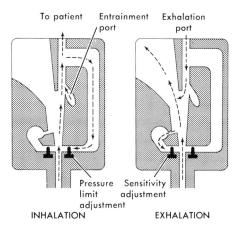

Fig. 8-33. Diagram of fluidic respirator. (Modified from Mine Safety Appliances product data, Pittsburgh, Pa.)

patient can exhale. When the patient is ready for his next breath, he generates a negative pressure, which is reflected on the right side of the gas stream, tending to draw the stream to the right. The *sensitivity* control on the left adjusts the flow of gas supplying the feedback channel from the main flow of gas leaving the unit from the exhaust port. The *greater* this flow is, the more the stream is inclined to *switch back* to the right, and therefore, the *more sensitive* the unit is. Both the sensitivity and pressure limit controls consist of small adjustable orifices. The larger the orifice size is, the greater will be the feedback mechanism. Examples of these types of units on the market are those produced by Mine Safety Appliances and the Retec models by Burton Division of Cavitron.

VENTILATORY MODIFICATIONS

There are several modifications to the basic intermittent (inspiratory) positive-pressure breathing (IPPB) pressure waveform, and some examples are shown in Fig. 8-34. When used continuously for ventilatory support, the title is often changed to intermittent positive-pressure ventilation (IPPV).[8,9]

The alterations to the basic inspiratory pressure curve called *inspiratory holds* or *plateaus*[10] include pressure hold and volume hold. With a pressure hold, the preset pressure is reached and held for some period of time. An example of this type of curve could exist with a manually limited, Venturi-powered unit if the manual control were not released when the peak pressure is reached. Volume hold exists when the predetermined volume is delivered and then held for a period of

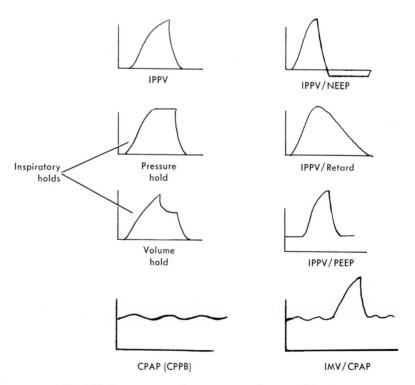

Fig. 8-34. Pressure curves for common ventilatory modifications.

time. The result is a notch in the pressure curve as the circuit and patient pressures approach equilibration.

Expiratory modifications to the curve have become increasingly prevalent in recent years. Negative (end) expiratory pressure (NEEP) was designed to counterbalance the increase in mean intrathoracic pressures caused by IPPB in hopes of returning one of the normal mechanisms (negative intrathoracic pressure) for venous return to the right atrium. Generally, negative pressure is applied to the circuit on exhalation by utilizing a Bernoulli jet or Venturi to entrain circuit gas. The resulting subatmospheric pressure is applied to the patient's airways (Fig. 8-35).

Considerations in using NEEP include (1) expiratory airway collapse causing air-trapping and (2) usage when congestive left ventricular failure is present where increased venous return to the right heart would increase the pulmonary capillary pressure, which would not be desirable.

Expiratory retard affords a resistance to expiratory gas flow by incorporating a restriction on the expiratory outflow tract. The basic objective of resistance to expiratory gas flow is to maintain a positive intra-airway pressure to prevent flaccid airways from collapsing in chronic obstructive disorders; this modification is similar

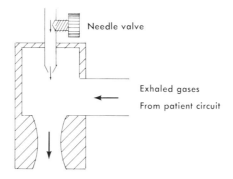

Fig. 8-35. Example of negative end expiratory pressure mechanism.

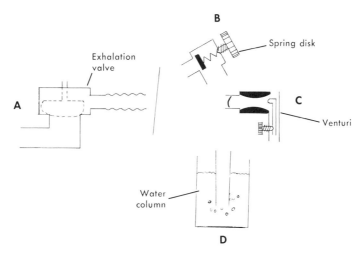

Fig. 8-36. Devices for applying PEEP.

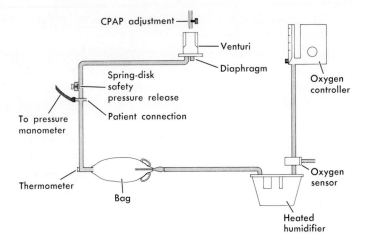

Fig. 8-37. Example of circuit used for CPAP.

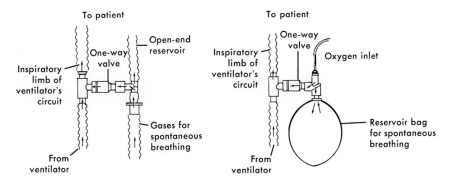

Fig. 8-38. Two common types of IMV attachments for ventilator circuits. (Modified from Desautels, D. A., and Bartlett, J. L.: Respir. Care **19:**187, 1974.)

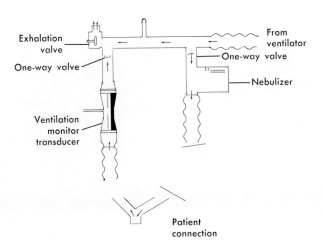

Fig. 8-39. Circuit used for continuous flow ventilation (CFV). (Modified from McPherson, S. P., et al.: Respir. Care **20:**261, 1975.)

to pursed-lip breathing.[11] Considerations in the use of expiratory retard include (1) increased mean intrathoracic pressures, which may decrease return of venous blood to the right heart to a greater degree than IPPV alone and (2) longer expiratory times.

Positive end expiratory pressure (PEEP) is a threshold-like resistance applied after active exhalation.[11,12] When inhalation ends, the circuit pressure drops to a set positive pressure level. Usually expiratory retard and PEEP differ in that pressure drops to atmospheric more slowly as expiratory gas flow ceases in retard, and pressure is held at an elevated baseline above atmospheric when flow ceases with PEEP. This difference has been compared as an orificial resistance to a threshold resistance.[9]

Some resistance to active expiratory gas flow can occur when PEEP is used, depending on the type of device used to accomplish PEEP. Fig. 8-36 shows some methods of providing PEEP. By trapping a pressure in an exhalation diaphragm, *A*, that pressure will also be held in the patient circuit unless leaks are present. A spring and disk at the exhalation port, *B*, can provide PEEP by utilizing spring tension. Applying the forward force from a Venturi (or Pitot) tube system, *C*, against a valve or diaphragm in the exhalation tube will in turn trap that pressure in the circuit. A simple water column, *D*, with a tube from the exhalation port of a circuit placed under the water will trap pressure equal to the height of the water column. Of these four examples, *A*, *B*, and *D* are the least flow dependent or resistant. The spring-disk devices usually apply some expiratory flow resistance as well as PEEP when used.

The objective of IPPV/PEEP is to increase the functional residual capacity by maintaining a positive pressure throughout the ventilatory cycle and to aid in the prevention of atelectasis by improving gas distribution.[1] A decrease in inspired oxygen fraction (FI_{O_2}) when PEEP is used can also be an advantage. Considerations with the use of PEEP include the effects of increasing mean intrathoracic pressure. Constant positive-pressure breathing (CPPB) or constant positive airway pressure (CPAP) refers to a patient breathing spontaneously at an elevated baseline pressure.[10,11,13] The objective of CPPB or CPAP is to increase FRC as with PEEP, for the same reasoning. The considerations are similar as for PEEP except that ventilatory back-up may be inadequate or absent. Fig. 8-37 illustrates a typical CPAP circuit. CPAP has been used in combination with a ventilator[14] sometimes as a weaning mechanism.[15]

Intermittent mandatory ventilation[16] (IMV) was designed as a weaning mechanism by providing a source of gas to the patient for spontaneous breathing, with the ventilator providing controlled breaths intermittently. Fig. 8-38 diagrams common IMV circuits. IMV can also be combined with CPAP-like breathing.[14,15]

Continuous-flow ventilation (CFV) was also designed as a weaning method and is able to utilize (1) IMV, (2) CPAP, and (3) continuous gas flow near ambient pressure, all with one circuit for versatility.[17] The circuitry allows for both monitoring the patient's expired volumes as well as reducing the circuit's compressibility factor to 0.5 cc/cm H_2O subtracted from the measured exhaled gases. This reduction is possible because the ventilator's and tubing circuitry's compressed gas volume exists the exhalation valve without passing through the monitoring device.[17] Fig. 8-39 diagrams a CFV circuit for a volume ventilator.

REFERENCES

1. Egan, D. F.: Fundamentals of respiratory therapy, ed. 3, St. Louis, 1977, The C. V. Mosby Co.
2. Vidyasagar, D.: Physiological basis and clinical implications of continuous negative chestwall pressure in hyaline membrane disease. In Keuskamp, D. H. G., editor: Neonatal and pediatric ventilation, Int. Anesthesiol. Clin., Winter, 1974.
3. Mushin, W. W., et al.: Automatic ventilation of the lungs, ed. 2, Oxford, England, 1969, Blackwell Scientific Publications, Ltd.
4. Pulmonary terms and symbols—a report of the American College of Chest Physicians—American Thoracic Society Joint Committee on Pulmonary Nomenclature, Chest 67:583, 1975.
5. McPherson, S. P., and Roads, J. S.: History of respiratory therapy. (To be published.)
6. Petty, T. L., and Broughton, J. O.: A new simple IPPB device for hospital and home care, J.A.M.A. 203:871, 1968.
7. Smith, R. K.: Respiratory care applications for fluidics, Respir. Ther. 3:29, May-June, 1973.
8. Safar, P., editor: Respiratory therapy, Philadelphia, 1965, F. A. Davis Co.
9. Young, J. A., and Crocker, D., editors: Principles and practice of respiratory therapy, ed. 2, Chicago, 1976, Year Book Medical Publishers, Inc.
10. Pulmonary terms and symbols—A report of the American College of Chest Physicians—American Thoracic Society Joint Committee on Pulmonary Nomenclature, Chest 67:583, 1975.
11. Barach, A. L., Bickerman, H. A., and Petty, T. L.: Perspectives in pressure breathing, Respir. Care 20:627, 1975.
12. Petty, T. L.: Intensive and rehabilitative respiratory care, ed. 2, Philadelphia, 1974, Lea & Febiger.
13. Gregory, G. A., et al.: Treatment of the idiopathic respiratory distress syndrome with CPAP, N. Engl. J. Med. 284:1333, 1971.
14. Kirby, R. R., et al.: A new pediatric volume ventilator, Anesth. Analg. 50:533, 1971.
15. Spearman, C. B.: Control of inspired oxygen concentration and addition of PEEP or CPAP with the Bourns Pediatric Ventilator, Respir. Care 18:405, 1973.
16. Downs, J. B., et al.: Itermittent mandatory ventilation—a new approach to weaning patients from mechanical ventilation, Respir. Care 18:405, 1973.
17. McPherson, S. P., et al.: A circuit that combines ventilator weaning methods using continuous flow ventilation (CFV), Respir. Care 20:261, 1975.

9 Bird respirators

THE BIRD MARK 7

The Bird Mark 7[1,2] (Fig. 9-1) will be the first of the ventilators to be discussed in this chapter. Several other models presented utilize the same principles and similar controls.

Most respirators are designed with features that function on the principle of two opposing forces. One of the primary principles of Bird respirators incorporates *magnetism versus gas pressure*. First, the effect of gas pressure on the diaphragm will be reviewed. As seen in Fig. 9-2, a box is divided into two halves by a simple *diaphragm*. On both sides are communications to the outside. The left side will remain exposed to *atmospheric pressure*, and changes in pressure on the right side will be introduced. When both sides are subjected to atmospheric pressure, A and D, the diaphragm is straight. In B, as gas volume is added to the right side, the pressure increases. The increased pressure causes a pressure gradient to be exerted to the left, causing the diaphragm to move in that direction. In C, gas is removed from the right side, and the pressure becomes subatmospheric. In this case, the pressure gradient is from left to right (from atmospheric to subatmospheric), and the diaphragm moves in that direction.

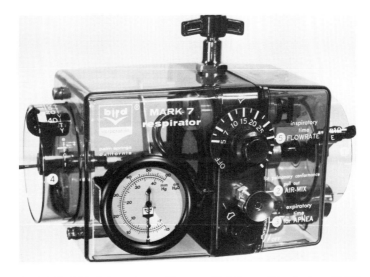

Fig. 9-1. Bird Mark 7 respirator. (Courtesy Bird Corp., Palm Springs, Calif.)

Two *magnets* are added to the same box, one on each side, and *metal clutch plates* are attached on either side of the diaphragm (Fig. 9-3). When the pressure is atmospheric on both sides of the diaphragm, *A,* the net forces on either side are equal. The forces attracting each plate to their respective magnets are equal if both of the magnets and corresponding clutch plates are equal distances from each other and if the pressures on both sides are equal and the diaphragm is straight. This situation does not actually occur in the Bird during normal operation, but the point to be made is that when both magnetic forces and gas pressures are equal, an equilibrium exists.

As gas volume is removed from the right side (Fig. 9-3, *B*), the pressure decreases to below atmospheric, and the diaphragm moves to the right, taking with it the metal plates. The clutch plate on the right is now in close proximity to the magnet on the right; the diaphragm will be *held to the right* side even though the pressure of the right chamber may return to atmospheric pressure, *C.* The diaphragm will remain there until sufficient gas volume is added, *D,* to the right side to cause an increased pressure to overcome the attraction of the magnet on the right magnet side to the right metal plate. Once that positive pressure has caused a sufficient pressure gradi-

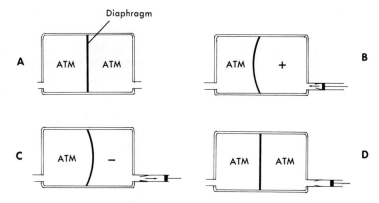

Fig. 9-2. Pressure changes across diaphragm. *ATM,* Atmospheric pressure. (Modified from Bird Corp., Palm Springs, Calif.)

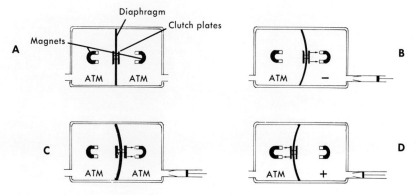

Fig. 9-3. Pressure changes across diaphragm with magnetic force. (Modified from Bird Corp., Palm Springs, Calif.)

ent toward the left to overcome the magnetic attraction, the diaphragm will be pushed to the left, where again it will remain, A.

To incorporate these principles of opposing forces just described into the Bird Mark 7 itself, some additional mechanisms will be required (Fig. 9-4). An incoming gas source near 50 psig passes through a *brazed-brass inlet filter*. The first structure through which the source gas will pass is a *flow rate control*, A. The next structure is basically a switching mechanism, B. The clutch plates are placed on either end of this device. This *ceramic switch* allows gas flow into the respirator if the *diaphragm and clutch plates* are to the right (inspiratory position). If the clutch plates and diaphragm are to the left, gas cannot pass through the switch. Gas next travels through the switch, and the line splits. One passageway leads to the *jet of a Venturi, C*. That Venturi supplies the initial main flow of gas to build pressure in the Bird Respirator. The second line travels to the *nebulizer* jet for creating aerosol, D, as well as to the *exhalation valve, E*, closing it during the inspiratory phase.

Fig. 9-5 diagrams the normal beginning of the inspiratory phase on the Bird Mark 7. Negative pressure generated by the patient's inspiratory effort causes the diaphragm to be pushed to the right by atmospheric pressure on the left. In Fig. 9-6, gas flow is allowed to pass through the ceramic switch and then splits, traveling in the left side to the jet of the Venturi, and passing to the line powering the nebulizer and exhalation valve. The Venturi jet then *entrains air* and passes these gases through the *Venturi gate* and on to the patient. This gas enters the patient system, and pressure begins to build on the right side of the Bird Mark 7. Thus, at the *beginning* of inspiration, gas flow into the circuit comes from (1) the Venturi jet, (2) the air that the Venturi jet entrains, and (3) the nebulizer jet. As *terminal inhalation* approaches, the pressure rises on the right side of the Bird, equaling the Venturi's *forward pressure*, and the Venturi gate closes (Fig. 9-7). The gas from the

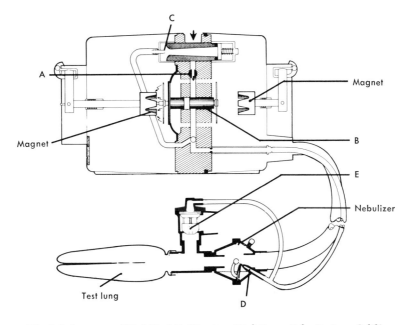

Fig. 9-4. Structure of Bird Mark 7. (Courtesy Bird Corp., Palm Springs, Calif.)

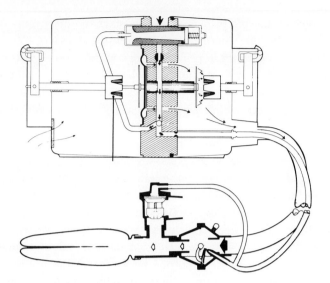

Fig. 9-5. Begin inhalation. (Courtesy Bird Corp., Palm Springs, Calif.)

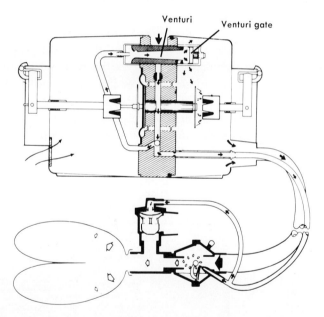

Fig. 9-6. Inhalation. (Courtesy Bird Corp., Palm Springs, Calif.)

jet of the Venturi then simply is forced into the left side of the machine, flushing that compartment with source gas. Once the Venturi gate has closed, the *only* gas flow during the remainder of inspiration into the patient system comes from source gas through the nebulizer jet. Once this jet has added enough gas to build the pressure up to a point so that it exceeds the magnetic attraction of the right (pressure-control) magnet, the diaphragm, clutch plate, and ceramic switch are then forced to the left, occluding gas flow into the respirator and starting exhalation. Then, with no

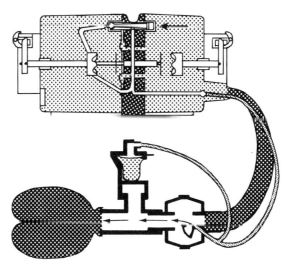

Fig. 9-7. End inhalation. (Modified from Bird Corp., Palm Springs, Calif.)

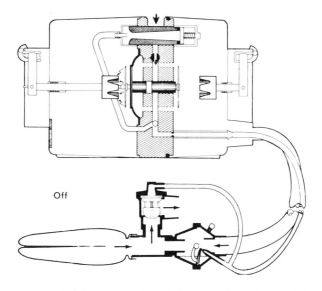

Fig. 9-8. Exhalation. (Courtesy Bird Corp., Palm Springs, Calif.)

gas flow into the Bird, the gas in the lines below the ceramic switch simply exits through their corresponding jets. The diaphragm and exhalation valve are now uncharged, and the existing positive pressure in the patient's circuit simply pushes the exhalation valve gate open (Fig. 9-8), allowing gas to escape. The unit is now ready to begin another ventilatory cycle.

The Bird Mark 7 contains a *pneumatic expiratory timing device,* which can be used to provide an automatically cycled breath in case the patient's ventilatory rate

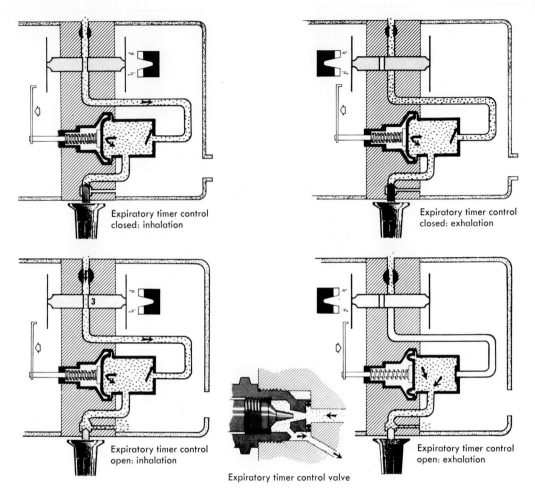

Expiratory timer control
closed: inhalation

Expiratory timer control
closed: exhalation

Expiratory timer control
open: inhalation

Expiratory timer control valve

Expiratory timer control
open: exhalation

Fig. 9-9. Exhalation timer and control. (Courtesy Bird Corp., Palm Springs, Calif.)

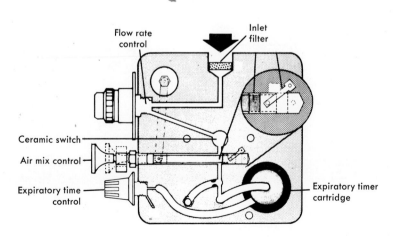

Flow rate
control

Inlet
filter

Ceramic switch

Air mix control

Expiratory time
control

Expiratory timer
cartridge

Fig. 9-10. Center body for Bird Mark 7. (Courtesy Bird Corp., Palm Springs, Calif.)

should drop or periods of apnea occur. The expiratory timer can be used to time-cycle the Bird into inhalation when used in the control or assist-control mode. The timer is a *pneumatic cartridge with a controlled leak* out of it (Fig. 9-9). On inhalation, the cartridge is charged by source gas, which enters by means of the one-way valve. The gas pushes the diaphragm to the left, depressing the *spring* and moving the *plunger and arm* to the left. The leak out of the cartridge around the *needle valve control* is reasonably small in comparison to the incoming gas flow, so once inhalation has begun, the unit is charged completely until inhalation ends. On end inhalation, no source gas is supplied to the cartridge, and the one-way entrance valve closes. The only path for gas to leave the cartridge is the leak past the needle valve on the outflow track. As gas leaks out, pressure decreases, and the diaphragm is pushed to the right by the spring. As that occurs, the plunger and its attached arm are moved slowly to the right. Once the arm has reached a point where it touches the clutch plate, the clutch plate is *physically pushed away* from the magnet, and the ceramic switch is mechanically maneuvered into the *on* position. Thus the *length* of expiratory time is controlled by this expiratory-time control *needle valve*. The greater the leak past the needle valve, the faster the cartridge will become discharged and the shorter the exhalation time will be.

Since the basic principle of operation of the Bird Mark 7 has been covered, the controls will be discussed independently, starting where the gas source enters.

1. The oxygen inlet is a brazed *brass filter* that acts as a high pressure inlet filter (Fig. 9-10). It removes any dust or debris that may have entered the incoming line.

2. The *flow rate control* (Fig. 9-11) is simply a needle valve. By turning the knob to a higher, *arbitrary* number, the orifice size is increased, and the flow of gas through the needle valve is higher. Therefore the flow of gas powering the jet of the Venturi and the jet of the nebulizer is also increased. The result is an increased total flow into the unit and increased nebulization. In addition to the higher flow rate setting, the end point of flow during inhalation from the nebulizer jet is higher. Peak flows from 0 to 80 L/min can be set by the flow rate control when the Venturi system is used (Fig. 9-14) and about 0 to 50 L/min on 100% source gas setting.

3. Next, gas passes to the *ceramic switch* (Fig. 9-12). If the clutch plate and ceramic switch are held to the right, gas is allowed to flow past the shaft of the switch, around the smaller center portion, and on to the rest of the respirator. If the ceramic shaft is held to the left, the larger-diameter outer portion blocks the incoming gas, and gas does not flow to the remainder of the respirator.

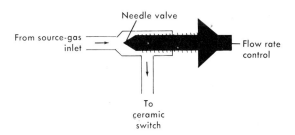

Fig. 9-11. Bird flow rate control.

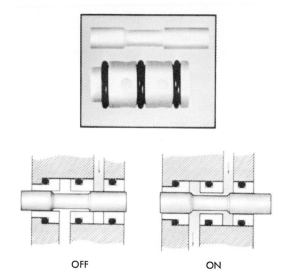

Fig. 9-12. Ceramic switch. (Courtesy Bird Corp., Palm Springs, Calif.)

4. Directly below the ceramic switch is the *Air-Mix control*. The Air-Mix control is a two-position switch (Fig. 9-13). When pushed in, the *O rings* seal the incoming source gas and direct it out the reed-covered *bleed hole* in the center body, providing a *constant flow* during the inspiratory phase. When the control is pulled out, the bleed hole is blocked by the top O ring, and gas is directed to the jet of the Air-Mix Venturi. The *decompression port* above the bleed hole is there simply to allow the plunger to be pushed in without compressing gas behind it. It functionally plays no part in the Air-Mix control itself. In the *100% setting* (*in* position), there are *two* constant sources of gas flow throughout inhalation into the respirator. One is the flow through the *bleed hole*, and the second is the flow through the *nebulizer*. There-fore, during inhalation, the two constant flows produce a *square wave* or a constant-flow pattern (Fig. 9-13). On *Air-Mix* (*out* setting), inhalation begins with gas flow sources from (1) the jet of the Venturi, (2) the air that the Venturi system en-trains, and (3) the jet of the nebulizer. At the end of inhalation, when the Venturi gate has closed, the only remaining flow is that from the *nebulizer*.

5. The *Venturi gate* contains a spring that is preset at approximately 2 cm H_2O. This is done so that when a patient exerts a slight negative pressure through the circuit and on that side of the ventilator, the Venturi gate is not opened, which would prevent the generation of sufficient negative pressure on the right side needed to open the ceramic switch. In addition, this gate provides a 2 cm H_2O opposition to Venturi gas flow. If, for example, the *peak forward pressure* of the Venturi is 14 cm H_2O with a certain gas flow to the jet, the Venturi actually becomes nonfunc-tional at near 12 cm H_2O because the gate spring contributes to the gas pressure opposing the Venturi. Therefore, at a pressure *above* 12 cm H_2O on the right side of the Bird, the gate will close, and Venturi jet gas will simply *accumulate* on the ambient side of the case. On the next breath, *oxygen is entrained* with the ambient air contributing to a higher oxygen concentration delivered to the patient as seen graphically in Fig. 9-14. The graph not only shows that the oxygen percentage starts

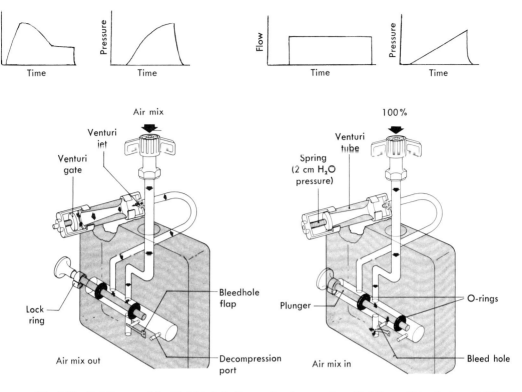

Fig. 9-13. Air-Mix control for Bird Mark 7. (Lower drawings courtesy Bird Corp., Palm Springs, Calif.)

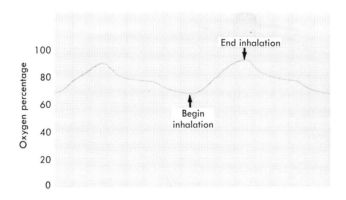

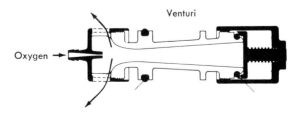

Fig. 9-14. Oxygen delivery percentage change during inhalation from Mark 7 driven with 100% oxygen and on air-mix mode. (Cross-sectional drawing modified from Bird Corp., Palm Springs, Calif.)

above 60% at begin inhalation but also that end inhalation is over 90%. This is caused by the Venturi system entraining less and less during the breath due to back pressure in the right side as well as the patient circuit. Changes in the patient's airway resistance and lung compliance would result in a different delivered oxygen concentration.

6. Two more controls are of importance on the Bird, but they do not directly adjust gas flow. These are the *pressure* and *sensitivity* adjustments. Basically, they adjust the *relative position* of each magnet to its corresponding metal plate (Fig. 9-15). The closer the magnet is to the plate, the stronger the magnetic attraction is and the more the force must be in terms of a greater pressure gradient across the diaphragm to overcome it. For example, the closer the magnet is to the plate on the right side (refer to Figs. 9-4 to 9-6), the higher the *positive* pressure must be on that side of the diaphragm to overcome the magnetic attraction and shut off the machine. Therefore *increased pressure-limit* values are acquired by simply moving the right-hand magnet closer to the metal plate. Pressure limit can be adjusted up to near 60 cm H_2O with the Mark 7 (also the Mark 8 and 10) ventilator.

On the left side, the force needed to move that clutch plate away from its magnet is the *negative pressure* generated by the patient on the right side of the diaphragm. The closer the magnet is moved to the clutch plate, the higher the pressure gradient across the diaphragm must be to move the diaphragm and clutch plate away from the magnet. This would be reflected by a *greater* negative pressure, requiring *more effort* to be generated by the patient.

7. The Bird's circuit *tubing* and *manifold* (Fig. 9-16) consists of (a) *a large bore,*

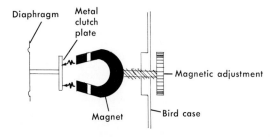

Fig. 9-15. Magnet adjustment for sensitivity or pressure control.

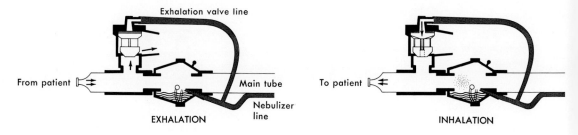

Fig. 9-16. Bird tubing circuit and manifold. (Modified from Bird Corp., Palm Springs, Calif.)

mainstream tube, through which gas from the respirator passes and (b) *the small-bore line*, carrying high-pressure source gas to a *nebulizer and exhalation valve*. The main gas stream passes *through* the nebulizer, picking up aerosol created by the source gas at the nebulizer jet and passing on to the patient. At the nebulizer, the small high-pressure line splits, supplying both the nebulizer jet and exhalation valve with gas. The Bird *nebulizer* can be utilized in either a *side* or *mainstream* configuration (Fig. 9-17). The expiratory *retard* cap, which covers the exhalation valve, provides various port sizes through which expired gas can pass (Fig. 9-18). The smaller the port is which is exposed to the exhalation valve's notch, the greater will be the resistance to exhalation.

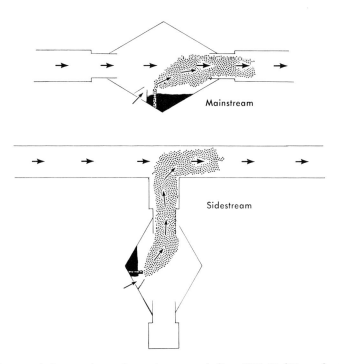

Fig. 9-17. Bird micronebulizer can be used as mainstream nebulizer. With Bird Tee and nebulizer cap, it can also be utilized as sidestream device.

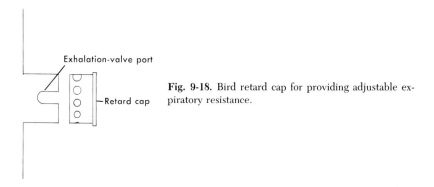

Fig. 9-18. Bird retard cap for providing adjustable expiratory resistance.

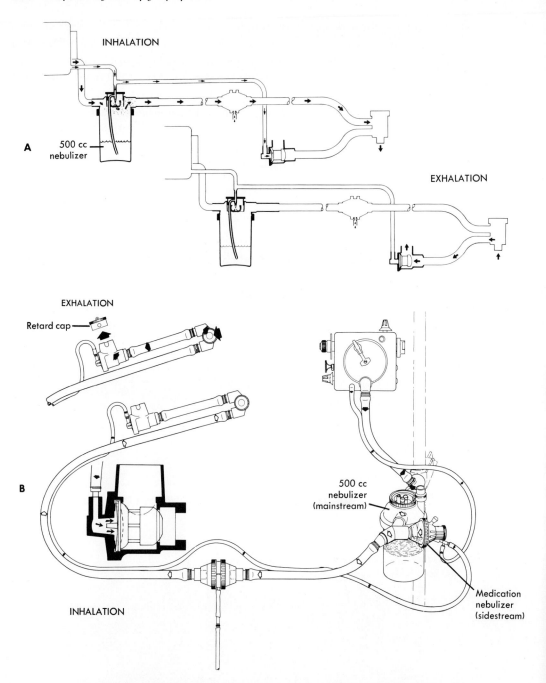

INHALATION

A

500 cc
nebulizer

EXHALATION

EXHALATION

Retard cap

B

500 cc
nebulizer
(mainstream)

INHALATION

Medication
nebulizer
(sidestream)

Fig. 9-19. Bird (positive) Q circle. (Courtesy Bird Corp., Palm Springs, Calif.)

8. The Mark 7 (positive) *Q circle* is a special Bird circuit that provides for *small mechanical dead space* for use with the respirator (Fig. 9-19).[1] With the Y arrangement, inspiratory gas flow travels through the top line to the patient. On exhalation, all gas leaves through the bottom line. Therefore the rebreathed gas volume is limited only to the small connecting piece. Note that in *A*, the 500 cc nebulizer

(Chapter 4) is being utilized in a *mainstream* fashion in this circuit. In *B*, the medication nebulizer is added next to the 500 cc unit and is placed in a *sidestream* fashion.

The newest series of the Mark 7 provides the following functional changes to the unit just described. (1) An external filter is used on the ambient (entrainment) side. (2) The Air-Mix control has been removed so that the unit is always on air-mix mode. (3) A pressure release (pop-off) valve is added to the pressure side. (4) Nebulizer flow rate is independent of the inspiratory flow rate setting. (5) Controlled rate is available against CPAP or PEEP pressures of up to 35 cm H_2O.

The Bird Mark 7A is essentially the same as the new Mark 7 with the addition of *apneustic flow* (see description under *Minibird II*, pp. 212 to 215) and time-limiting capabilities.

THE BIRD MARK 8

The Bird Mark 8[2,3] (Fig. 9-20) is functionally the same as the Mark 7 except that it comes with the capability of providing a flow of source gas during the expiratory phase, usually used for *negative expiratory pressure* (Fig. 9-21). The negative-pressure system (Fig. 9-22) consists of a *needle valve* and a *flow interrupter switch*. This switch is a pneumatic cartridge containing a plunger, spring, and diaphragm. During inhalation, gas flow passes through the ceramic switch and then charges a cartridge and blocks the flow of 50 psig source gas to the negative-pressure Venturi. During exhalation, gas is allowed to flow to the Venturi, and gases in the circuit and from the patient are entrained.

The *needle valve* adjusts the flow of gas to the jet of the negative-pressure Venturi, which is *located in the exhalation* valve of the circuit. The higher the gas flow to the jet, the greater the forward velocity of gas will be through it, and the greater the lateral negative pressure will be, as well. Therefore the greater the flow to the negative-pressure Venturi, the lower the negative pressure applied to the patient

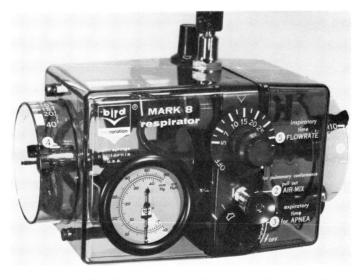

Fig. 9-20. Bird Mark 8. (Courtesy Bird Corp., Palm Springs, Calif.)

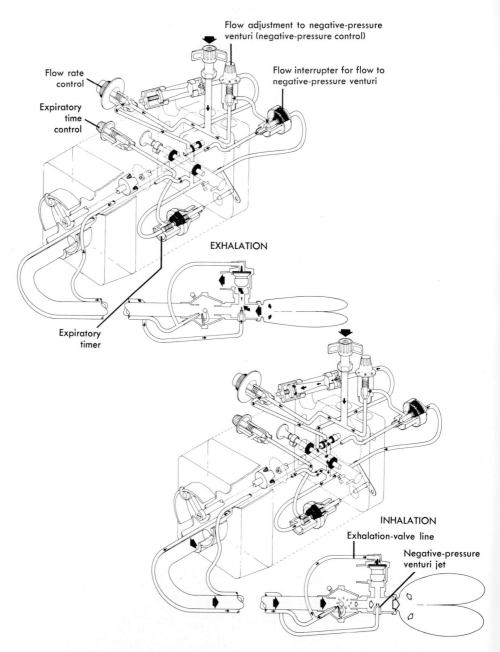

Flow adjustment to negative-pressure
venturi (negative-pressure control)

Flow rate
control

Flow interrupter for flow to
negative-pressure venturi

Expiratory
time
control

EXHALATION

Expiratory
timer

INHALATION

Exhalation-valve line

Negative-pressure
venturi jet

Fig. 9-21. Bird Mark 8 flow diagram. (Courtesy Bird Corp., Palm Springs, Calif.)

circuit. When negative pressure is utilized, the left (sensitivity) magnet must be moved *closer* to the metal clutch plate to counterbalance the subatmospheric pressure on the right side of the diaphragm. This adjustable gas flow during exhalation can also be used for providing PEEP, gases for spontaneous breathing during IMV, and expiratory nebulization when used with appropriate systems.

The Mark 8 circuit and manifold (Fig. 9-23) includes the negative-pressure Ven-

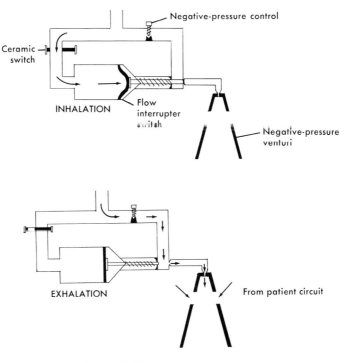

Fig. 9-22. Negative pressure system.

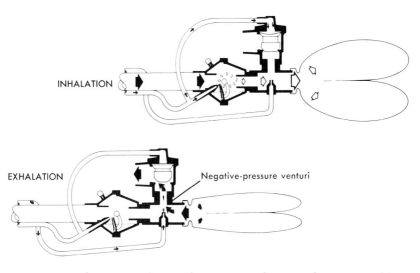

Fig. 9-23. Mark 8 circuit and manifold. (Courtesy Bird Corp., Palm Springs, Calif.)

turi. The Mark 8 (*positive/negative*) *Q circle* (Fig. 9-24) also includes the negative-pressure Venturi. In all other aspects this circuitry is the same as found on the Mark 7.

The newest series of the Mark 8 provides the same basic changes as described for the new Mark 7 as well as retaining the system for providing expiratory flow.

The Bird Mark 8A also encompasses the apneustic flow and time-limiting capabilities of the Mark 7A.

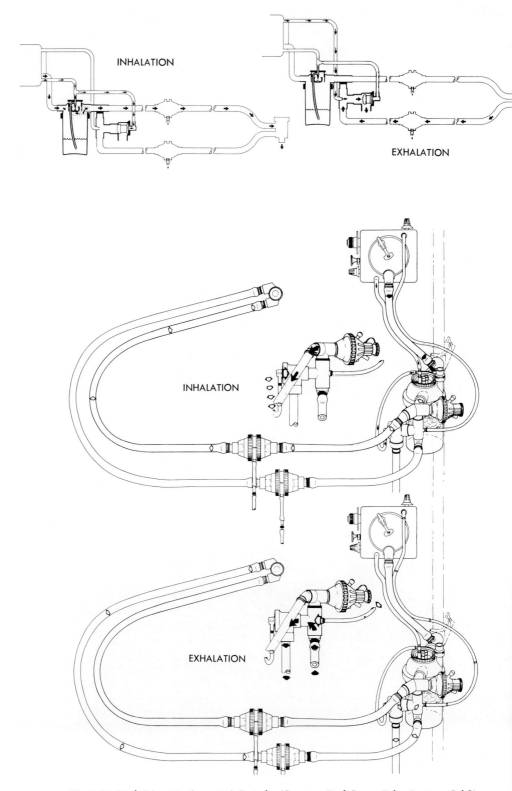

INHALATION

EXHALATION

INHALATION

EXHALATION

Fig. 9-24. Mark 8 (positive/negative) Q circle. (Courtesy Bird Corp., Palm Springs, Calif.)

THE BIRD MARK 9

The Bird Mark 9[4] (Fig. 9-25) is basically the same as the Mark 8 with two important exceptions: (1) the pressure limit magnet is larger and provides pressures up to 200 mm Hg and (2) it has a dual-flow range system for providing high flow rates through its double-jet Venturi system. The Mark 9 is generally used in veterinary medicine.

THE BIRD MARK 10

The *Bird Mark 10*[2,5] (Fig. 9-26) contains all the features of a Mark 7 except that it is permanently set on Air-Mix (no Air-Mix control externally), and it has an added

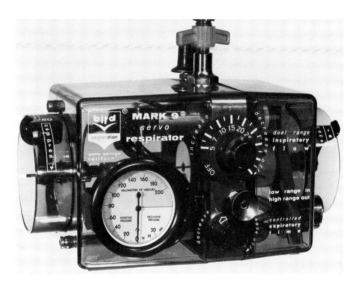

Fig. 9-25. Bird Mark 9. (Courtesy Bird Corp., Palm Springs, Calif.)

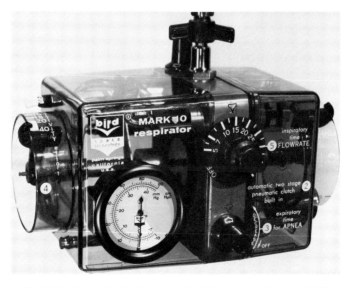

Fig. 9-26. Bird Mark 10. (Courtesy Bird Corp., Palm Springs, Calif.)

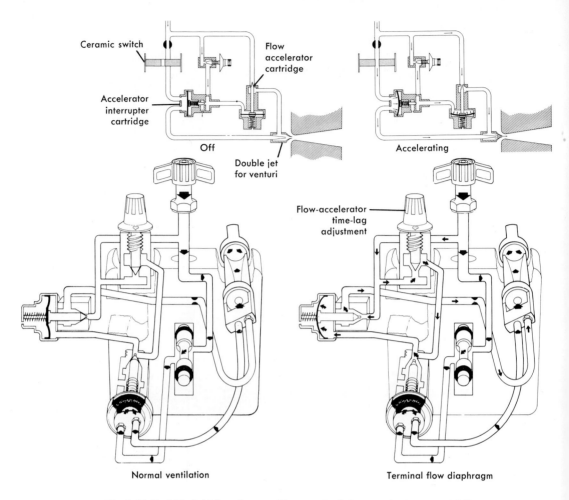

Fig. 9-27. Bird Mark 10 flow diagram (Courtesy Bird Corp., Palm Springs, Calif.)

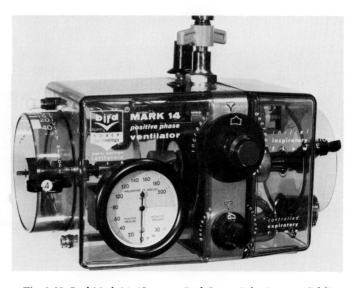

Fig. 9-28. Bird Mark 14. (Courtesy Bird Corp., Palm Springs, Calif.)

feature of an inspiratory *flow accelerator* generally used for leak compensation. The flow accelerator actually kicks in an *extra flow of gas* at a specific time so that if inspiration has not yet ended, pressure needed to cycle off the unit will be built up *rapidly* because of the sudden increased flow of extra gas through the circuit. The adjustment of when the flow acceleration is to occur is accomplished by a needle valve and two pneumatic cartridges (Fig. 9-27). The first cartridge, which is the *accelerator interrupter cartridge,* phases the accelerator to be functional on inhalation only. When the ceramic switch is closed, source gas does not flow to the left cartridge, and gas from the needle valve leaks out of a port in the cartridge. When the ceramic switch is open, the leak is blocked by a plunger in the left cartridge, allowing source gas from the needle valve to travel to a second cartridge, the *flow accelerator cartridge.* Once sufficient gas flow from the needle valve has entered the right cartridge to depress its diaphragm, a plunger opens the source gas line to the *second jet* in the Mark 10's Venturi, causing sudden increased gas flow. As the gas flow past the needle valve is *increased,* the right cartridge allows flow to the second jet sooner, and the flow acceleration occurs earlier in the inspiratory phase.

One model of the Mark 10[6] was originally designed to provide a more simplified

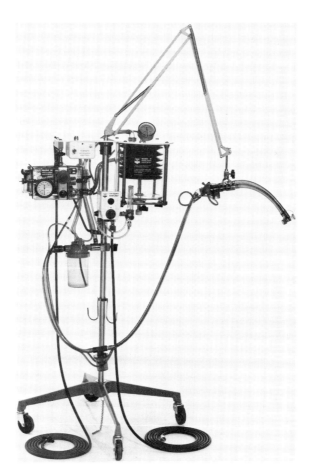

Fig. 9-29. Bird Mark 6 minute volume ventilator system. (Courtesy Bird Corp., Palm Springs, Calif.)

version of the basic Mark 7 respirator for use by less trained individuals. First, the flow control was provided with just an *on* and an *off* setting. The *on* setting basically corresponded with the *no. 15* on the flow rate control of the standard Bird Mark 7. The pressure gauge was provided with a green area of *good ventilation*, which basically meant that the pressure had reached a point that was potentially sufficient for *average*, normal ventilation. The unit also had a preset leak compensation, flow-accelerator mechanism which could be altered or calibrated to a different point. It was an automatic flow-acceleration device with a built-in constant delay.

THE BIRD MARK 14

The Mark 14[2,5] (Fig. 9-28) has the pressure capabilities of the Mark 9 and a flow accelerator like the Mark 10, but it has no negative-expiratory pressure mechanism. The Mark 14 is basically a Mark 10 with a *larger pressure limit magnet* to acquire higher delivery pressures. The unit also utilizes a *finer* sensitivity adjustment called a *vernier*.

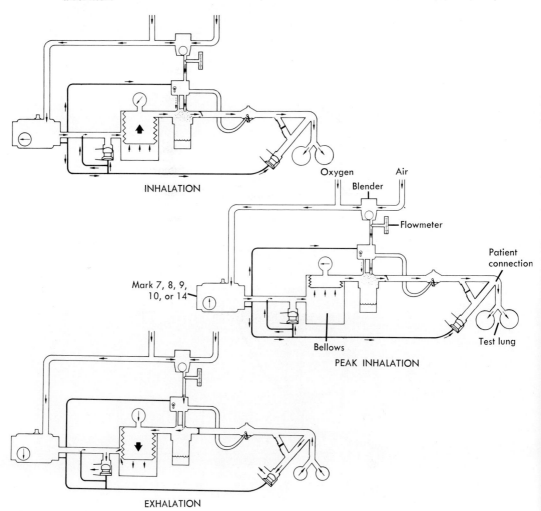

Fig. 9-30. Mark 6 minute volume ventilator flow diagram. (Courtesy Bird Corp., Palm Springs, Calif.)

Two new ventilators from Bird that utilize a metal center-body similar to the Mark 7, 8, 9, 10, and 14 units are The Bird Ventilator and The Bird Ventilator with Demand CPAP. These units are similar to the other new Mark 8A unit, but they can also provide inspiratory flow acceleration with slope control and well over 100 cm H_2O pressure limiting. The unit with demand CPAP also provides a system for spontaneous breathing at an elevated baseline pressure.

THE BIRD MARK 6

The Mark 6[7] (Fig. 9-29) actually consists of a *bellows* housed in a transparent cylinder. It is driven (compressed) by some other Bird ventilator, such as a Mark 7, 8, 9, 10, or 14. Fig. 9-30 diagrams its function. Minute volume is set on the *blender's flow meter* from 2 to 25 L/min and is collected in the *bellows* between breaths. During inhalation, the *Mark 7, 8, 9, 10, or 14* compresses the bellows, which ventilates the patient. At peak inhalation, the bellows is empty, and the ventilator compressing the bellows abruptly reaches its preset pressure limit and exhalation begins. During exhalation, gases from the blender are again collected in the bellows chamber. As long as the flow from the blender remains constant, *tidal volume* will be a result of that flow divided by the respiratory rate. If the rate increases, as in a patient who begins to assist, the *tidal volume* would decrease and vice versa. Because the bellows contains the patient's gases and the Mark 7, 8, 9, 10, or 14 is only used to compress the bellows, this system is an example of a *double-circuit* device. The Bird Mark 2 time-cycled, time-limited ventilator (to be described later in this chapter) has also been used with the Mark 6 system.

THE BIRD MARK 1

The Mark 1 incorporates the same principle of operation as is found in the Mark 7. It is a design attempt to produce a simplified and compact unit. Instead of using metal clutch plates with two magnets, *only one magnet* is used with the metal plates lying on either side (Fig. 9-31 and 9-32, *A*). The sensitivity and pressure calibration are accomplished by *moving the plates* closer or further from the magnet, rather than by moving the magnets, as in the Mark 7. The unit functions characteristically the same, since the movements of magnets and plates are just reversed. The diaphragm works functionally in the manner of the one in the Mark 7. When the patient takes a breath and establishes a slight negative pressure in the circuit, the *master diaphragm* is pulled to the *right (start)*. This moves the clutch plates and shaft to the right, opening the on/off switch at the left of the unit. This *on* position allows gas to flow through the flow rate needle valve to (1) the jet or nebulizer and (2) to the jet of the Venturi. The Venturi then supplies gas flow to the patient, and the nebulizer jet produces an aerosol (inhalation). Once enough pressure has been exerted in the circuit and on the diaphragm to overcome the magnetic attraction of the top right (pressure-adjustment) plate for the magnet, the whole assembly is pushed to the left, closing the on/off switch. The patient then exhales out of the unit past the exhalation diaphragm. The basic design of the Mark 1 is also incorporated into both the Minibird and Portabird (Fig. 9-32, *B* and *C*). Pressure limits are externally adjustable, but sensitivity is internal only. These devices provide pressures up to 25 cm H_2O.

The Bird integrated Mark 1 sequencing servo[8] was introduced in 1973.[9] It allows for independant, external adjustment for sensitivity *and* pressure and a pressure limit range normally up to 60 cm H_2O with a 100 cm H_2O option. A new generation of Bird ventilators incorporates the Mark 1 sequencing servo system.

THE MINIBIRD II

The Minibird II[10] (Figs. 9-33 and 9-34) uses the Mark 1 sequencing servo. It also has a new feature called *apneustic flow time*.

The ball valve in the Mark 1 of the Minibird II acts as the main on/off switch.

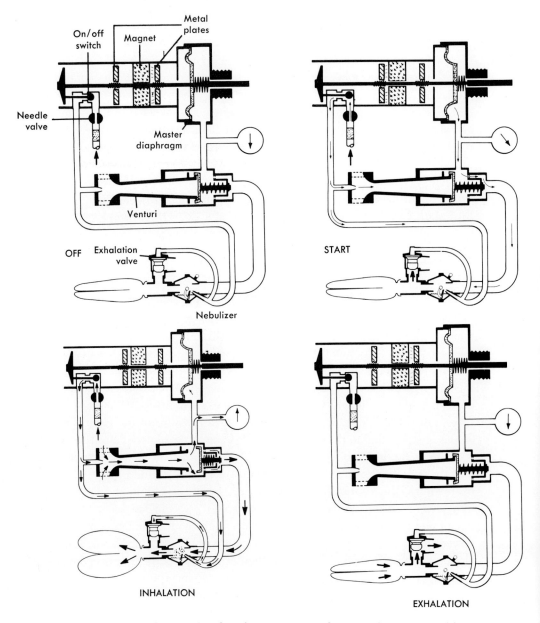

Fig. 9-31. Flow diagram of Bird Mark 1. (Courtesy Bird Corp., Palm Springs, Calif.)

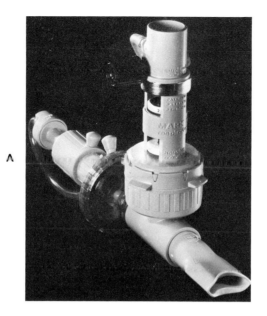

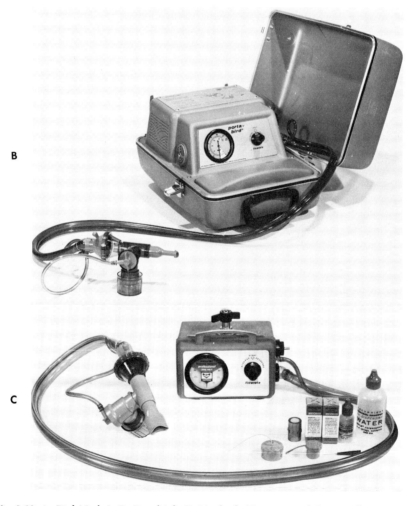

Fig. 9-32. **A**, Bird Mark 1. **B**, Portabird. **C**, Minibird. (Courtesy Bird Corp., Palm Springs, Calif.)

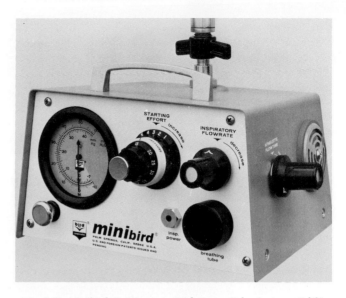

Fig. 9-33. Minibird II. (Courtesy Bird Corp., Palm Springs, Calif.)

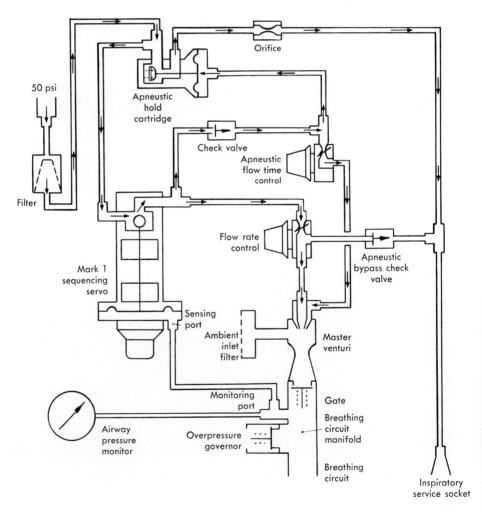

Fig. 9-34. Flow diagram for Minibird II ventilator. (Courtesy Bird Corp., Palm Springs, Calif.)

When the unit is in the inspiratory phase, this ball valve opens and allows source gas to flow (1) to the *flow rate control* (needle valve) and (2) to *apneustic hold cartridge* and *apneustic flowtime control* (needle valve). Gas flow from the flow rate control also splits to feed the *master Venturi* (which entrains filtered ambient air) to feed the patient's breathing circuit, and also to the *inspiratory service socket*, which feeds the nebulizer in the tubing circuit.

Gas pressure in the apneustic hold cartridge opens this normally closed device during inhalation and allows source gas to be added to the line leading to the inspiratory service socket and nebulizer. When the pressure limit (set on the Mark 1) is reached, the ball valve closes, and gas flow to the flow rate control and the apneustic hold cartridge ceases. The line between the apneustic hold cartridge and the ball valve must empty its pressure through the apneustic flow time control's needle valve and out the outside jet of the master Venturi. While this pressure release is occurring, the hold cartridge is "slowly" closing (at a rate proportional to the apneustic flowtime control setting). During this time, some source gas continues to flow out the inspiratory flow service socket and to the patient by way of the nebulizer. The amount of this apneustic flowtime is therefore set by the amount of opening of the apneustic flowtime control's needle valve. This time can be set up to 3 seconds following normal pressure limit. To protect the patient from excessive airway pressures and volumes, a spring-loaded relief valve, the *overpressure governor*, opens at pressures 65 cm H_2O normally or 100 cm H_2O as an option.

THE THERAPYBIRD

The Therapybird[9,11] (Figs. 9-35 and 9-36) incorporates the Mark 1 sequencing servo, has apneustic flowtime, and also has a system for flow acceleration.

The *source inlet manifold* feeds several systems within the Therapybird. They

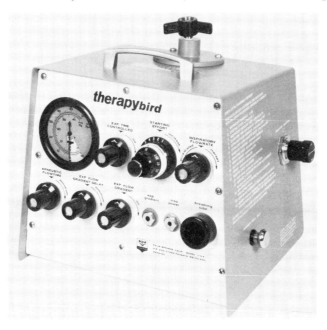

Fig. 9-35. Therapybird. (Courtesy Bird Corp., Palm Springs, Calif.)

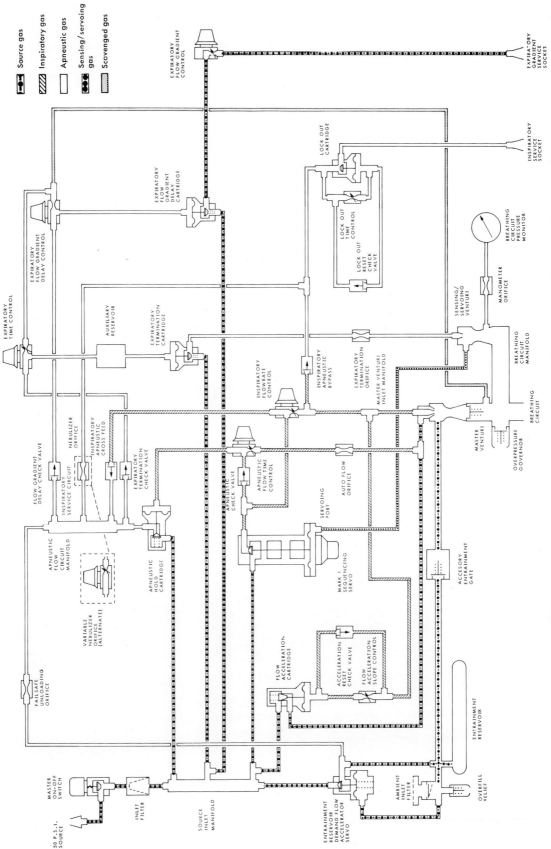

Fig. 9-36. Flow diagram for Therapybird ventilator. (Courtesy Bird Corp., Palm Springs, Calif.)

include the *entrainment reservoir demand flow accelerator servo, the apneustic hold cartridge, the expiratory termination cartridge, the expiratory flow gradient delay cartridge, and the flow acceleration cartridge.* The apneustic flowtime system works in a similar fashion to that of the Minibird II.

The demand valve in the entrainment reservoir demand flow accelerator servo system keeps the *entrainment reservoir* supplied with source gas. During inhalation, the master Venturi entrains gases from this reservoir and demand valve; therefore 100% source gas concentration is delivered to the patient throughout the breath. Ambient air can be entrained through the *ambient inlet filter* only if the entrainment flows exceed the capabilities of reservoir and demand valve.

An accelerating flow pattern can be achieved with the Therapybird. The *inspiratory flow rate control* (needle valve) controls the amount of gas going to the master (inside) jet of the *master Venturi* throughout inspiration. It also controls the amount of gas *pressure* that is exerted on the diaphragm of the *flow accelerator cartridge* through a restriction at the *flow acceleration slope control.* A spring opposing the diaphragm in the acceleration cartridge requires the diaphragm to exert about 18 psig to open a seat in the cartridge, which would allow source gas to flow through the cartridge and to the second jet of the master Venturi. If this second jet were powered during inspiration, flow to the patient could potentially "accelerate." The "therapy range" on the inspiratory flow rate control does not allow enough pressure to the diaphragm of the acceleration cartridge to open this second source of gas and thus no acceleration occurs. When the flow rate control knob is set beyond the "therapy range" and into the "accelerated range," then pressures in the acceleration cartridge can open this source gas to the master Venturi's jet for additional total flow to the patient. Time delays are from about a second into inhalation to nearly immediately during inhalation for gradual and rapid acceleration settings, respectively. During the expiratory phase, pressure in the flow acceleration system falls rapidly as gases vent out the master Venturi jet into the breathing circuit. Flows of up to 100 L/min against a back pressure of over 20 cm H_2O can be obtained.

The *expiratory termination cartridge* in conjunction with the *expiratory timer control* function in a fashion similar to that of the expiratory timer in the Mark 7. During inhalation, gases from the ball valve of the Mark 1 feed the *apneustic flow circuit manifold*, which in turn charges the expiratory termination cartridge. During exhalation, pressure in the cartridge drops gradually as it leaks its gas through the expiratory time control (needle valve). When pressure in the cartridge is low enough, its spring opens a line from source gas. The line from source gas feeds the jet of the *sensing/servoing Venturi*, creating a momentary flow through the jet and a corresponding negative pressure near the jet. It is this negative pressure that is sensed by the Mark 1 by its *sensing port* that triggers inhalation automatically. When inhalation begins, the expiratory termination cartridge is once again charged, closing off the line from source gas to the sensing/servoing Venturi. If the needle valve in the expiratory timer control is very open, then the leak it creates will cause a *short* expiratory time and vice versa. The patient may interrupt and shorten the preset expiratory time whenever he creates sufficient negative pressure in the Mark 1 first.

A flow of gas during the expiratory phase is available with the Therapybird for powering a PEEP Venturi, NEEP Venturi, or any other device in the patient circuit.

The *expiratory flow gradient delay cartridge* functions in a similar fashion to the expiratory timer cartridge in that it is charged during inhalation and may be open during exhalation. The *expiratory flow gradient delay control* determines how fast from end inhalation that the expiratory flow is available to the *expiratory gradient service socket*. The delay controls adjust the leak from the delay cartridge into the breathing circuit. Once the leak is sufficient to allow the cartridge spring to open a line from source gas, then flow rate out the socket is set by the *expiratory flow gradient control* (needle valve). When this control is wide open, maximal expiratory gas flow will drive the devices attached and vice versa.

The *lockout cartridge* in conjunction with the *lockout time control* comprise a maximum inspiratory time safety system. If inspiratory time ever lasts long enough (usually 10 seconds) to allow gas pressure across the lock-out time control (needle valve), the diaphragm in the cartridge will push its plunger to a closed position, thus stopping flow to the *inspiratory service socket*. Pressure and flow from the inspiratory service socket leads to the nebulizer and exhalation valve in the patient's breathing circuit. When this line is closed, the exhalation valve opens, and the patient is allowed to exhale. If, due to other malfunctions, there continues to be gas flow to the master Venturi, the spontaneously breathing patient can inhale from these gases and exhale out the exhalation valve. If all gas flow has stopped (mechanical expiration with a lockout condition), the patient can draw ambient gases in through the ambient inlet filter by way of the *accessory entrainment gate* and master Venturi.

An *overpressure governor* near the breathing circuit connection provides a safety pressure relief. It is usually set to open at 65 cm H_2O with an option of 100 cm H_2O available.

THE BIRD MARK 2

The Mark 2 (Fig. 9-37) consists of two pneumatic cartridges that provide timing of the inspiratory delivery of source gas and timing of how long the absence of that flow exists. It provides a *timed flow of 50 psig gas* and a timed lack of gas flow by adjusting two controls. A third control then adjusts the *actual flow rate* during the inspiratory (flow) phase. Fig. 9-38 provides a flow diagram for the Mark 2. The Mark 2 source gas enters the unit and divides into two branches. The left inlet branch, A, goes to a chamber that is sealed by an O-ring. The other branch, B, supplies a needle valve. The needle valve adjusts the quantity of gas that can pass into the chamber on right side of the *upper* pneumatic cartridge. Once sufficient gas has leaked into the cartridge, its diaphragm bows to the left, depressing the spring and plunger over to the left. As the plunger moves to the left, gas is allowed to flow through the left branch, A, to the flow rate control. This cartridge acts as the *expiratory timer* of the Mark 2. It adjusts how much time passes until inspiratory gas flow *starts*. Once gas is flowing around the shaft into the flow rate control, it branches, C, just before the flow control to supply another needle valve. This needle valve also adjusts a leak of gas into another diaphragm chamber. Once enough gas has leaked into the left-hand side of the *bottom* cartridge, the spring and plunger are pushed to the right. As this occurs, the gas from the upper cartridge is allowed to escape out a *dump port*, stopping the flow of gas for inspiration. This control acts

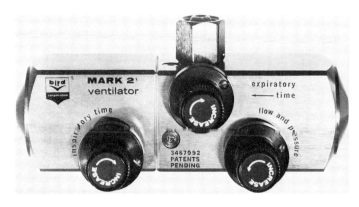

Fig. 9-37. Bird Mark 2 ventilator. (Courtesy Bird Corp., Palm Springs, Calif.)

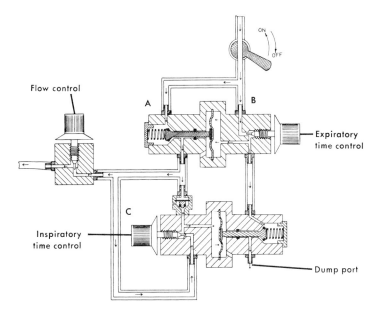

Fig. 9-38. Flow diagram for Bird Mark 2 ventilator. (Courtesy Bird Corp., Palm Springs, Calif.)

as the *inspiratory time control* mechanism of the Mark 2 and adjusts how long inspiratory flow lasts. The Mark 2 can be used for a variety of things, although one of the unit's main uses has been to power a Venturi to compress a ventilatory bag for anesthesia. The basic design of the Mark 2 is also incorporated into the structure of the Babybird.

THE BABYBIRD

The Babybird[12,13] (Fig. 9-39) is a time-cycled, time-limited, constant-flow pediatric ventilator. Because inspiratory time and flow are both constant, volume delivery can also be constant. A pressure relief system can create a pressure plateau or hold during inhalation until time limiting occurs. Volume delivered, then, is determined by the length of inspiratory time, the amount of pressure limit set, and the patient's resistance and compliance parameters. The device is generally used as an IMV unit

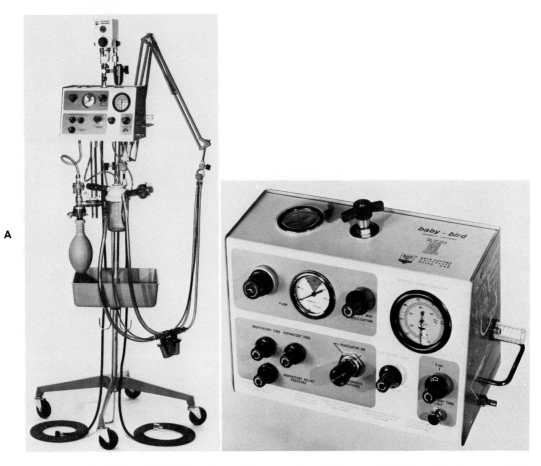

Fig. 9-39. A, Babybird ventilator. **B,** Its control panel. (Courtesy Bird Corp., Palm Springs, Calif.)

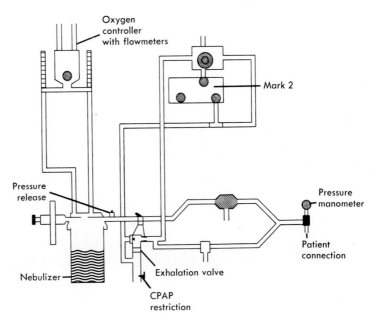

Fig. 9-40. Original Babybird design. (Modified from Kirby, R. R., et al.: Anesth. Analg. **50:**533, 1971.)

(ventilator on mode) with or without CPAP or for CPAP alone (spontaneous breathing mode).

The Babybird was designed originally[13] from a (1) Mark 2, (2) an adjustable system-pressure release, (3) a 500 cc nebulizer, (4) a Bird Blender, (5) two flow-meters, (6) an exhalation valve mechanism, and (7) a CPAP restriction (Fig. 9-40). The unit has two separate modes for ventilatory support: (1) *ventilator on* setting and (2) the *spontaneous breathing* mode. The control ("ventilator on") mode provided a flow of gas for a timed inspiratory phase with the exhalation valve closed and then released the pressure on the valve during a timed exhalation. During the timed inspiratory gas flow period, the exhalation valve was occluded and held gas in the system; this allowed the gas coming in through the nebulizer to build up pressure. Pressurization of the system ended because the Mark 2 stopped inspiratory flow to the exhalation valve. Pressure could be limited to a specific level by a *pressure release* until the Mark 2 shut off flow to the exhalation valve.

The production unit (Fig. 9-41) acquired additional refinements, but the Mark 2 is the basic component of the unit, the Bird Blender supplies set oxygen percentages, and the 500 cc nebulizer is the entry point for gas flows through the circuit.

The Mark 2 provides the first pathway for gas flow in the Babybird. The gas flow from the Mark 2 on the inspiratory phase travels through the *compound lockout cartridge* to a *Venturi* (Fig. 9-41). The pressure that this Venturi will achieve is adjusted by a leak out of the *inspiratory relief pressure control.* A portion of the maximum flow to the Venturi is allowed to leak out, decreasing the pressure that it will exert on the exhalation diaphragm. The greater the leak to the Venturi, the lower the pressure that opposes continuous gas flow through the circuit. Therefore, when the Mark 2 establishes inhalation, it exerts pressure against the exhalation diaphragm. Once the gas pressure in the patient circuit has reached the value set by the Venturi and inspiratory relief, all but the excess pressure is held in the circuit, and a pressure plateau is generated until time ends the inspiratory phase of the Mark 2. A *time-limiting* mechanism (compound lockout cartridge) below the Mark 2 in the schematic (Fig. 9-41) provides a safety device so that if some malfunctions were to occur in the Mark 2, inhalation would end due to the action of this cartridge. Gas flows into the cartridge from the top through the small *duckbill check valve* during the expiratory phase. The *inspiratory interrupter switch* stops the flow into the cartridge when the Mark 2 establishes inhalation, and the gas in the cartridge then leaks out slowly through a needle valve, the *inspiratory time limit.* Once gas has leaked out of the cartridge completely and the diaphragm becomes straight up and down, the unit occludes flow to the Venturi by a line on the right side, stopping inhalation, and a line on the left side opens gas flow to an *audible alarm.* The higher the leak out of the cartridge, the shorter the time limit. The unit may be returned to operation by depressing the *reset button,* which will open the inspiratory interrupter switch so that the compound lockout cartridge can be recharged with gas.

The second pathway for gas flow in the unit is the continuous gas flow supplied to the 500 cc nebulizer, which then travels on to the patient. The *nebulizer control* directs this gas to either the jet of the nebulizer or simply routes it straight through the nebulizer. The *flow regulator* of the Babybird is simply a pressure-reducing valve that sets a pressure gradient across set-sized restrictions in the patient circuit. It

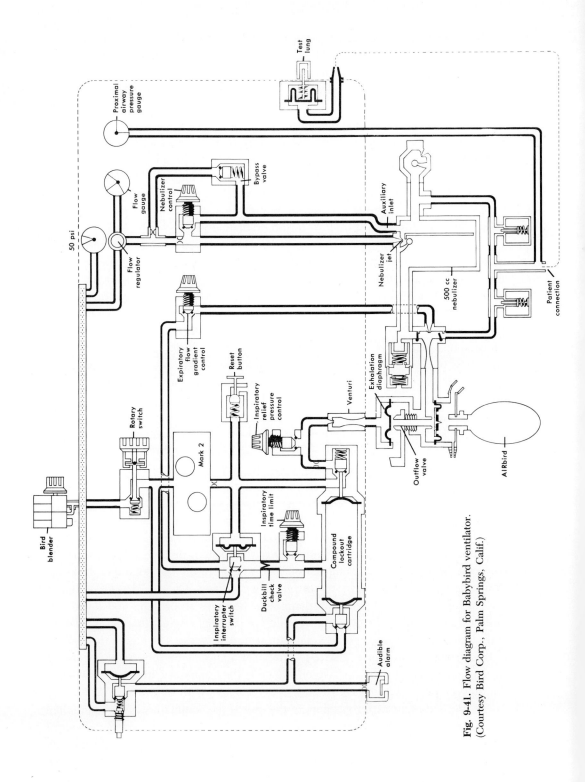

Fig. 9-41. Flow diagram for Babybird ventilator. (Courtesy Bird Corp., Palm Springs, Calif.)

functions in a manner similar to that of a Bourdon regulator. The unit provides control of gas flow by adjusting the pressure at the restrictions. This adjustment is read on the front of the machine on a *flow gauge* that actually measures pressure but is calibrated in liters per minute. The unit appears to be accurate in normal clinical use, since ventilation pressure does not approach the pressure supplied to the orifices, rendering the alteration in pressure gradient across the restrictions insignificant. Once this flow into the system has been established, the nebulizer control directs flow to either the jet of the nebulizer or into the nebulizer itself. Basically, on maximum nebulization, the majority of gas flow is directed to the jet of the nebulizer to produce the highest aerosol delivery possible, with the smaller portion bypassing this and going directly into the nebulizer. On minimum nebulization, the flow bypasses the jet almost exclusively and goes directly into the nebulizer. In both cases, or no matter what the control setting of the nebulizer is on, the *total flow* that is provided into the 500 cc nebulizer is the same as the flow that is set on the front of the machine and read on the flow gauge. The nebulizer control simply divides the flow between the two places. Therefore gas flow into the Babybird circuitry comes from (1) the nebulizer jet and (2) from an auxiliary port on the top of the 500 cc nebulizer. This gas then passes to the patient en route to the exhalation valve, where it exits.

The *expiratory flow gradient control* is provided simply to overcome resistance to gas flow through the exhalation valve. At reasonable flows, it is impossible without this control to get a CPAP pressure below approximately 2 to 4 cm H_2O. The expiratory negative pressure, then, provides a mechanism where during exhalation, the gas in the circuitry can be *entrained;* therefore pressure during exhalation or spontaneous breathing can be lowered to zero or below if desired. The inspiratory interrupter switch blocks the flow of gas to this Venturi during the inspiratory phase.

Intermittent manual inflation can be accomplished with the compression of the *Airbird* as well. Compression of the Airbird sends gas flow through a one-way valve to the 500 cc nebulizer and on to the patient through the inspiratory tubing. Then, when the bag is released, gas flows back from the patient through the expiratory side and out the exhalation valve. Normally, patient gas flow in the Babybird comes through either the nebulizer jet or directly through the nebulizer ports. When the Airbird is compressed, however, *additional gas* is sent through the one-way valve, through the nebulizer itself, and on to the patient. Therefore it should be remembered that gas flow still enters from the nebulizer jet and ports even as the bag is compressed if a flow has been set on the flow regulator.

The flow curve from the Babybird is a constant flow square wave. With pressure limiting utilized, the pressure curve initially inclines linearly and then plateaus at the pressure-limit level until time ends inhalation (Fig. 9-42), and then the curve drops to baseline pressure.

The *spontaneous breathing mode* sends a continuous flow of gas through the circuit. As this flow meets resistance in the exhalation valve, a CPAP effect is encountered. The level of CPAP desired is adjusted by a red-handled retard mechanism. The retard simply adjusts the size of the restriction through which expiratory gas flow passes. This makes the CPAP system flow dependent; in other words, at a set-size restriction on the expiratory outflow tract, increased flow through the system would also increase the expiratory resistance and cause an increased CPAP level.

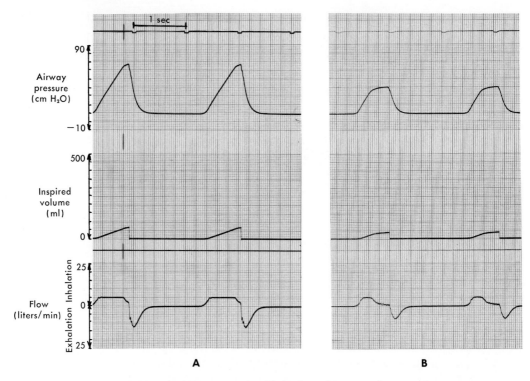

Fig. 9-42. Pressure, volume, and flow curves for Babybird ventilator using lung simulator. Lung compliance equals 1 ml/cm H_2O, and approximate resistance equals 50 cm H_2O/L/sec. Graph **A** shows unit volume limiting without pressure relief. Graph **B** shows same setting with pressure relief set for 40 cm H_2O.

THE IMVBIRD

The IMVbird[14] (Fig. 9-43) is a time-cycled, time-limited adult and pediatric ventilator capable of providing spontaneous breathing on patient demand between ventilator breaths. The device has no direct pressure-limiting device for terminating the inspiratory phase, nor does it have a volume limit per se. Tidal volume is determined primarily by inspiratory time and flow and by the patient's resistance and compliance characteristics. Mechanical respiratory rates from one breath every 3 minutes to thirty breaths per minute can be set.

Fig. 9-44 diagrams the pattern of gas flow through the ventilator. Source gas (generally from an oxygen controller) enters past the *on/off switch* to the *reduction regulator* (reducing valve) set for 45 psig. This gas then feeds the *source manifold*, the *auxiliary nebulization control*, and the *autophase reset*.

The IMVbird's operation can be divided into mechanical inspiratory phase, mechanical expiratory phase, and spontaneous breathing phases (which occur during mechanical exhalation).

During spontaneous breathing, pressure in the patient circuit is monitored through the *airway pressure monitoring socket*, one leg of which connects to the *demand flow accelerator servo*. When the demand flow servo senses a drop in pressure (patient effort), it opens a line connecting source gas to the center jet of the *master Venturi*, which in turn feeds the patient circuit with the demanded flow. The patient exhales normally through an exhalation valve in the breathing circuit.

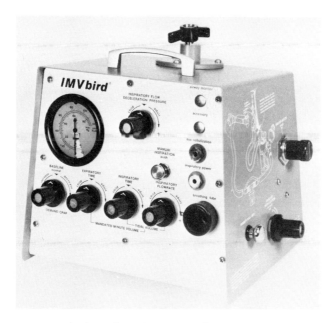

Fig. 9-43. IMVbird ventilator. (Courtesy Bird Corp., Palm Springs, Calif.)

During *mechanical* inhalation and exhalation, several circuits of pneumatic cartridges and controls are utilized. The *starting autophase cartridge* is programmed to allow gas flow through the cartridge into a timing circuit for about a second when source gas is initially turned on. This charges the circuit containing the *master cartridge, inspiratory time control*, and *balance reservoir*, as well as the *expiratory time control*. The timers (needle valves) then servo the master cartridge to start and stop the inspiratory phase. When first charged, the autophase cartridge starts the ventilator in the expiratory phase by charging the master cartridge through the balance reservoir. This closes the normally open master cartridge and stops all flow to the inspiratory flow circuitry. This initial charge of gas also pressurizes the expiratory timer through the *expiratory time accumulator*. The expiratory time control adjusts a bleed out of the expiratory time circuit, which slowly relieves pressure on the master cartridge's diaphragm and eventually allows the cartridge to open, starting inhalation (mechanical). This inspiratory time control now regulates gas pressure in the reverse direction, slowly *building* pressure against the master cartridge, eventually closing it, which starts mechanical exhalation again.

Inspiratory flow from the master cartridge feeds several systems. The *lockout time control* and *lockout cartridge* provide for a maximum allowable inspiratory time in a similar fashion to that described for the Therapybird. The *inspiratory service socket* feeds the nebulizer and exhalation valve in the patient breathing circuit during the inspiratory phase (mechanical).

The *inspiratory flow rate* adjusts the flow of gas passing through it to the dual jet system of the *master Venturi*. It also meters gas flow to the *entrainment reservoir refill servo* system and the *entrainment reservoir*. The reservoir itself is fed by source gas (through the flow rate control) so that normally all gases leaving the master Venturi are of the same concentration. The *ambient inlet filter* allows for entrainment of ambient air by the Venturi should the entrainment reservoir refill servo be inade-

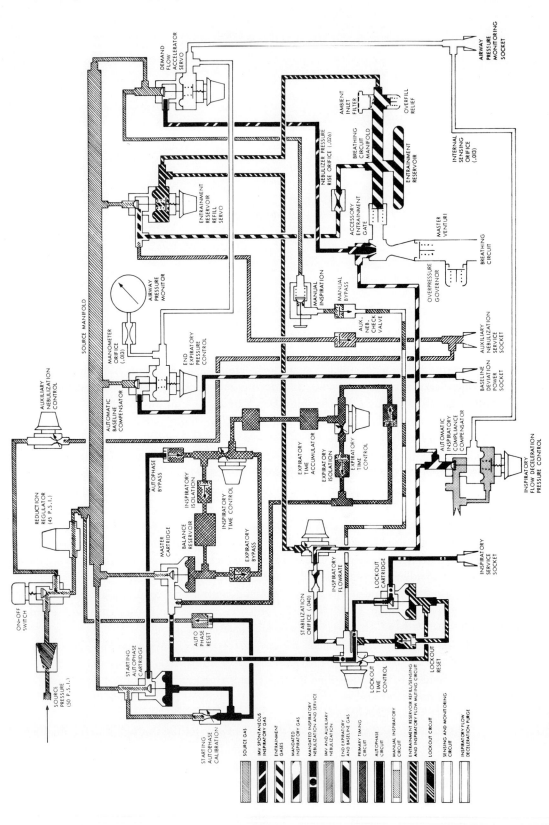

Fig. 9-44 Flow diagram for IMVbird. (Courtesy Bird Corp., Palm Springs, Calif.)

Table 9-1. Summary of Bird ventilator characteristics

Model	Pneumatic powered	Pressure limited	Time limited	Patient-cycled on	Time-cycled on	NEEP available	PEEP available	Pressure relief	Accelerated flow available	IMV system	Apneustic flowtime	Lockout system	Air-Mix mode	100% source mode
Mark 1	X	X		X									X	
Mark 2	X	X	X		X									X
Mark 7	X	X		X	X								X	X
Mark 8	X	X		X	X	X	X						X	X
Mark 9	X	X		X	X	X	X						X	
Mark 10	X	X		X	X				X				X	
Mark 14	X	X		X	X				X				X	X
Babybird	X		X		X	X	X	X	X	X		X		X
Minibird	X	X		X				X					X	
Minibird II	X	X		X				X			X		X	X
Therapybird	X	X		X	X	X	X	X	X		X	X		X
IMVbird	X		X		X	X	X	X		X		X		X
New Mark 7	X	X		X	X	X		X					X	
New Mark 8	X	X		X	X	X	X	X					X	
Mark 7A	X	X	X	X	X	X	X	X			X		X	
Mark 8A	X	X	X	X	X	X	X	X			X		X	
Bird Ventilator	X	X	X	X	X	X	X	X	X		X		X	
Bird Ventilator with demand CPAP	X	X	X	X	X	X	X	X	X	X	X		X	

quate. It can also supply a source for spontaneous breathing should source gas fail or be absent.

During mechanical inspiration, the *inspiratory flow deceleration pressure control* senses pressure in the patient circuit by the *airway pressure monitoring socket*. As pressure rises, the deceleration control opens the line leading to the dual jet of the master Venturi to the atmosphere, causing a decreasing jet pressure and, therefore, a decelerating flow to the patient. The inspiratory service socket is powered on inhalation by the master cartridge and, in turn, powers the nebulizer and exhalation valve in the patient circuit. The *auxiliary nebulizer control* (needle valve) adjusts constant flow to an auxiliary port on the nebulizer in the patient tubing system through the *auxiliary nebulization service socket*. This outlet is also fed by source gas when the entrainment reservoir refill servo is open.

The *manual inspiration* button can be depressed to cause source gas from it to feed the jets of the Venturi if desired.

The *end expiratory pressure control* adjusts the amount of available gas flow through the *baseline deviation power socket* to which a NEEP or PEEP Venturi can be attached.

The maximum pressure obtainable with the ventilator is about 110 cm H_2O, above which the *overpressure governor* (relief valve) opens.

Since flows through the master Venturi can vary during mechanical inhalation depending on resistance met in the patient circuit, exact tidal volumes cannot be set. Rather, a *range of* available tidal volume is set by a combination of the set inspiratory time and range of potential flow rates set by the inspiratory flow rate control.

The characteristics of the Bird ventilators discussed in this chapter are summarized in Table 9-1.

REFERENCES

1. Specifications, Bird Mark 7 positive phase medical respirator, Form L714, Bird Corp., Palm Springs, Calif.
2. Instructions for operating the Mark 7 respirator, Mark 8 respirator, Mark 10 and Mark 14 ventilators, Form L716, Bird Corp., Palm Springs, Calif.
3. Specifications, Bird Mark 8 positive/negative phase medical respirator, Form L718, Bird Corp., Palm Springs, Calif.
4. Specifications for the visible Bird Mark 9 simplex positive/negative phase servo respirator, Form 9,101, 1966, Bird Space Technology, Palm Springs, Calif.
5. Specifications for the Bird Mark 10 and Mark 14 ventilators with automatic flow acceleration, Form 722, 1971, Bird Corporation, Palm Springs, Calif.
6. Instructions, Bird Mark 10 automatic/cycling leak compensating respirator, Form 10,201, 1965, Bird Corp., Palm Springs, Calif.
7. Specifications for Bird Mark 6 minute volume ventilator, Form 6.1, 1971, Bird Corp., Palm Springs, Calif.
8. Understanding the Bird Mark 1 sequencing servo, Form L847, 1974, Bird Corp., Palm Springs, Calif.
9. Therapybird, Form L873, Bird Corp., Palm Springs, Calif.
10. Understanding the Minibird II with the Bird apneustic flowtime, Form L856, 1974, Bird Corp., Palm Springs, Calif.
11. Understanding the Therapybird, Form L886, 1975, Bird Corp., Palm Springs, Calif.
12. Babybird Ventilator Specifications, Form L795, 1974, Bird Corp., Palm Springs, Calif.
13. Kirby, R. R., et al.: A new pediatric volume ventilator, Anesth. Analg. (Cleve.) **50:**533, 1971.
14. Understanding the IMVbird, Form L876, 1975, Bird Corp., Palm Springs, Calif.

10 Bennett respirators

THERAPY MODELS

The therapy models of Bennett ventilators[1] are pneumatically powered, pressure limited at low terminal flow, and patient cycled (assistor). They have a relatively low pressure capability and cannot be automatically cycled on.

The two basic components of the various models of Bennett pressure-limited ventilators are similar. Each will be presented independently and then tied together in the operation of the basic therapy units.

The *diluter regulator* is the unit responsible for much of the operational characteristics of the Bennett units. It is functionally an *adjustable reducing valve* (Fig. 10-1). The black knob on the face of a Bennett adjusts spring tension against the right side of a diaphragm while gas pressure equalizes the spring tension on the left side, A. If gas pressure drops on the left, the spring pushes the diaphragm to the left, causing the *poppet assembly* to pivot, opening the valve gate, B. When the valve gate opens, source gas is allowed to enter the diluter regulator and will continue to enter until the pressure on the left of the diaphragm again equals the spring tension and returns the diaphragm to a straight up-and-down position. When the diaphragm is straight, the poppet assembly closes, and no source gas enters the diluter regulator. From the diluter regulator gas passes through to the Bennett valve.

Gas first enters the top of the *Bennett valve* (Fig. 10-2), where it is exposed to the

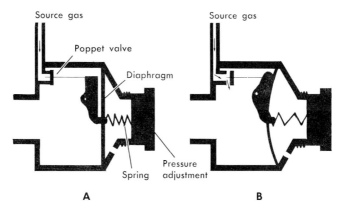

Fig. 10-1. Bennett diluter regulator. **A,** Pressure equals spring tension. **B,** Pressure is below spring tension.

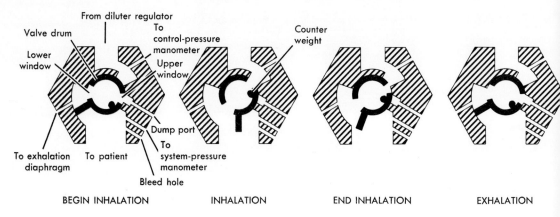

Fig. 10-2. Bennett valve.

valve drum. The drum itself is a hollow cylinder closed at both ends, and there are two *windows* cut into its sides. One window is located on the *upper* side and the other is on the *lower* side. When the valve is rotated to the open position (inhalation), gas can flow from the top of the valve through the drum and out the bottom. When the valve is rotated closed (exhalation), gas is blocked from entering the valve, and it is held above the valve drum.

The *dump port* serves to allow gas from within the drum to dump to atmospheric pressure (exhalation). In the Bennett valve there are also two manometer ports; one is for *control* pressure from the diluter regulator, and the second pressure gauge monitors the pressure in the *patient* circuit. The bleed hole is there simply to allow a *small leak* out so that when the valve opens, it does not recoil backward and start to flutter.[2]

The operation of the Bennett valve also requires a *drum vane.* This vane sets up a barrier between atmospheric pressure and circuit pressure. When the patient starts to take a breath, volume reduction in the tubing circuitry below the valve causes a subatmospheric pressure. When the pressure gradient across the valve is about 0.5 cm H_2O pressure, the gradient's force will rotate the valve counterclockwise (begin inhalation). Once the valve has rotated sufficiently so that the upper drum window communicates with the inflow tract from the diluter regulator, gas flows through the center of the Bennett valve drum (inhalation). A small flow of gas out of the valve travels out the exhalation valve line and inflates an exhalation *diaphragm* so that gas does not escape through the exhalation port of the tubing circuit during the inspiratory phase. Gas also flows on through the Bennett valve, holding the valve in its far counterclockwise position. As pressure builds up in the patient tubing, flow continually *drops* because of the reduced pressure gradient between the pressure set in the diluter-regulator and the patient's circuit pressure. This reduced flow against the vane allows the *counterweight* (a pin set off center) to pull the valve toward the closed (clockwise) position due to the force of gravity. Once the valve has a flow through it of approximately 1 to 3 L/min, gravity swings the valve shut.[3] At that point, the exhalation valve line is communicated with the center of the Bennett valve and opens to the dump port, so that its gas empties to atmospheric pressure.

Next, the function of the diluter regulator and the Bennett valve are discussed in

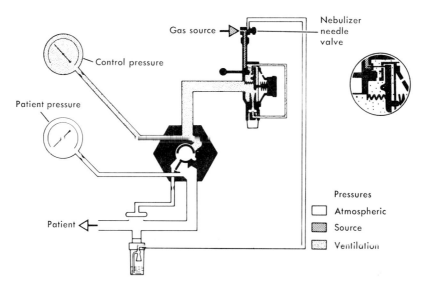

Fig. 10-3. Therapy unit connected to source pressure. (Courtesy Bennett Respiration Products, Inc., Santa Monica, Calif.)

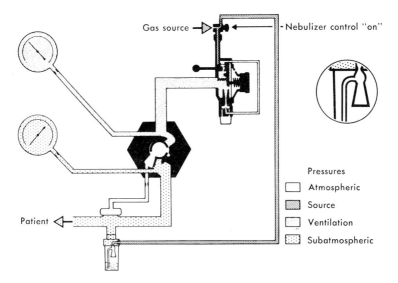

Fig. 10-4. Therapy unit at begin inhalation. (Courtesy Bennett Respiration Products, Inc., Santa Monica, Calif.)

operation together as seen in the therapy models (Fig. 10-3). The *nebulization control* is actually a *needle valve*. A line of source gas goes directly to it, and when it is on, flow to the nebulizer is continuous throughout the ventilatory cycle. Once the Bennett is connected to source pressure, gas flows to the nebulization control and the diluter regulator. Flow to the diluter regulator provides gas at ventilation pressure to the upper side of the Bennett valve. This pressure is monitored on the *control pressure* manometer. Inhalation begins as the patient starts to inhale through the circuit, and gas is removed from the tubing leading to the valve (Fig. 10-4). The

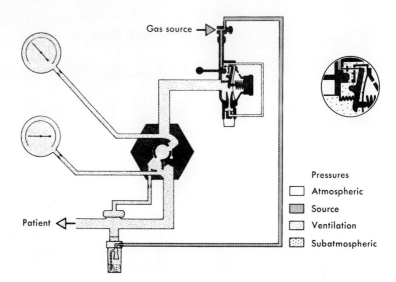

Fig. 10-5. Therapy unit at initial inhalation. (Courtesy Bennett Respiration Products, Inc., Santa Monica, Calif.)

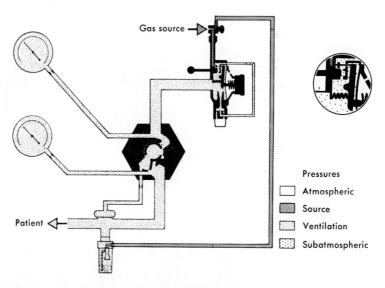

Fig. 10-6. Therapy unit at terminal inhalation. (Courtesy Bennett Respiration Products, Inc., Santa Monica, Calif.)

resultant negative pressure causes a pressure gradient from left to right across the lower drum, and the valve rotates open. Once the valve is in the open position (Fig. 10-5), gas flows from the diluter regulator, and the poppet valve opens to provide flow to the Bennett valve. The Bennett valve is held completely open by the force of forward gas flow against the left side of the drum vane. During *inhalation,* as pressure within the patient's system starts to increase, the pressure gradient between ventilation pressure and the pressure in the circuit drops, causing flow through the Bennett valve to drop also. Near the *end of inhalation* (Fig. 10-6), once this flow has dropped to approximately 1 to 3 L/min against the lower drum vane, a counterweight

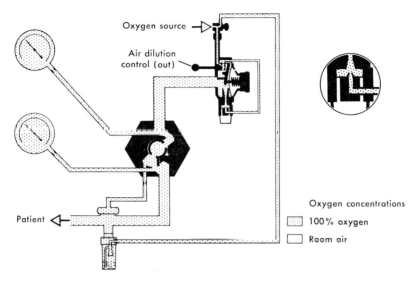

Fig. 10-7. Therapy unit using 100% oxygen. (Courtesy Bennett Respiration Products, Inc., Santa Monica, Calif.)

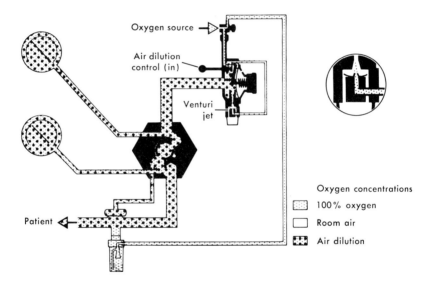

Fig. 10-8. Therapy unit using air dilution. (Courtesy Bennett Respiration Products, Inc., Santa Monica, Calif.)

in the Bennett valve allows gravity to rotate the valve shut, starting *exhalation.* Once the valve is closed, the exhalation valve is allowed to dump, and gas from the patient circuit flows out into the room.

The diluter regulator provides for either *air-diluted source gas* or *100% source gas* to be delivered to the patient circuit. With the *air dilution control* pulled *out* (Fig. 10-7), source gas takes the path of least resistance and enters the diluter regulator directly. Therefore the gas supplying pressure to the left side of the diaphragm of the diluter regulator is *100%* source gas. When the control is pushed *in*, on *air dilution* (Fig. 10-8), gas flow is directed through a line to the *jet of the Venturi.* The Venturi

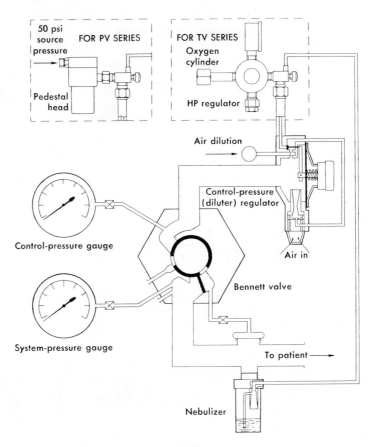

Fig. 10-9. Flow diagram for Therapy model Bennett ventilator. Bennett valve is shown from *behind* device. (Courtesy Bennett Respiration Products, Inc., Santa Monica, Calif.)

entrains room air and thus provides a flow of mixed air and source gas into the diluter regulator. Functionally, flow characteristics are the same for both 100% and air dilution settings.

The units described up to this point have been the standard Bennett *Therapy* units. These units are divided into two groups. The *PV* (pedestal ventilator) series (Fig. 10-9) utilizes a pedestal mount that is supplied by source gas from a *wall outlet.* The *TV* (tank ventilator) units (Fig. 10-9) are mounted on *cylinders* and have a *reducing valve* to lower the pressure to 50 psi and then supply gas to the unit itself. The *TV-2P* (Fig. 10-10, *A*) is mechanically the same unit as the *PV-3P* (Fig. 10-10, *B*), except that it is cylinder mounted. The *TV-4* (Fig. 10-10, *C*) is provided with air dilution *only* (control removed). Since the Bennett acts functionally as a *demand valve* on both the air dilution and 100% settings (Fig. 10-11), the *flow curve* tends to *increase sharply* at first and then gradually *taper* as it reaches the peak pressure point. A demand valve *automatically* adjusts flow, as a reducing valve does, to increase pressure in the system quickly. Therefore it would increase flow into a large-volume system or in response to patient demand.

THE PR-2

The Bennett PR-2[4] ventilator (Fig. 10-12) is pneumatically powered, pressure limited at low terminal flow, time limited, patient cycled (assistor), and time cycled

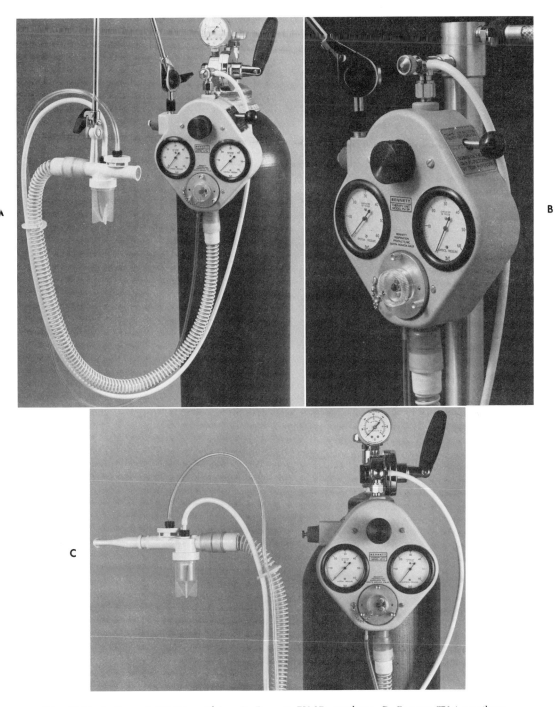

Fig. 10-10. A, Bennett TV-2P ventilator. **B,** Bennett PV-3P ventilator. **C,** Bennett TV-4 ventilator. (Courtesy Bennett Respiration Products, Inc., Santa Monica, Calif.)

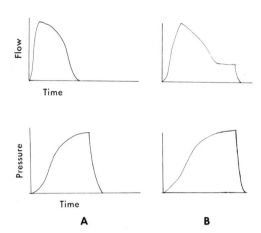

Fig. 10-11. Bennett flow and pressure curves, **A,** without using nebulizer, and **B,** when nebulizer is on.

(controller). It has controls for adjusting sensitivity, peak flow, independent inspiratory and expiratory nebulizer gas flows, negative expiratory pressure, terminal flow for minor leak compensation, and an automatic rate with adjustable I:E ratios. Either 100% source gas or air-diluted source gas can be delivered through the device.

The Bennett PR-2 contains a diluter regulator and Bennett valve, which act principally the same as those found in the therapy units. There are structural changes in both of these devices to accommodate other controls, which will be discussed separately.

The *pressure switch* is designed to allow a flow of gas from the 50 psig source inlet to one group of *controls* when the machine is in the *inspiratory* phase and to a different group of controls when the machine is in the *expiratory* phase (Fig. 10-13).[2] When the machine is in the expiratory phase, all three compartments of the pressure switch (Fig. 10-13) are charged with 50 psig source gas, and the spring around a plunger pushes it to the *left, occluding* the outflow tract to the *inspiratory controls.* At the same time, the outflow tract to the *expiratory controls* is open, making gas accessible to them. When inhalation starts and the Bennett valve opens, gas flow from the Bennett valve inflates the diaphragm at the top to the pressure switch. The inflated diaphragm moves the small lever on top of the pressure switch up, which allows the gas to escape in the center compartment. Now there is 50 psig gas on the left side of the left diaphragm with well below 50 psig on the right side of it because the center compartment has been emptied. Since there is a restriction on the inflow tract to the center compartment, the gas pressure remains well below 50 psig. This pressure gradient across the diaphragm moves the plunger to the *right,* compressing the spring. As a result, the inspiratory controls are opened and the expiratory ones are occluded. Once inhalation has ended, the Bennett valve closes, the balloon in the switch collapses, and the lever falls, allowing the center compartment to repressurize. This places equal pressure on both sides of the diaphragm, and the spring pushes the plunger to the left, occluding the outflow tract to inspiratory controls and opening the outflow tract to the expiratory controls. In the body of the pressure switch, the expiratory and inspiratory *nebulization* controls are located. They work only on their respective phase of the ventilatory cycle, since gas flow is being supplied to them only on the appropriate phase of ventilation by the pressure switch. Each nebulizer control is a needle valve that adjusts the quantity of gas going to the nebulizer jet. The expiratory nebulization control is generally opened just *slightly* to provide an accumulation of a modest quantity of aerosol in the circuitry between breaths. Inspiratory nebulization is usually adjusted to deliver a given quantity of medication or solution in the amount of time desired

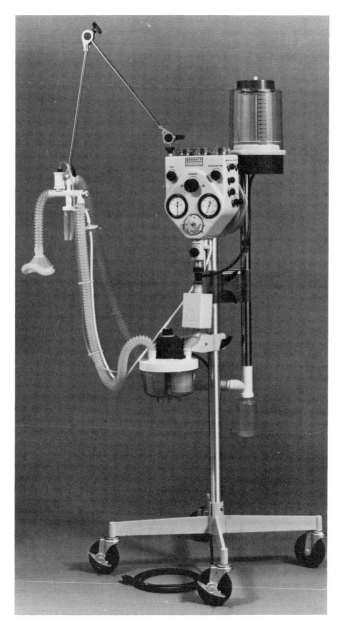

Fig. 10-12. Bennett PR-2 ventilator. (Courtesy Bennett Respiration Products, Inc., Santa Monica, Calif.)

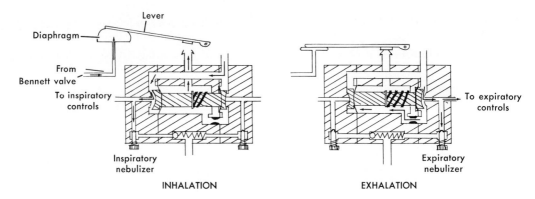

Fig. 10-13. PR-2 pressure switch. (Courtesy Bennett Respiration Products, Inc., Santa Monica, Calif.)

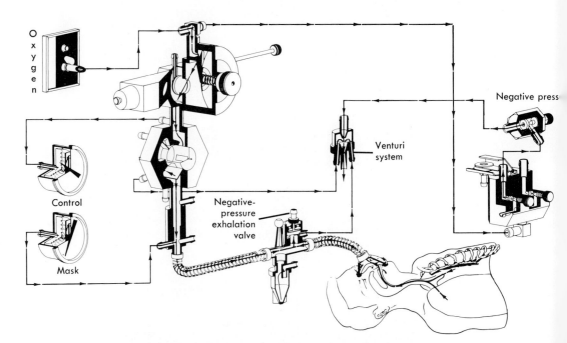

Fig. 10-14. Functional diagram of negative pressure control system of PR-2 ventilator during exhalation. (Courtesy Bennett Respiration Products, Inc., Santa Monica, Calif.)

On the expiratory side of the pressure switch, another line comes off the top and supplies a needle valve that controls a flow of 50 psig source gas during the expiratory phase. This needle valve adjusts the flow of gas to the *jet of a Venturi* inside the Bennett, which attempts to *entrain* gas from two lines. One line goes to the exhalation manifold and tends to generate a *negative pressure* in the circuit itself (Fig. 10-14). The other line communicates above the upper side of the *lower* drum vane of the Bennett valve in an attempt to *equalize* negative pressure applied through the circuitry to the lower side of the drum vane. This double line accomplishes two things: (1) it prevents the negative expiratory pressure applied to the circuitry from prematurely cycling the ventilator to the inspiratory phase and (2) it equalizes the

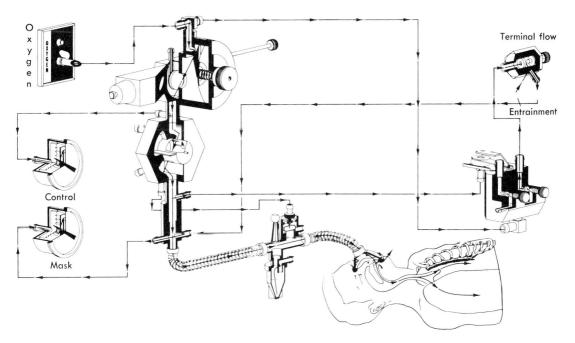

Fig. 10-15. Functional diagram for PR-2's terminal flow control during inhalation. (Courtesy Bennett Respiration Products, Inc., Santa Monica, Calif.)

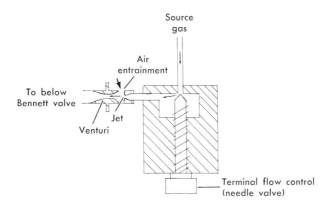

Fig. 10-16. Terminal flow control.

pressure across the drum vane exerted by the negative pressure control to retain the necessary 0.5 cm H_2O pressure drop to turn the Bennett valve to the *on* position without further sensitivity adjustment.

From the inspiratory side of the pressure switch is a line traveling to the *terminal flow control*. The terminal flow control is a simple needle valve supplied with source gas only on the *inspiratory* phase. This flow of gas passes to the jet of a small *Venturi* (Fig. 10-15), which adds an *additional flow of diluted* gas below the Bennett valve. This added flow is necessary because of the increased quantity of leaks that exist in the PR-2 in comparison to the therapy units. A minor leak exists in the PR-2's internal circuitry, and when the pressure is set *above* 20 to 25 cm H_2O pressure, the terminal flow control can offset this or other minor leaks in the patient circuit and allow the flow past the Bennett valve to decrease to a level low enough so that the valve can close. Fig. 10-16 shows a functional diagram of the terminal flow control. It should also be noted that terminal flow does add air-diluted source gas that will be a factor when the oxygen percentage control is on the 100% source setting.

The balance of the controls on the PR-2 require timing accumulators. The *accumulators* are supplied with gas from the *low-pressure reducing valve*, which reduces 50 psig incoming source gas to 60 cm H_2O (Fig. 10-17). The 60 cm H_2O pressure gas supplies not only the accumulators but also the remainder of the controls working in conjunction with the accumulators.[5] The accumulators are actually *pneumatic timing mechanisms* that, when inflated (Fig. 10-18), cause the piston shaft to move *down*. There are three *grooves* in the shaft of the accumulators. When the accumulators are in the *up* position, the odd-numbered ports (*1, 3,* and *5*) are *open*,

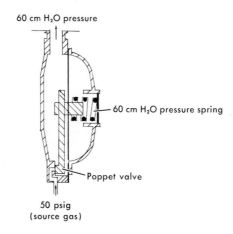

Fig. 10-17. Low-pressure reducing valve. (Courtesy Bennett Respiration Products, Inc., Santa Monica, Calif.)

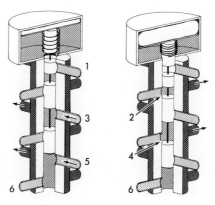

Fig. 10-18. Function of accumulator used as timing mechanism. (Courtesy Bennett Respiration Products, Inc., Santa Monica, Calif.)

and gas can flow on through around the grooves. When the accumulator reaches the *bottom*, the odd-numbered ports are occluded, and the even-numbered ports (*2* and *4*) are *opened* so that gas can pass through them. Port *6* on all of the accumulators is the *inflating* port. As gas travels up the center, hollow portion of the shaft, it inflates the balloon and pushes the plunger down.

There are three accumulators on the PR series ventilators. The left accumulator is considered no. *1*, the middle one no. *2*, and the right one no. *3*.

The *master accumulator* (no. *2*) is in the center, and it receives gas flow to its inflation port (no. *6*) from a line originating directly *below* the Bennett valve; the center accumulator *always* moves down (inflated) on inhalation. This center accumulator also establishes *phasing* of inhalation to exhalation, on which the other accumulators can base their function.

The *left* accumulator (no. *1*) must be phased to function during *exhalation*, and the *right* accumulator (no. *3*) must be phased to work during *inhalation*. To accomplish this, lines (Fig. 10-19) from the low-pressure regulator pass through the rate

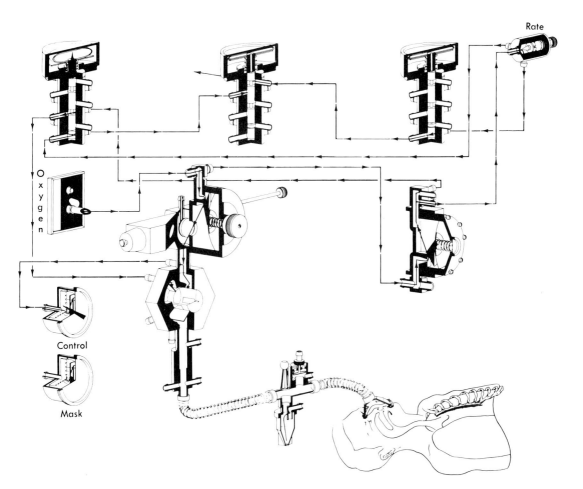

Fig. 10-19. Functional diagram of the rate control at begin inhalation. (Courtesy Bennett Respiration Products, Inc., Santa Monica, Calif.)

control to port 6 of both the right and left accumulators. The *rate control* is a needle
valve that adjusts the flow of gas out of it to port 6 of the right and left accumulators.
The gas entering port 6 of the right and left accumulators is directed to the middle
accumulator for phasing. The line from port 6 of the right accumulator is connected to
an odd-numbered port (no. *1* in diagram) of the center accumulator. The line from
port 6 of the left accumulator is attached to an even-numbered port (port *2* in
diagram) of the middle accumulator. Since the center accumulator is in the *up*
position in the expiratory phase, the even-numbered ports are blocked. The even-
numbered port, from which gas flow from port 6 of the left accumulator is connected,
is *blocked* and allows only one pathway for gas flow from the rate control to travel.
Thus, gas flows up the hollow shaft, inflates the balloon, and moves the piston of the
left accumulator downward. The flow of gas through port 6 of the right accumulator,
which is connected to port *1* of the center accumulator, can continue straight on
through and *escape* into the back of the machine. Therefore, in this instance, the

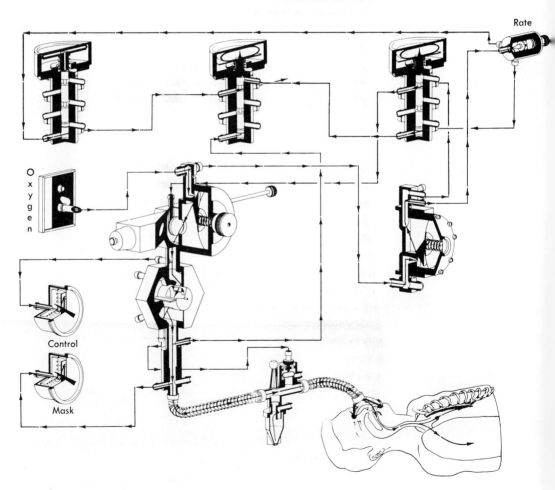

Fig. 10-20. Functional diagram of rate control at begin exhalation. (Courtesy Bennett Respiration
Products, Inc., Santa Monica, Calif.)

right accumulator does nothing and the left accumulator, moving down on exhalation, finally reaches the bottom. A second line coming from the low-pressure reducing valve passes through the even-numbered port (no. *4*). Once the left accumulator has reached the bottom, this second line's gas can flow through. This gas is supplied to a port above the *upper drum vane* of the Bennett valve. This flow then pushes the upper drum vane *downward*, rotating the valve counterclockwise into the *open position*, which causes gas from the diluter regulator to flow to the patient (inhalation). By adjusting gas flow to the left accumulator, the rate control adjusts *how quickly* it moves down and, therefore, the time that exhalation can last. Functionally, the left accumulator is the expiratory time accumulator and *time cycles* inhalation *on* when it reaches the bottom.

On inhalation, a flow of gas from below the Bennett valve travels to port 6 of the center accumulator and inflates it, moving its shaft down (Fig. 10-20). This *reverses* the ports that will be open. Now, the right accumulator's flow through port 6 is

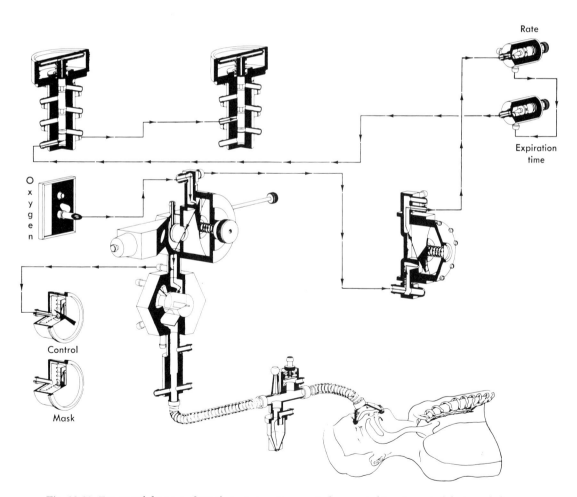

Fig. 10-21. Functional diagram of PR-2's expiratory time control connected to rate control during exhalation. (Courtesy Bennett Respiration Products, Inc., Santa Monica, Calif.)

blocked, since it is connected to an odd port (port *1*) of the center accumulator. The flow from port *6* of the left accumulator is open, and this accumulator is temporarily nonfunctional. Next, the right accumulator *3* starts to move down as its diaphragm is inflated. The speed at which accumulator *3* moves down is based on the amount of flow coming through the needle valve of the rate control. Once the diaphragm reaches the bottom, a line coming directly from the low-pressure reducing valve goes through an even port (no. *2* in the diagram). The flow passes through and inflates a *diaphragm* in the outflow tract of the diluter regulator. This *stops* flow out of the diluter regulator. With no flow to the Bennett valve, it swings shut, and exhalation occurs. Therefore the right accumulator moves down *only* on inhalation, lagging behind the center accumulator, making the right one the *time-limiting* accumulator. The Bennett has a built-in I:E ratio of 1:1.5. This is accomplished by adjusting the height of the accumulator shaft body and how far down the shafts have to travel. In other words, the left accumulator must travel one and a half times as far as the right accumulator does to reach the bottom position.

The *expiratory time control* is a needle valve (Fig. 10-21) placed in the line from the rate control to port *6* of the left accumulator. This control can decrease the

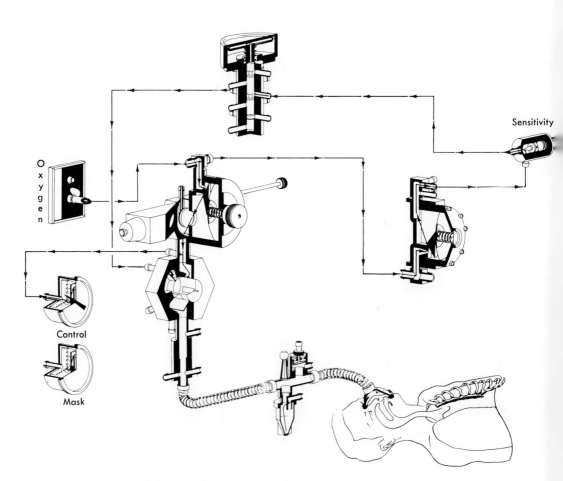

Fig. 10-22. Functional diagram of sensitivity control's operation during exhalation. (Courtesy Bennett Respiration Products, Inc., Santa Monica, Calif.)

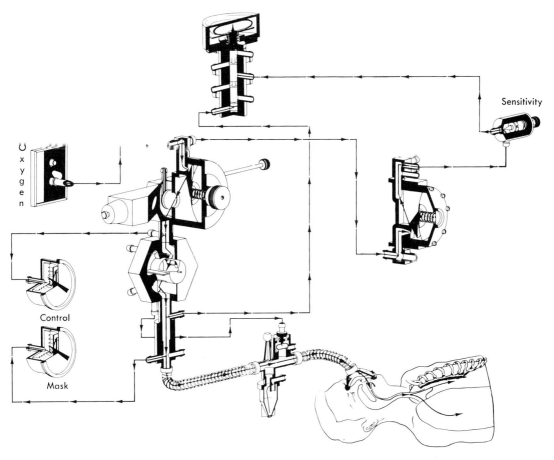

Fig. 10-23. Functional diagram of sensitivity control during inhalation. (Courtesy Bennett Respiration Products, Inc., Santa Monica, Calif.)

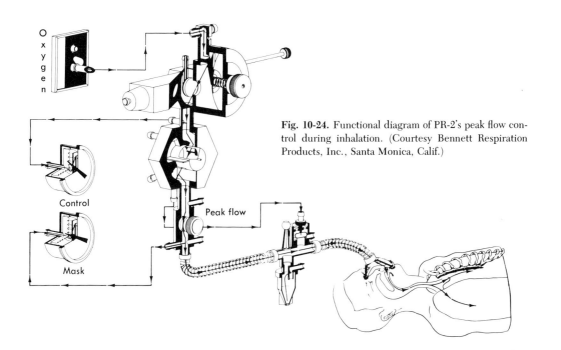

Fig. 10-24. Functional diagram of PR-2's peak flow control during inhalation. (Courtesy Bennett Respiration Products, Inc., Santa Monica, Calif.)

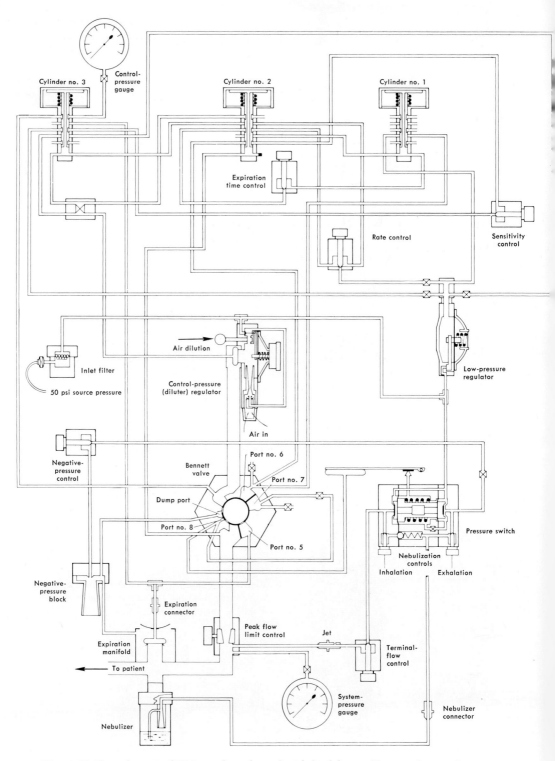

Fig. 10-25. Flow schematic of PR-2 ventilator shown from *behind* device. (Courtesy Bennett Respiration Products, Inc., Santa Monica, Calif.)

amount of gas flow even further when it is turned on, so that the accumulator's inflation occurs more slowly, making exhalation time *longer*. The control is a reverse *needle valve*, since turning it on makes the orifice progressively smaller and smaller.

The *sensitivity control* (Fig. 10-22) is also supplied with gas from the low-pressure reducing valve. This control is simply a needle valve with its line attached to an odd-numbered port of the center accumulator. During the expiratory phase, gas flow through the center accumulator travels to a port with an outflow restriction *above* the upper drum vane. The more the sensitivity needle valve is opened, the *higher* the flow is into the compartment above the upper drum vane. This higher flow tends to push the upper drum vane *downward*, rotating the valve slightly toward the inspiratory position. Thus *less effort* is required on the part of the patient to turn

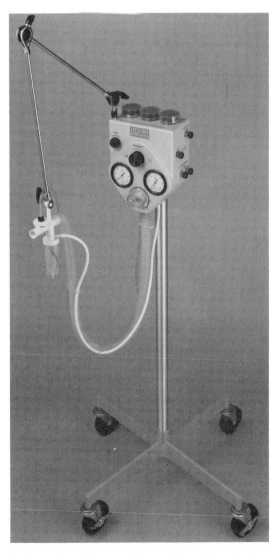

Fig. 10-26. Bennett PR-1 ventilator. (Courtesy Bennett Respiration Products, Inc., Santa Monica, Calif.)

the unit on. Once the Bennett valve opens (inhalation), the flow from below the Bennett valve drives the middle accumulator down and occludes the flow of gas from the sensitivity control (Fig. 10-23).

There is one other control on the PR-2, and it is not related to either the pressure switch or the low-pressure reducing valve. This is the *peak flow control*. The control is a *variable-size restriction* to gas flow out of the Bennett valve (Fig. 10-24). In its full-open position, *maximum* peak flow is available. In the full-closed position, the maximum flow out of the Bennett valve is decreased to about *15 L/min*. The peak flow control does not act functionally as a flow rate control, such as in the Bird Mark series ventilators, because it limits only the *maximum* flow that can be delivered from the unit.

Fig. 10-25 shows a flow schematic of the PR-2 with all controls connected. This diagram is shown from the *back* of the ventilator (mirror image).

THE PR-1

The Bennett PR-1[6] ventilator (Fig. 10-26) is pneumatically powered, pressure limited at low terminal flow, time limited, patient cycled (assistor), and time cycled (controller). It has controls for adjusting sensitivity, inspiratory and/or continuous nebulization, and an automatic rate at a preset I:E ratio. Either 100% source gas or air-diluted source gas can be delivered through the device.

The PR-1 is basically a PR-2 unit with some controls removed or modified. First, the PR-1 does not have an *expiratory time control* to prolong the expiratory phase of the ventilatory cycle during automatic cycling. Second, the PR-1 does not have a *peak flow control*. Third, there is *no negative pressure capability*. Fourth, there is *no terminal flow* control. The PR-1 pressure switch is slightly altered (Fig. 10-27) so that in place of an expiratory nebulizer, there is a *continuous nebulizer*. Functionally, the pressure switch and nebulizers work the same as the PR-2 except that the inspiratory nebulization is a *composite* of the continuous nebulizer and the inspiratory nebulizer flows, whereas in the PR-2, the nebulizer flow is *independently* controlled during inspiratory and expiratory phases. Fig. 10-28 shows the flow schematic for the PR-1 drawn from *behind* the ventilator.

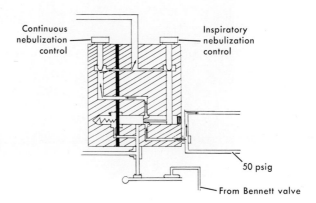

Continuous nebulization control

Inspiratory nebulization control

50 psig

From Bennett valve

Fig. 10-27. PR-1's pressure switch. (Courtesy Bennett Respiration Products, Inc., Santa Monica, Calif.)

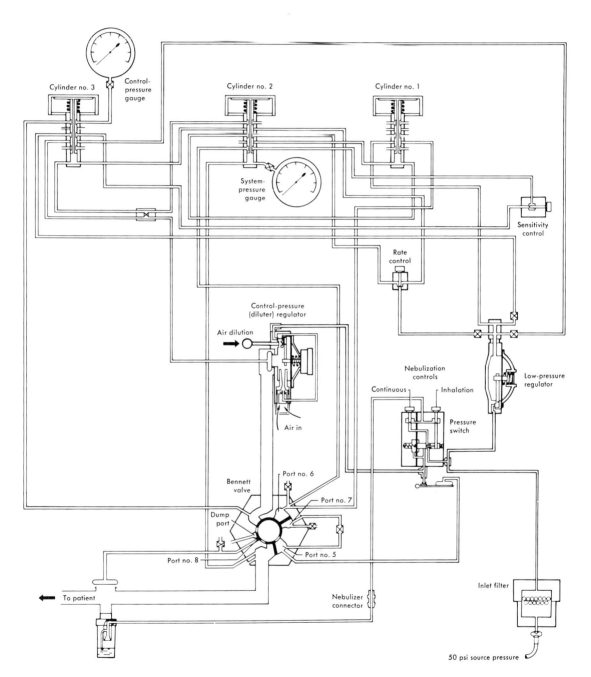

Fig. 10-28. Flow schematic for PR-1 ventilator shown from *behind* device. (Courtesy Bennett Respiration Products, Inc., Santa Monica, Calif.)

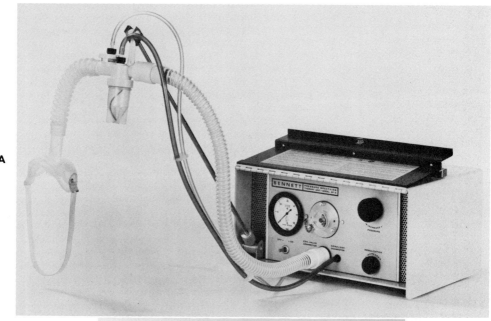

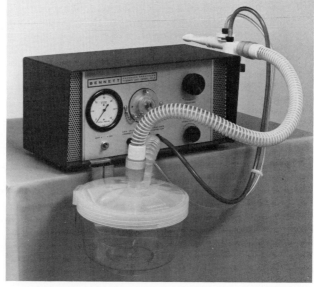

Fig. 10-29. A, Bennett AP-4. **B,** Bennett AP-5. Both units are air-compressor–driven ventilators. (Courtesy Bennett Respiration Products, Inc., Santa Monica, Calif.)

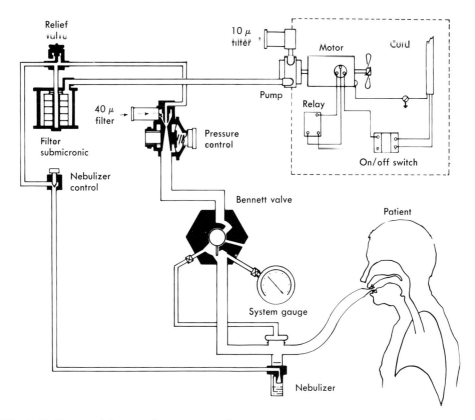

Fig. 10-30. Functional diagram of AP series ventilators. (Courtesy Bennett Respiration Products, Inc., Santa Monica, Calif.)

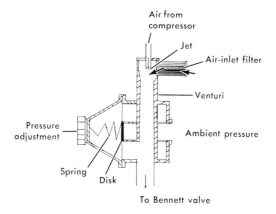

Fig. 10-31. Pressure control for AP series ventilators. (Courtesy Bennett Respiration Products, Inc., Santa Monica, Calif.)

THE AP SERIES

The Bennett AP series ventilators[7] (Fig. 10-29) are electrically powered, compressor driven, pressure limited at low terminal flow, and patient cycled (assistor). Continuous flow for nebulization can be adjusted.

The AP series provides a *compressor driven unit*, primarily for home use. As diagramed in Fig. 10-30, air from the compressor (pump) passes through a *filter* and then divides. Air flows to the jet of the Venturi in the *pressure control* and to a needle valve that acts as a nebulization control for the jet of the nebulizer. The jet of the Venturi entrains additional air through an intake filter (Fig. 10-31). In place of the diluter regulator, there is a *spring and disk release valve*. When the gas pressure in the system's control unit *exceeds* that of the spring tension, the pressure pushes the disk to the left, allowing the excess pressure to vent to *ambient pressure*. With all gas venting through the release valve, the Bennett valve rotates shut, starting exhalation. When the Bennett valve opens, gas flows from the control unit to the patient (Fig. 10-30). Other Bennett therapy units have peak flow and pressure poten-

Table 10-1. Summary of Bennett pressure-breathing therapy and respiration units

	AP-4, AP-5	PV-3P	TV-2P	TV-4	PR-1	PR-2
Table mounted	X					
Pedestal mounted	X	X			X	X
Cylinder mounted			X	X		
Pneumatic powered		X	X	X	X	X
Electric powered	X					
Time-cycled "on"					X	X
Time-limited "off"					X	X
Pressure/flow limited	X	X	X	X	X	X
Assistor	X	X	X	X	X	X
Controller					X	X
Inspiratory nebulizer					X	X
Expiratory nebulizer						X
Continuous nebulizer	X	X	X	X	X	
100% setting (source gas)		X	X		X	X
Air dilution		X	X	X	X	X
Compressed air	X					
Negative-pressure control						X
Terminal-flow control						X
Sensitivity control					X	X
Rate control					X	X
Expiratory-time control						X
Peak-flow control						X
3 L/min terminal flow	X	X	X	X		
1 L/min terminal flow					X	X
0 to 35 cm H_2O pressure range		X	X	X		
0 to 50 cm H_2O pressure range					X	X
Flow sensitive	X	X	X	X	X	X
0 to 30 cm H_2O	X					

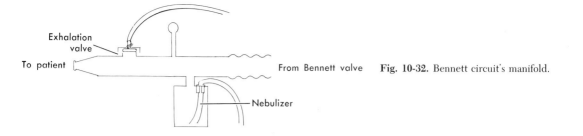

Exhalation valve

To patient

From Bennett valve

Nebulizer

Fig. 10-32. Bennett circuit's manifold.

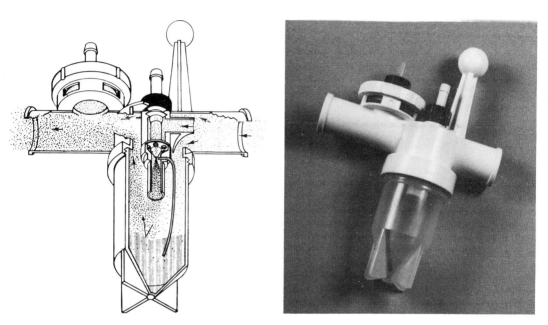

Fig. 10-33. Bennett Slip/stream nebulizer. (Drawing courtesy Bennett Respiration Products, Inc., Santa Monica, Calif.)

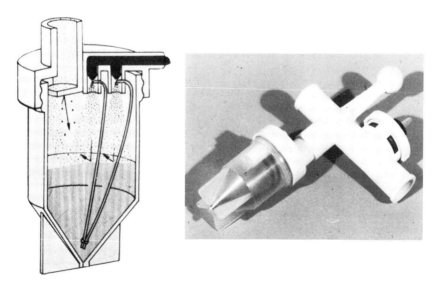

Fig. 10-34. Bennett Twin jet nebulizer. (Drawing courtesy Bennett Respiration Products, Inc., Santa Monica, Calif.)

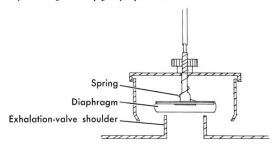

Spring

Diaphragm

Exhalation-valve shoulder

Fig. 10-35. Bennett retard exhalation valve.

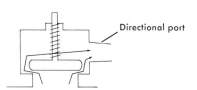

Directional port

Fig. 10-36. Bennett gas collector exhalation valve.

tials similar to those of the AP series. The *maximum* pressure potential is generally about *30 cm H₂O* pressure. The AP-4 and AP-5 are basically the same with the only difference being that the AP-4 has a support arm mounted in a carrying case with a cover, and the AP-5 does not. Functionally, the pressure and flow curves of the AP units are the same as in other Bennett units. Table 10-1 provides a summary of the characteristics of all the Bennnett units presented.

BENNETT CIRCUITS

The basic Bennett circuit is comprised of a *nebulizer* and *exhalation valve* (Fig. 10-32). The exhalation valve receives *ventilation-pressure* gas from the Bennett valve. The nebulizer receives source gas. Two types of nebulizers are available. The Bennett Slip/stream acts as a *mainstream* nebulizer (Fig. 10-33), and the Bennett Twin is a *sidestream* unit (Fig. 10-34).

The Bennett *retard exhalation valve* consists of a spring that is compressed as the diaphragm nut is tightened (Fig. 10-35). When the nut is loosened, the spring pushes the diaphragm *closer* to the shoulder of the exhalation valve, causing a *resistance* to expiratory gas flow.

The *gas collector exhalation valve* (Fig. 10-36) allows for measurement of expired gases through a single *directional port*.

The *tracheostomy circle* provides a flexible *minimum dead space circuit* (Fig. 10-37). On inhalation, gas passes through the inspiratory line to the patient, and on exhalation the exhaled gases and gas compressed in the circuit pass through the expiratory line and out the exhalation valve.

The *minimum dead space* (MDS) manifold is structured so that the exhalation valve is *on top* of the patient connection (Fig. 10-38). On exhalation, both the gas that is compressed within the circuit and exhaled gas from the patient exit directly above the patient connection. A gas collector or retard top can be used with the MDS unit.

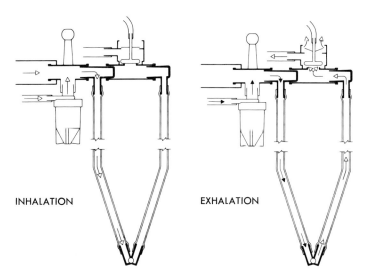

INHALATION   EXHALATION

Fig. 10-37. Bennett tracheostomy circle. (Courtesy Bennett Respiration Products, Inc., Santa Monica, Calif.)

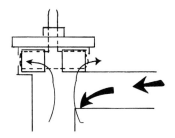

Fig. 10-38. Bennett minimum dead space (MDS) exhalation valve.

REFERENCES

1. Operating instructions, IPPB Therapy Unit Models TV-2P, PV-3P, and TV-4, Form 1008B, Santa Monica, Calif., 1969, Bennett Respiration Products, Inc.
2. Beven, R., Bennett Respiration Products, Inc.: Personal communication, 1974.
3. Persels, J. B., Bennett Respiration Products, Inc: Personal communication, 1974.
4. Operating instructions, Bennett PR-2 Respiration Unit, Form 2131H, Santa Monica, Calif., 1975, Bennett Respiration Products, Inc.
5. Gage, B., Bennett Respiration Products, Inc.: Personal communication, 1974.
6. Operating instructions, Bennett PR-1 Respiration Unit, Form 1693G, Santa Monica, Calif., 1975, Bennett Respiration Products, Inc.
7. Operating instructions, Pressure Breathing Therapy Unit Models AP-4, AP-4B, AP-5, AP-5B, Form 2768E, Santa Monica, Calif., 1972, Bennett Respiration Products, Inc.

11 Piston ventilators

THE MÖRCH VENTILATOR

The Mörch Ventilator (Fig. 11-1), produced in 1945 by Dr. E. Trier Mörch,[1] is an electrically powered, rotary-driven piston,[2] single-circuit, time-cycled, time- and volume-limited controller. Referring to Fig. 11-2, the *piston* pulls in air and oxygen on its return stroke (exhalation). As the *motor* rotates the piston into its forward stroke (inhalation), the piston moves gases from the cylinder into the patient system through a *humidifier* and exhalation valve. The ball in the exhalation valve (Fig. 11-3) is lifted by flow during inhalation occluding the exhalation port. When inspiratory flows cease, the ball falls, allowing exhalation by the patient to occur.

Mörch built this unit to be used with a tracheostomy tube system that was purposely cuffless, providing air leaks around the tube[3,4] (Fig. 11-4). That is, more

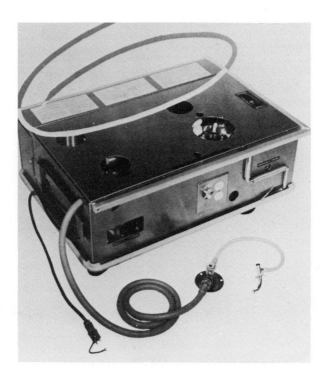

Fig. 11-1. Mörch Piston Ventilator. (Courtesy V. Mueller, Chicago, Ill.)

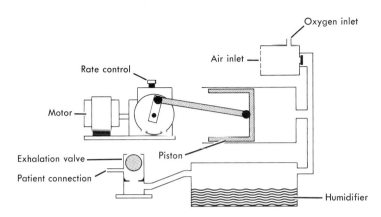

Fig. 11-2. Mörch Ventilator schematic. (Modified from Mushin, W. W., et al.: Automatic ventilation of the lungs, ed. 2, Philadelphia, 1969, F. A. Davis Co.)

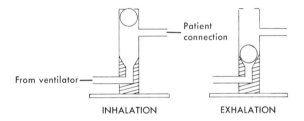

Fig. 11-3. Mörch exhalation valve.

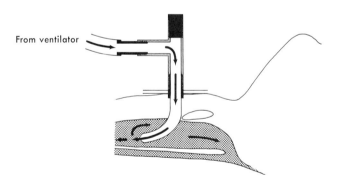

Fig. 11-4. Mörch tracheostomy tube with swivel connector.

than the necessary volume is set, and large quantities of gas leak out around the tube. This method of ventilation accomplished several things. (1) It allowed the patient to talk while on the ventilator and thus communicate with his environment. (2) The flow of gas past the tracheostomy tube may move secretions above the tube upward to be expelled or suctioned. (3) Not using a cuff to provide a seal tended to minimize the problem of tracheal necrosis.

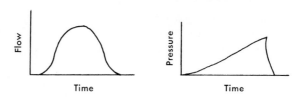

Fig. 11-5. Typical flow and pressure patterns for Mörch ventilator.

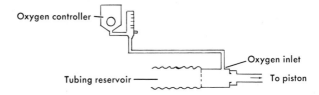

Fig. 11-6. Mörch oxygen system modified.

Drive mechanism and flow characteristics. The piston is driven by a rotary motor and the flow and pressure patterns (Fig. 11-5) are consistent with single-circuit, rotary-driven piston units described in Chapter 8.

Volume control. Tidal volume is adjustable up to 2.5 liters[3] per breath. The unit has a variable compressibility factor varying from about 2 to 3 cc/cm H_2O, depending on the tidal volume set (stroke distance of the piston). When the humidifier is empty, approximately 0.8 cc/cm H_2O can be added to the compressibility factor. At the minimum stroke volume, maximum volume remains in the piston's cylinder at the end of inhalation, and therefore the compressibility factor is the greatest.

Rate mechanism. The rate control is a gear box adjustment for setting the *speed* of the piston's travel.

I:E ratio. The inspiratory to expiratory time ratio on the Mörch is 1:1,[2] based on the drive mechanism, and it is fixed at that value.

Oxygen system. The oxygen concentration for the Mörch is controlled by a simple *oxygen addition* (Fig. 11-2) system that will vary oxygen percentage with rate and volume changes.[2] A reservoir and oxygen controller can be added to stabilize the oxygen percentage (Fig. 11-6).

Humidification system. A simple blow-by type humidifier was used to add some moisture to the inspired gases.

Specifications for the Mörch ventilator are as follows: tidal volume, 0 to 2500 cc; rate, 0 to 35 breaths/min.

THE EMERSON 3-PV VENTILATOR

The Emerson 3-PV Post-Op (Fig. 11-7) was devised and produced by John Emerson in 1965. It is an electrically powered, time- or patient-cycled on, rotary-driven piston, single-circuit ventilator that was designed to be volume-limited.

Referring to Fig. 11-8, gas is drawn from a *reservoir* and an *oxygen inlet* by the *piston* on its down (or return) stroke. On its upward (or forward) stroke the piston moves its content out of the *cylinder* through a one-way valve, through the *humidifier, past the pressure manometer* connection and a spring-loaded *pressure release valve* to the *patient connection*. The *exhalation valve* is also inflated by pressure from the cylinder during inhalation.

Drive mechanism and flow characteristics. The drive mechanism is a motor-driven wheel that moves the piston by means of a *lever*.[2] Because the rotary wheel moves the lever, which in turn moves the piston, the Emerson provides flow and pressure patterns similar to those of the Mörch ventilator. Examples are shown in Fig. 11-9.

Volume control. The location of the piston's rod on the lever (Fig. 11-8) provides for stroke volume adjustments.[2] The *closer* the rod is to the *pivot* of the lever, the *smaller* the stroke (tidal) volume set. The *volume adjustment* knob simply moves the pivot closer or further away from the rod.

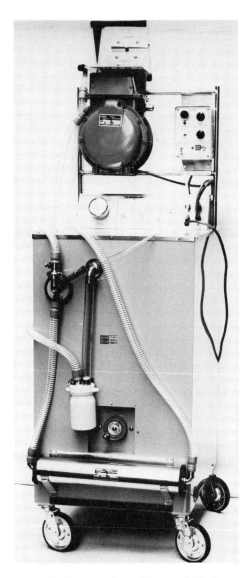

Fig. 11-7. Emerson 3-PV (Post-Op) volume ventilator. (Courtesy J. H. Emerson Co., Cambridge, Mass.)

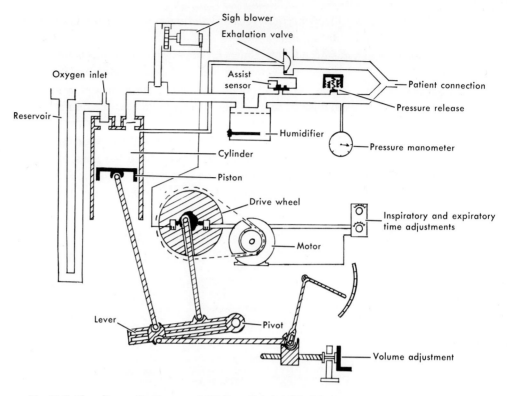

Fig. 11-8. Flow diagram for Emerson 3-PV (Post-Op). (Modified from Mushin, W. W., et al.: Automatic ventilation of the lungs, ed. 2, Philadelphia, 1969, F. A. Davis Co.)

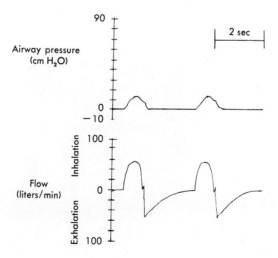

Fig. 11-9. Example of flow and pressure curves for Emerson 3-PV ventilator against compliance of 50 ml/cm H_2O and resistance of 5 cm H_2O/L/sec set on a lung simulator (redrawn from actual curves).

The compressibility factor of the Emerson varies from about 3.2 to 4.2 cc/cm H_2O pressure with a full humidifier dependent on stroke volume. About 2 cc/cm H_2O pressure should be added when the humidifier is empty.

Rate and I:E ratio mechanisms. Rate is achieved by the Emerson by independent inspiratory and expiratory timers. The circular *cam* on the inside of the larger *drive wheel* (Fig. 11-10, A) is beveled to a smaller diameter on half of its circumference. Two *microswitches* placed 180 degrees from each other on the cam are either depressed or allowed to be open, depending on which portion of the cam they are exposed.[5] The top microswitch has two positions allowing current flow to one of two *potentiometers.*[5] One potentiometer adjusts *inspiratory* current flow on one phase (inhalation) of the piston cycle, and the other adjusts current flow to the motor during

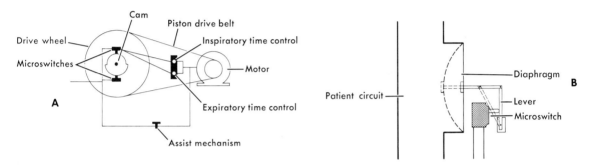

Fig. 11-10. **A,** Emerson inspiratory and expiratory time controls. **B,** Assist mechanism.

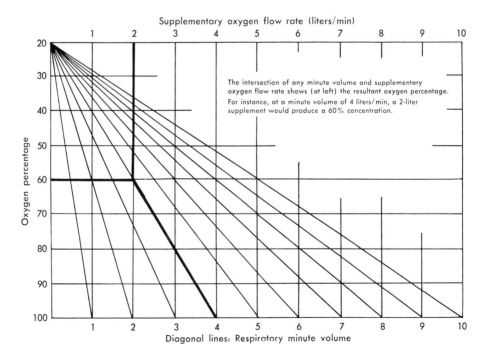

Fig. 11-11. Emerson oxygen percentage chart. (Courtesy J. H. Emerson Co., Cambridge, Mass.)

the *expiratory* phase (return stroke) of the piston. The current flow changes the motor speed and allows for the *adjustable* I : E ratio.

Assist mechanism. An optional assist mechanism is available for the 3-PV ventilator (Fig. 11-10, *B*). When the patient generates a negative (subatmospheric) pressure within the tubing circuit, the diaphragm in the assist mechanism bows to the left, triggering the assist microswitch. Once this microswitch is triggered, *maximum current* is supplied to the motor (Fig. 11-10, *A*) for the remainder of the piston's return stroke (exhalation). This causes the piston to return as rapidly as possible to move forward again to begin inhalation. The maximum *delay* between the assist signal and inhalation is in the neighborhood of 600 msec. Generally, the delay time will be dependent on the piston's position when the assist signal is created.

If positive end expiratory pressure (PEEP) is used, the patient must exert enough effort to cause the pressure in the tubing circuit to drop from the PEEP level and then to become negative to cause an assisted breath.

There is *no* provision on the Emerson's optional assist attachment for adjusting the negative pressure needed to provide an assist signal.

Oxygen system. Oxygen is *added* into a convoluted pipe resembling a trombone, which supplies gas to the piston during its refill[2] (Fig. 11-8). The volume of this reservoir is larger than the stroke volume of the piston. The oxygen percentage delivered can be calculated if the volume per minute leaving and the oxygen flow entering the reservoir are known. The chart shown in Fig. 11-11 can be used by intersecting the line opposite the desired oxygen percentage with the minute volume set on the Emerson (tidal volume × respiratory rate). The value directly above this intersection represents the flow of oxygen to be added (in liters per minute) to the reservoir.

The formula for finding the needed oxygen flow when minute volume and desired oxygen percentage are known is as follows:

$$O_2 \text{ flow} = \frac{\text{Total flow} \times (F_{IO_2} - 0.2)}{0.8}$$

where

$$\text{Total flow} = \text{Minute volume in liters per minute (L/min)}$$

$$F_{IO_2} = \text{Fraction of inspired oxygen}$$

$$O_2 \text{ flow} = \text{Oxygen flow to be set in L/min}$$

EXAMPLE: Known − Total flow (minute volume) = 10 L/min

$$F_{IO_2} = 0.6 \, (60\% \, O_2)$$

$$O_2 \text{ flow} = \frac{10 \times (0.6 - 0.2)}{0.8}$$

$$= \frac{10 \times 0.4}{0.8}$$

$$= \frac{4}{0.8}$$

$$= 5 \text{ L/min}$$

For both the chart and the formula, a nonfluctuating minute volume is assumed. If the minute volume varies, such as when the patient initiates breaths by assisting at a variable rate, the oxygen percentage predicted will not be produced.

Controlling oxygen concentrations with the Emerson can be simplified by using an oxygen controller (Fig. 11-12) and flushing the trombone with the desired oxygen mixture.

Sigh system. The Emerson's optimal sigh mechanism is a *rotary blower* (Fig. 11-13). This blower adds air during the inspiratory phase. The amount of air added by the blower can be adjusted somewhat by increasing speed of the blower's rotation. The faster the blower turns, the greater forward force (pressure) it can exert. The maximum pressure that can be set on the sigh unit is about 50 to 55 cm H_2O. Once the available force set on the blower is reached in the patient circuit during inhalation, the sigh system no longer adds air to that breath. Usually, the sigh system adds room air (Fig. 11-14) to the circuit, diluting the oxygen from the piston.

This process can be modified by having the sigh mechanism draw its gas directly

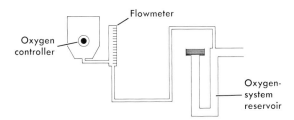

Fig. 11-12. Emerson oxygen system modified with oxygen controller. Flow from controller must exceed minute volume delivered by ventilator to maintain stable oxygen percentage.

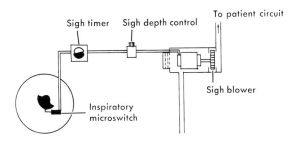

Fig. 11-13. Emerson sigh system diagram.

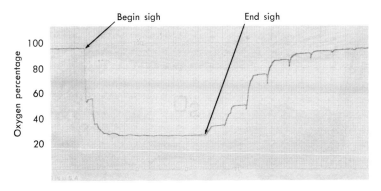

Fig. 11-14. Measured oxygen percentage during sigh mode with Emerson 3-PV ventilator showing rapid decrease in delivered oxygen concentration during sigh mode when sigh blower introduces room air into system.

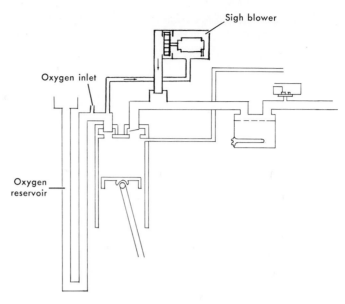

Fig. 11-15. Emerson sigh system modified by connection to oxygen system.

from the oxygen reservoir and by using an oxygen controller[6] (Fig. 11-15). This is done so that when a sigh breath occurs, the gas drawn into the blower comes from the trombone at the same preset oxygen concentration as the piston system is utilizing.

Humidification system. On the forward stroke of the piston, gas moves through a heated *blow-by* humidifier (made from a simple pressure cooker) and then through *copper mesh.*[2,5]

Specifications for the Emerson 3-PV Post-Op ventilator are summarized in the accompanying box.

Specifications for Emerson 3-PV Post-Op ventilator

Tidal volume:	0 to 2000 cc
Inspiratory time:	0.4 to 3 seconds (approximate)
Expiratory time:	0.4 to 3 seconds (approximate)
Approximate rate range:	10 to 50 breaths/min
Assist effort:	−1 cm H_2O pressure (approximate)
Pressure limit:	40 to 160 cm H_2O pressure on relief valve
Sighs:	Various sigh systems available on request

THE ENGSTRÖM VENTILATORS
Engström 150 and 200 Series

In response to the 1956 polio epidemic in Sweden, Dr. C. G. Engström developed and produced the Engström model 150. The Engström units are electrically powered, rotary-driven piston, double-circuit, time-cycled, time- and volume-limited controllers.

Referring to Fig. 11-16, the basic component of the Engström is a *piston* that incorporates *leak channels* in the driving rod to allow decompression within the piston's *cylinder* during parts of the piston's forward and backward strokes. During the forward stroke (piston moving to the right in Figs. 11-16 and 11-17), gas within the cylinder is not initially pressurized on the right side because of the communication that a leak channel provides in the shaft, A. Once the piston is moved to the right sufficiently to occlude that leak channel, positive pressure builds in the right

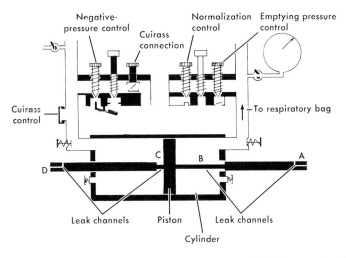

Fig. 11-16. Functional diagram of Engström 150 piston system. (Modified from Mushin, W. W., et al.: Automatic ventilation of the lungs, ed. 2, Philadelphia, 1969, F. A. Davis Co.)

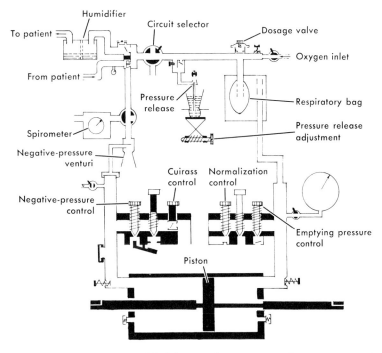

Fig. 11-17. Engström 150 schematic. (Modified from Mushin, W. W., et al.: Automatic ventilation of the lungs, ed. 2, Philadelphia, 1969, F. A. Davis Co.)

side of the piston, which then sends gas to compress the *respiratory bag* (Fig. 11-17). Pressure continues to be generated in the right side of the chamber as the piston travels forward until the next leak channel on that side (*B* in Fig. 11-16) is exposed, which then expels the pressure in the right side of the piston to atmospheric pressure. During the *forward* stroke of the piston, gas is compressed only 67% of the time.[2] This leaves the remaining 33% plus 100% of return stroke time for the expiratory phase, thus providing a 1:2 I:E ratio[2] (Fig. 11-18). On the reverse stroke, the same percentage of time is spent with *negative pressure* being exerted in the right side of the delivery system. It is this negative pressure that *refills* the *respiratory bag* (Fig. 11-18). There are two *throttle needle valve adjustments* on the 150, which provide for leaks in or out of their respective sides of the piston (Figs. 11-17 and 11-18). During the forward stroke, gas can leak out the *emptying pressure control* (Fig. 11-17), thereby limiting the amount of positive pressure that can be exerted around the respiratory bag. On the left side of the piston, a suction or negative pressure can be applied by the *cuirass control.*

On the reverse stroke of the piston, positive pressure is developed on the left side of the piston. This positive pressure is used to power the jet of the *negative-pressure Venturi,* which can entrain gas out of the patient circuit (Fig. 11-17). This system also has a throttle to adjust the leak out of the left side and, therefore, the peak positive pressure developed to power the jet.[2] The higher the pressure powering the jet, the *lower* the negative pressure that will be generated to entrain circuit gas. The Engström's negative pressure does *not* establish itself *immediately* on expiration.[2] Fig. 11-18 outlines the phases of ventilation (inhalation or exhalation) and the pressures (positive or negative) exerted by the piston. It shows that there is a definite lag before negative expiratory pressure is exerted in the system. This was designed in hopes of reducing *air trapping* so that the patient would have time to exhale normally before the negative pressure was applied.[7]

On the right side of the piston during the reverse stroke, the closing of the leak channels now causes a negative pressure to be applied on the respiratory bag (Fig. 11-17) by the *normalization control.* This control is set so that when the respiratory bag is filling, a red-line pressure of −30 cm H_2O is seen on the driving circuit's pressure manometer.

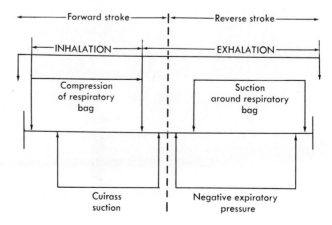

Fig. 11-18. Engström piston cycle.

Drive mechanism and flow characteristics. The piston is rotary driven for the Engström ventilators. However, because the units are double circuit devices and because of the leak channels just described, the typical sine-wave–like pattern of other piston ventilators is modified. Because the respiratory bag within the patient circuit will normally be empty before the forward stroke of the piston is completed, usually only the first part of the compression period for the piston is actually sending gases to the patient. The result is an *accelerating* flow pattern and a pressure pattern that has a notch indicative of a volume hold. Both the 150 and 200 series units have flow and pressure patterns similar to the 300 series (shown later in this chapter).

Volume control and oxygen system. The Engström ventilators control *minute volume* primarily. *Tidal volume* is a result of the set minute volume divided by the set *respiratory rate*.

The controls dictating both *oxygen concentration* and *minute volume* are the *dosage valve* and a set of *rotameters*[2] (uncompensated Thorpe tube flowmeters) shown in Fig. 11-19. The dosage valve basically acts as an air flowmeter, although, in actuality, it is an air-entrainment port (Fig. 11-20). It establishes the *minute volume* of *air* delivered to the patient and has a range of *0 to 30* L/min.

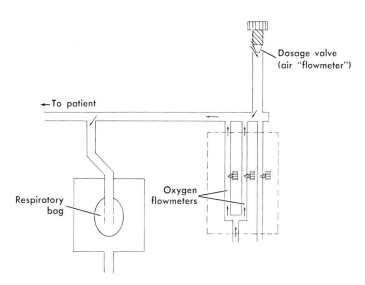

Fig. 11-19. Dosage valve and flowmeter system for Engström ventilators. This system provides air and oxygen to respiratory bag.

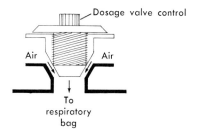

Fig. 11-20. Engström dosage valve.

The pressure gradient supplied for the dosage valve is from atmospheric to -30 cm H_2O pressure, set by the normalization control on the bag refill phase of the reverse stroke of the piston. Since bag refill lasts only a third of the ventilatory cycle, the flow across the valve is actually *three times* the value indicated on the dial. For example, if it is set on 10 L/min for a third of the ventilatory cycle, the flow is actually 30 L/min through the dosage valve. The net result is a third of 30 L/min, or 10 liters, collected in the respiratory bag per minute. As long as the calibration of the orifice adjustment is accurate as well as the normalization pressure actually being -30 cm H_2O, the unit is accurate. Two oxygen flowmeters establish the minute volume of oxygen delivered. The ranges on the two oxygen flowmeters are from 0 to 5 L/min on one and from 0 to 15 on the other. The formula, described previously, can be used to calculate the setting of the oxygen flowmeter. The total of the settings of the dosage valve and the oxygen flowmeters sets the minute volume. That is, if 3 L/min were set on the dosage valve and 3 liters on the oxygen flowmeter, the set minute volume to the patient would be 6 L/min of mixed air (dosage valve) and oxygen.

The setting on the rate control would then determine the tidal volume. The following illustrations are used to show an important concept for the Engström ventilators.

Normally on *tidal-volume*–controlled ventilators, if it is desired to decrease the patient's alveolar minute ventilation, it can be done by decreasing the rate, leaving the set tidal volume the same. Doing this (decreasing the set rate only) on the Engström causes the *reverse* to happen, as shown in the practical examples below.

$$\begin{array}{rl} \text{Setting for air dosage valve:} & 6 \text{ L/min} \\ \text{Setting for oxygen rotameter:} & +6 \text{ L/min} \\ \hline \text{Set minute volume:} & 12 \text{ L/min} \end{array}$$

Given: A patient with 0.1 liters anatomic dead space

EXAMPLE A:

Setting for rate (f) = 24 breaths/min

$$\frac{\text{Minute volume } 12}{f} = \frac{12}{24} = 0.5 \text{ liter tidal volume}$$

$$\begin{array}{l} 0.5 \text{ liter tidal volume} \\ -0.1 \text{ liter anatomic dead space} \\ \hline 0.4 \text{ liter } \textit{alveolar} \text{ volume (tidal)} \end{array}$$

0.4 liter $\times$ 24 = 9.6 *alveolar* minute volume

EXAMPLE B:

Setting for rate *decreased* to 12 breaths/min

$$\frac{12}{12} = 1.0 \text{ liter tidal volume}$$

$$\begin{array}{l} 1.0 \text{ liter tidal volume} \\ -0.1 \text{ liter anatomic dead space} \\ \hline 0.9 \text{ liter } \textit{alveolar} \text{ volume (tidal)} \end{array}$$

0.9 liter $\times$ 12 = 10.8 liters *alveolar* minute volume

Thus a *decreased* rate with the same set total minute volume will result in an *increased* alveolar minute volume with Engström ventilators.

The *compressibility factor* in the 150 is constant at about 5 cc/cm H_2O pressure unless the humidifier level changes. The normal fluid level change in the humidifier adds about 0.5 cc/cm H_2O pressure. Compressibility factors have to be altered and recalculated with tubing circuitry size changes.

Rate mechanism. The rate is controlled by adjusting the speed of the motor driving the piston, and this is accomplished by an adjustable hydraulic transmission. Increasing the motor's speed increases the number of piston cycles per minute.

I:E ratio. Because of the leak channels in the piston's rod described previously, the I:E ratio for the Engström ventilators is fixed at 1:2. Functionally, this ratio can be altered to close to 1:1.5 when the negative expiratory pressure control is used. Basically, on exhalation, once negative pressure is released on the patient's circuit, a flow of gas from the unit starts *before* gas flow from the piston is initiated because of negative pressure in the patient's airways. This functionally causes inhalation to start *early*, shortening exhalation and prolonging inhalation. The end result is a changed I:E ratio from a fixed 1:2 to a functional one of about 1:1.5.

Assist mechanism. There is no assist system for the Engström units. They are strictly controllers.

Other systems. The *circuit selector* directs the flow of gas through the system along a specific path. On *manual*, the unit allows for a *manual sigh* with a self-inflating bag. The respiratory bag is bypassed on this setting, and the expiratory circuit is operational. Regarding the other settings, there is a *spirometer on or off* position where the spirometer can be bypassed either to minimize the water condensation in it from exhaled air or when used when negative pressure is in use. There is a *filling position*, which is used for filling the respiratory bag in a rebreathing system for anesthetic gases.

The *pressure relief* designed on the unit is a combination of a *water column* and an *adjustable, spring-tension release* (Fig. 11-21).[2] Once the gas has overcome that tension, it simply bubbles through the water. The pressure release can be set up to

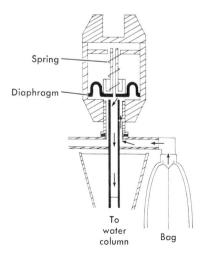

Fig. 11-21. Engström 150 pressure relief valve system.

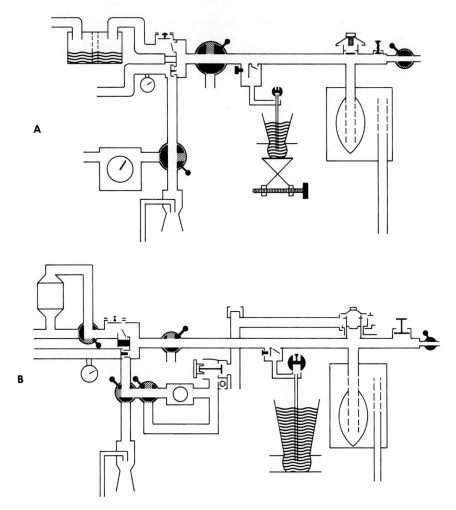

Fig. 11-22. Comparison of diagrams for **A,** Engström 150, and **B,** Engström 200, model ventilators. (Modified from Mushin, W. W., et al.: Automatic ventilation of the lungs, Philadelphia, 1969, F. A. Davis Co.)

35 cm H_2O pressure by adjusting the water level on a wedge-jack type of structure or to *70 cm H_2O* pressure with a spring-tension release device (Fig. 11-17).

The Engström 200 is principally the same as the 150 but has a circuit for re-breathing anesthetic gases (Fig. 11-22).

Engström 300 series

The Engström 300 series ventilator (Fig. 11-23) has now replaced the 150 and 200 series models. Several structural improvements were made over the 150 and 200 series that clinically provide improved stability and ease of operation. Instead of using leak adjustments on the piston, *spring disks* are used (Fig. 11-24). An adjusta-ble normalization control is no longer necessary because a 30 cm H_2O spring is positioned against the intake disk, so the pressure on the right side of the piston is maintained at −30 cm H_2O pressure during the bag refill phase (Fig. 11-25). The *emptying pressure* is now an adjustable spring-tension pressure release that adjusts

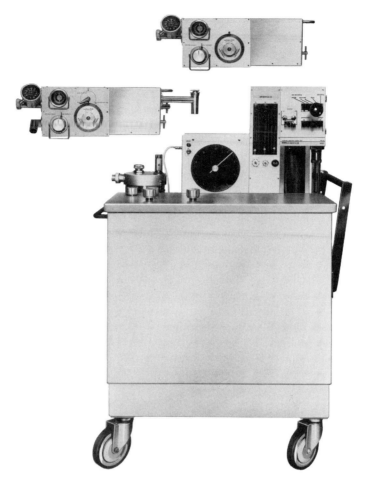

Fig. 11-23. Engström 300 series ventilator system. (Courtesy LKB Medical, Inc., Rockville, Md.)

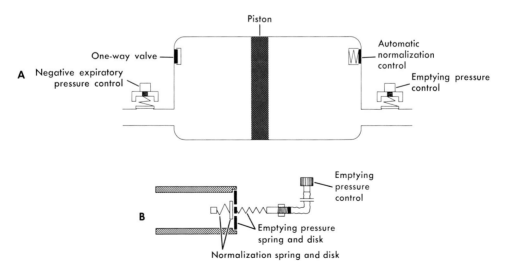

Fig. 11-24. A, Engström 300 series piston system. **B,** Emptying pressure and normalization control diagram.

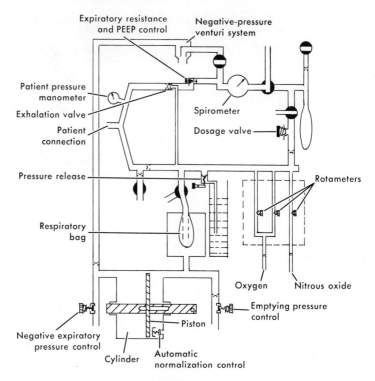

Fig. 11-25. Functional diagram of Engström 300 series ventilator. (Modified from LKB Medical, Inc., Rockville, Md.)

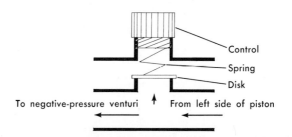

Fig. 11-26. Engström 300 series negative pressure system control.

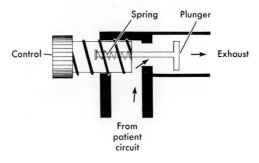

Fig. 11-27. Engström 300 series expiratory resistance and PEEP control.

the level to which peak pressure will be reached around the respiratory bag (Figs. 11-24 and 11-25). The *negative expiratory pressure* setting is also a spring-disk adjustment that changes the pressure powering the jet of the expiratory *negative-pressure Venturi system* (Fig. 11-26). Utilization of the spring disks makes their attained values *independent* of rate changes. There is no cuirass attachment on the 300, so a one-way valve serves to allow gas to flow into the left side of the piston during the forward stroke.

Volume control and oxygen system. These functions are similar to those of the 150 units previously described.

Rate mechanism. The rate mechanism is similar to that described for the 150 ventilator.

I:E ratio. The I:E on the 300 series is fixed at 1:2 in a manner similar to that of the 150 units. Again, negative expiratory pressure functionally alters the I:E ratio to about 1:1.5.

Expiratory resistance and PEEP control. The 300 series has a *dual-function* expiratory control knob (Fig. 11-27). Turned *clockwise*, the control provides *expiratory resistance* by narrowing the orifice through which expired gas flows. This functionally acts as an expiratory retard system. The expiratory retard is adjustable to *total* occlusion of the expiratory circuit. Total occlusion is used only to test for leaks in the system before patient connection.[7] Moving the control knob *counterclockwise* seats a disk on the expiratory valve outlet.[7] As the control knob is turned more, the spring tension is tightened on the disk. This adjusts the pressure necessary for expiratory gas flow to exit past the spring disk, thus *providing* PEEP. PEEP is adjustable up to about 20 cm H_2O pressure.

Other systems. The *pressure release* (Fig. 11-28) is an adjustable spring-disk pop-off device. When gas pressure in the circuit *exceeds* the spring tension, the disk is pushed away from its seat, and gas escapes through a water column.

A multifunction lever moves a rod with numerous O-ring seals along it. The *position* of the seals within the head of the 300 dictates which paths are open to gas flow. The *spirometer on* position directs expired gas to the spirometer for monitoring expired volumes. The *spirometer off* position bypasses the spirometer to either minimize condensation buildup or allow the use of negative expiratory pressure. The *manual* setting permits a manual sigh to be delivered to the circuit with a self-inflating bag *inline,* and, by blocking flow from the respiratory bag, gas is drawn in as the bag is released and allowed to refill. The *rebreathing* setting on the multifunction

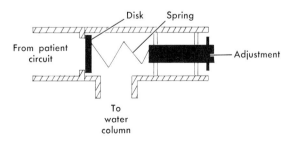

Fig. 11-28. Engström 300 series pressure release control.

lever provides a recirculating gas system through a carbon dioxide absorber. The inflation phase is accomplished manually with an anesthetic bag.

There is a *low-pressure alarm*[7] that operates on a *photoelectric cell in the manometer.* If the needle indicating system pressure does not break the light beam to a photoelectric cell in the manometer, the alarm goes off (Fig. 11-29). A power disconnect or *power loss alarm* is also present and is powered by cadmium batteries in the unit.[7]

The humidifier (Fig. 11-30) has a *sponge* that absorbs water. Gas passes through the sponge and is thus humidified on the way to the patient. A *heating plate* on the bottom of the humidifier's water reservoir heats the water to provide increased humidity.

The *compressibility factor* is constant at about *4.5 cc/cm H_2O* pressure. Changes in the tidal volumes will not change this factor, but different sizes of tubing circuits will.

Flow and pressure patterns for the 300 series are similar to those of the 150 and 200 series. Examples of these patterns are shown in Fig. 11-31 against relatively normal conditions. Fig. 11-32 shows a circumstance in which patient conditions are

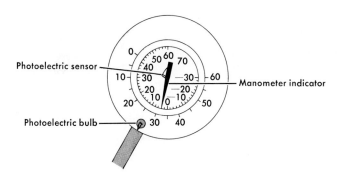

Fig. 11-29. Engström 300 series pressure manometer and low-pressure alarm.

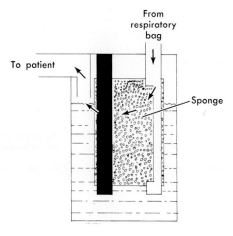

Fig. 11-30. Engström 300 series humidifier.

changed. Generally, the flow pattern for Engström ventilators is an *accelerating* pattern even though the device is driven by a rotary system somewhat like that in Emerson ventilators. As described in Chapter 8, the primary difference is that Engströms are *double-circuit* units. Gas delivered to the patient comes from the respiratory bag and the rotameters during inhalation. Since the bag is usually empty *before* the end of inspiratory time (67% of the piston's forward stroke), generally only the first part (acceleration) of the piston's movement affects the flow out of the bag.

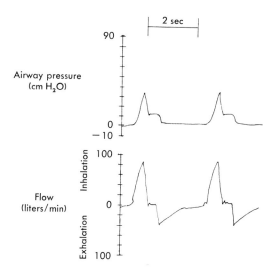

Fig. 11-31. Flow and pressure patterns common to Engström ventilators redrawn from actual curves taken using Engström 300 series ventilator and lung simulator set for compliance of 50 ml/cm H_2O and resistance of 5 cm H_2O/L/sec.

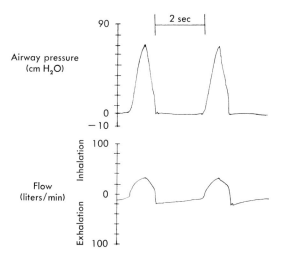

Fig. 11-32. Pressure and flow patterns redrawn from actual curves taken with Engström 300 series ventilator connected to a lung simulator. Compliance was set for 50 ml/cm H_2O and resistance to 50 cm H_2O/L/sec. Note sine wave–like appearance of flow pattern.

However, if the patient's airway resistance increases as in the example of Fig. 11-32, it will take more pressure and time to empty the bag. Thus a flow pattern more closely resembling a sine wave results.

Specifications for the Engström ventilators discussed are summarized in the accompanying box.

Specifications for Engström ventilators

Minute volume:	0 to 50 L/min
Rate:	12 to 36 (300 series)
	10 to 30 (150 and 200 series)
	(I:E ratio fixed at 1:2)
Pressure limit:	30, 60, or 90 cm H_2O pressure (300 series)
	To 35 or 70 cm H_2O pressure (150 and 200 series)
Emptying pressure:	50 to 110 cm H_2O pressure (300 series) (variable on 150 and 200)
Expiratory pressure:	-10 to $+20$ cm H_2O pressure (300 series)
Alarms:	Disconnect and low pressure

THE BOURNS LS104-150 INFANT VENTILATOR

The Bourns Infant Ventilator (Fig. 11-33) is the outgrowth of a research program conducted on the mechanical ventilation of neonates at Iowa State University in the early 1960s. The Bourns Corporation began production of the ventilator in 1966.

The unit was designated as a volume-limited ventilator with time-cycled or patient-cycled capabilities (assistor or assistor/controller) and is an electrically powered single-circuit unit.[8] Gas is supplied to the patient through a single circuit by a *linear-drive piston* (Fig. 11-34).[2] On the forward stroke (to the right in the diagram) of the piston, gas is pumped to the patient through a one-way check valve. Gases then pass through the humidifying device and to the patient connection. An electric *solenoid* serves as the exhalation valve and is closed during inhalation and open during exhalation. During exhalation (return stroke of the piston), patient and circuit gases flow past the open solenoid and the *expiratory* check leaf (one-way valve), through the *PEEP Venturi* and out the expired gas outlet. The piston fills with blended gases from the port marked *From mix box*.

Drive mechanism and flow characteristics. The piston is driven linearly by a gear-and-clutch mechanism (Fig. 11-35). The travel of the piston is accomplished at a nearly constant rate. This rate is regulated by an independent control called *Flow rate* (Fig. 11-33, *B*), which is calibrated in milliliters per second.

Because the drive mechanism is a linear type, the flow pattern produced is a relatively constant or square wave. The piston is sealed in its cylinder by a rolling diaphragm. During inhalation, this diaphragm may change its shape slightly with pressure changes in the cylinder, causing some bumps in the flow pattern. Examples of flow and pressure patterns achieved with a lung simulator are shown in Fig. 11-36.

Volume control. The piston stroke is controlled by a pair of magnetic position switches. The *tidal volume* is adjusted by changing the location of one of the position switches, thereby allowing the piston to stroke different lengths. The piston is driven by the motor when an electromagnetic clutch is engaged. After the forward stroke of the piston is complete, the rear clutch is engaged, driving the piston back to its resting position where it awaits the next forward clutch actuation, causing an inhalation.

Set tidal volumes from 5 to 150 ml are displayed on an analog meter that reflects the position of the piston after the return stroke (Fig. 11-33, *B*).

The Bourns allows for a low compressibility factor, generally about 0.3 to 0.5 cc/cm H_2O pressure depending on the size of the tubing circuit used. This factor should be calculated for each circuit, since volume lost in the circuit can play a significant role in infant ventilation.

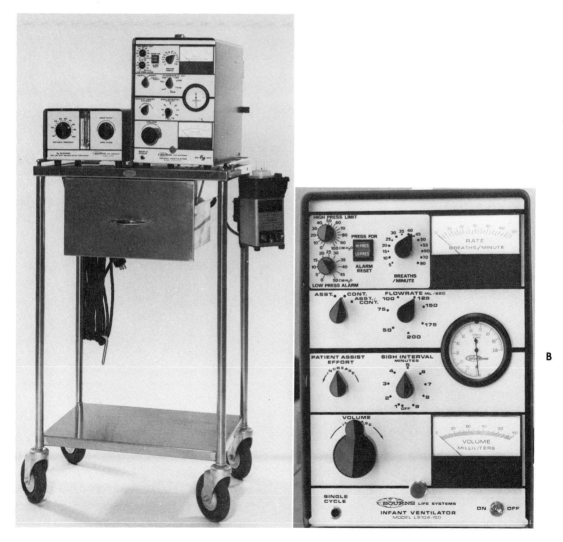

Fig. 11-33. Bourns LS104-150 Infant Ventilator. **A,** Ventilator system with oxygen blender and ultrasonic nebulizer on mobile cart. **B,** Front panel of ventilator. (Courtesy Bourns, Inc., Life Systems Division, Riverside, Calif.)

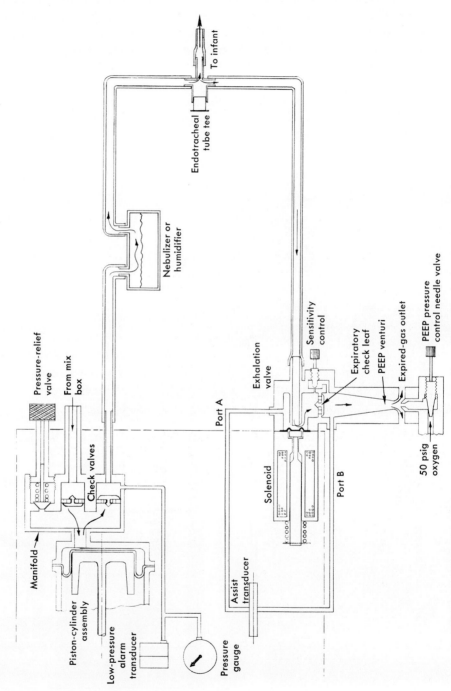

Fig. 11-34. Functional flow diagram for LS104-150 with PEEP attachment. (Courtesy Bourns, Inc., Life Systems Division, Riverside, Calif.)

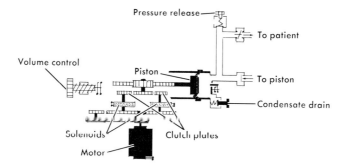

Fig. 11-35. Bourns drive mechanism. (Modified from Mushin, W. W., et al.: Automatic ventilation of the lungs, ed. 2, Philadelphia, 1969, F. A. Davis Co.)

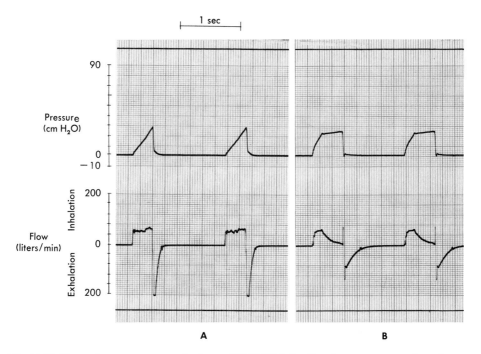

Fig. 11-36. Flow and pressure patterns for Bourns LS104-150 Infant Ventilator. **A,** Unit in volume-limiting mode with lung simulator set for compliance of 1 ml/cm H_2O and approximate resistance of 50 cm H_2O/ L/sec. **B,** Unit with pressure relief set to open near 20 cm H_2O with lung simulator settings of compliance of 1 ml/cm H_2O and approximate resistance of 200 cm H_2O/L/sec.

Rate mechanism. The *rate* is set on the LS104-150 by a single rate control that divides each minute into equal parts (ventilatory cycle time). It can be set for five to eighty breaths/min in five-breath increments. The average rate of the ventilator is displayed on the analog rate meter for all modes of operation (Fig. 11-33, *B*).

I:E ratio. The I:E ratio is a function of several controls for the LS104-150. It is determined by the tidal volume, inspiratory flow rate, and breathing rate. On control mode, the I:E ratio can be estimated either with the chart or slide rule provided by Bourns and shown in Fig. 11-37.

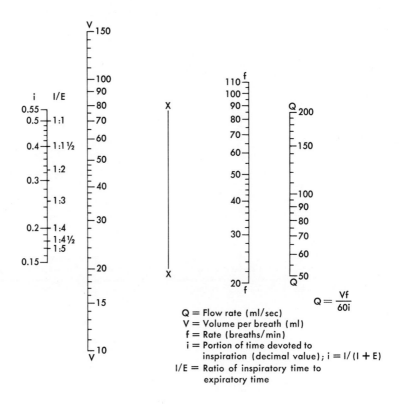

$$Q = \frac{Vf}{60i}$$

Q = Flow rate (ml/sec)
V = Volume per breath (ml)
f = Rate (breaths/min)
i = Portion of time devoted to
inspiration (decimal value); i = I/(I + E)
I/E = Ratio of inspiratory time to
expiratory time

To select Q, first select V and f. Connect these
points intersecting X axis at point P. Draw
line from desired i or I/E value through P to Q.

Set slide so that ventilator
tidal volume is directly above
breathing rate reading.

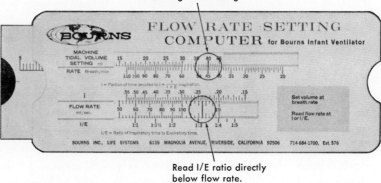

Read I/E ratio directly
below flow rate.

Fig. 11-37. Bourns I : E ratio chart and slide rule. (Courtesy Bourns, Inc., Life Systems Division, Riverside Calif.)

Assist and sensitivity mechanism. The assist and sensitivity mechanism uses an *electronic capacitance transducer*. The transducer senses inspiratory effort by detecting the motion of a metal strip attached to a diaphragm. As the patient generates a negative pressure in the circuit (Fig. 11-38), the deflection of the diaphragm moves the metal strip away from a metal plate. The resulting change in capacitance is electronically detected and reduced to a signal used to actuate engagement of the forward clutch plate, beginning the inspiratory phase. The sensitivity of the transducer may be varied through a front panel control (reference potentiometer), which allows variation for different patient efforts. It can be set to provide an assisted breath when a drop in pressure in the patient circuit of as little as 0.05 cm H_2O or up to 1 cm H_2O is seen by the assist transducer.[8] The response time of this system has been reported to be near 25 msec[10] and 36 msec[11] and will be somewhat dependent on tubing circuit size.

The assist mechanism is functional even when PEEP is applied as described on p. 285.

Since the return stroke of the piston occurs in about two thirds the time of inhalation, high assist rates can be achieved.

Oxygen system. An early Bourns oxygen system utilized a *mixing chamber* (Fig. 11-39) as described in Chapter 5. This system can be modified with a reservoir and controller (Fig. 11-40). A new oxygen system is presently available (LS145 oxygen blender) that blends pressurized air and oxygen to the concentration set on the control.[9] The new oxygen system (Fig. 11-41) incorporates two regulators to reduce and balance the pressures of the air and oxygen to 10 psig each. The proportioning of the gases is accomplished in the *differential area gas blending valve* (precision meter-

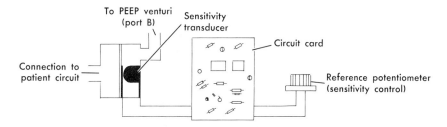

Fig. 11-38. Functional diagram of Bourns LS104-150 sensitivity mechanism.

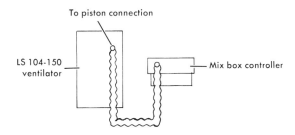

Fig. 11-39. Early Bourns oxygen control system (described in Chapter 5).

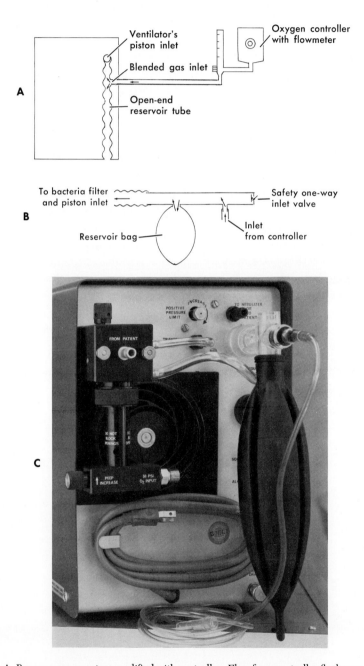

Fig. 11-40. A, Bourns oxygen system modified with controller. Flow from controller flushes open reservoir tube, and ventilator's piston draws from this preset oxygen concentration. **B,** Flow diagram for Bourns oxygen system modified for CPAP. **C,** Bourns model LS126 CPAP attachment connected to piston inlet of LS104-150 ventilator. (**C** courtesy Bourns, Inc., Life Systems Division, Riverside, Calif.)

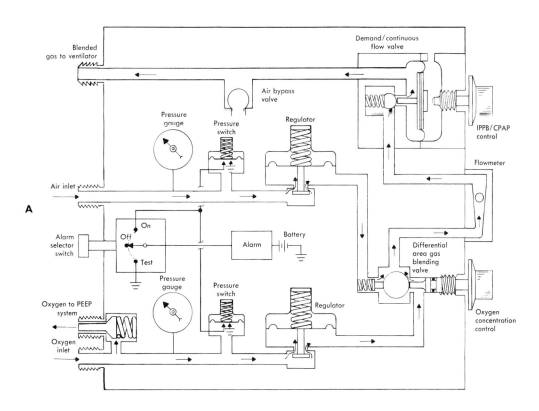

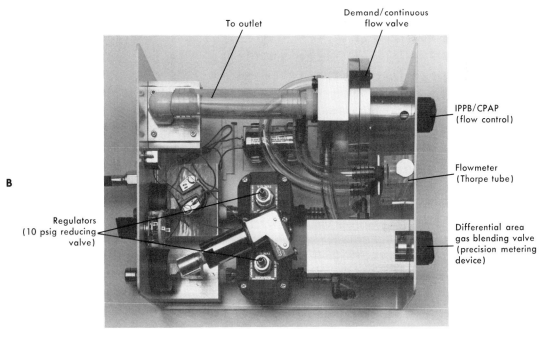

Fig. 11-41. A, Flow diagram for new Bourns oxygen system (model LS145). **B,** Components of Bourns LS145 oxygen blender. (Courtesy Bourns, Inc., Life Systems Division, Riverside, Calif.)

ing device). The differential area valve controls the oxygen concentration delivered by the blender by adjusting the size of the outlet for air and oxygen.

The proportionated gas is metered to the ventilator by a demand valve system. When the controller is on the *IPPB flow* mode, the piston draws gas from the demand valve as required.[9] Turning the demand valve control to the *CPAP Flow* position causes the controller to provide a continuous flow for CPAP or IMV operation.[9] Gas flow is indicated by the *flowmeter*.

Sigh system. The LS104-150 is equipped with a *sigh* capability that can be set for a sigh every 1 to 9 minutes or not at all.[8] When the sigh is activated, the exhalation solenoid does *not* open after the delivery of the set tidal volume. Instead, it remains

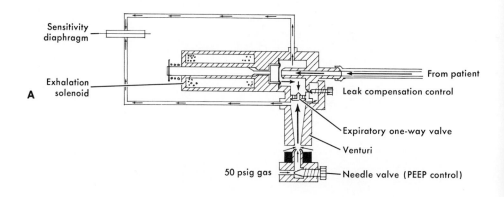

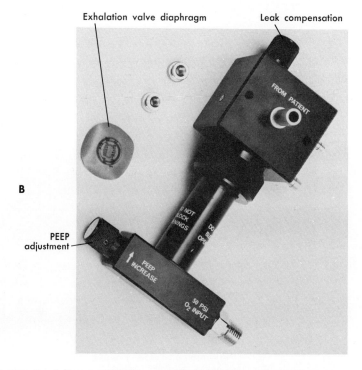

Fig. 11-42. A, Functional diagram of PEEP system for LS104-150 ventilator. **B,** Components of Bourns PEEP attachment. (**B** courtesy Bourns, Inc., Life Systems Division, Riverside, Calif.)

closed while the piston quickly refills and delivers a second tidal breath. Therefore the sigh volume is always double the set tidal volume when used and delivered within the pressure limits set.

PEEP system. Recently, a PEEP attachment (Fig. 11-42) has been released that provides the capabilities of PEEP on assist, control, and assist/control modes for this ventilator.[8,12] The unit consists of a *Venturi* supplied by 50 psig gas. A simple needle valve controls the flow of gas to the jet of the Venturi and therefore the forward pressure that the Venturi can exert. The forward pressure establishes a PEEP level against the *expiratory one-way valve*. As the patient circuit gas exits past the valve, the circuit pressure cannot drop below the PEEP pressure opposing it, unless there are leaks in the patient system. A second needle valve (the *leak compensation control*) is applied to maintain PEEP in the face of leaks in the patient circuit.[8] If the leak compensation control is set too high, the patient will have difficulty in triggering the ventilator.[8,12] This would be noticed clinically by an increased effort on the patient's part, such as increased depth of sternal retraction and no ventilator response. Too low a setting of the compensation mechanism would be made evident by the machine's *self-cycling* during the assist mode. This would be observed clinically by the ventilator's triggering without any obvious inspiratory effort on the part of the patient.

Other systems. Two types of pressure limits can be set on the LS104-150 Infant Ventilator. One is a pressure relief (pop off) valve (Figs. 11-34, 11-35,

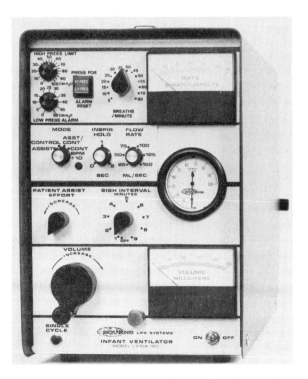

Fig. 11-43. Early D model of Bourns LS104-150. Note addition of breaths/min divided by 10, inspiratory hold control, and decreased flow rate range to 25 to 150 ml/sec. Newer units have flows from 25 to 200 ml/sec. (Courtesy Bourns, Inc., Life Systems Division, Riverside, Calif.)

Specifications for Bourns LS104-150 Infant Ventilator

Tidal volume:	5 to 150 cc
Rate:	5 to 80 breaths/min or ½ to 80 with ÷10 switch on D units
Flow rate:	50 to 200 ml/sec (3 to 12 L/min) or 25 to 200 ml/sec on D units
Pressure limit:	Up to 100 cm H_2O pressure on either pressure relief or high-pressure limit
Sensitivity:	Stable from −0.05 cm H_2O to −1.0 cm H_2O
Response time:	35 msec (average)
Sigh volume:	Double tidal volume set
Sigh interval:	Every 1 to 9 minutes or off
PEEP:	0 to 18 cm H_2O pressure
Oxygen concentration:	21% to 100% with LS145 blender
Flows for CPAP and IMV modes:	0 to 20 L/min
Audible and visual alarms:	High-pressure alarm (and limit) 0 to 100 cm H_2O pressure
	Low pressure alarm 0 to 50 cm H_2O pressure
	Apnea (on assist mode) lasts for 5 seconds while unit reverts to control mode after a drop in rate to 60% of control setting for 10 seconds.

---

and 11-40, *C*) located near the piston and exposed out the back panel of the unit. This control provides a pressure hold effect when its set pressure is reached while excess gases pass from the piston to the atmosphere (see Fig. 11-36, *B*, for examples of flow and pressure patterns). The other pressure limit is combined with the *high-pressure alarm* set on the front panel (Fig. 11-33, *B*). This is an electric pressure sensor that cycles the ventilator into exhalation immediately when its preset pressure is reached and provides an audible and visual alarm to indicate that occurrence.[8] Both pressure-limiting systems are adjustable up to 100 cm H_2O pressure and can be monitored on an aneroid pressure manometer.

A low-pressure system for alarm conditions allows for a disconnect or low-pressure condition to be monitored. This control, also on the front panel (Fig. 11-33, *B*) sets the *minimum* pressure allowed in the circuit to prevent an audible and visual alarm condition. If the condition lasts for longer than 15 seconds, the audible intermittent beep with each breath will change to a continuous, steady alarm.[8] The values are adjustable up to 50 cm H_2O pressure.

Another alarm condition can occur when the unit is set to assist mode. An audible alarm and automatic changeover to control mode will occur if the rate meter falls below 60% of the rate control setting for 10 seconds. The unit will stay on control for 5 seconds, then return to assist mode until the condition exists again.

Humidification system. Usually a modified (detuned) ultrasonic nebulizer is used for humidifying gases to be inhaled. An optional heated blow-by humidifier (modified from a pneumatic nebulizer) is also available.

D model. An updated version of the LS104-150 is the D version of that model (Fig. 11-43). This unit is functionally the same except that an *inflation hold* control and *rate-divided-by-ten* controls have been added. A new lower flow rate is also available. The inflation hold acts as a *volume* hold by delaying the exhalation solenoid's opening for a programable period up to 2 seconds after volume delivery. The BPM-divided-by-ten position on the mode control switch functionally allows the set rate control value to be divided by ten so that a second rate range of a half to eight breaths per minute is available primarily for use during weaning with IMV procedures. The new flow rate range is from 25 to 200 ml/sec instead of 50 to 200 ml/sec as on previous units.

Some specifications for the Bourns LS104-150 ventilators are summarized in the box on p. 286.

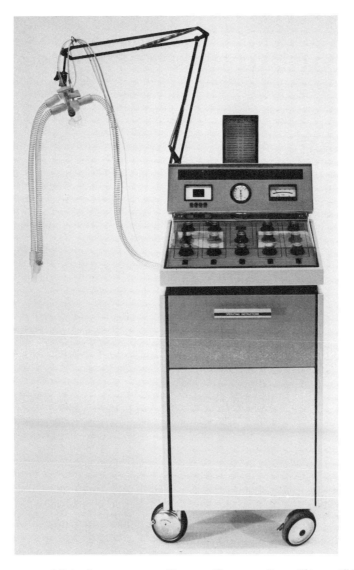

Fig. 11-44. Gill 1 volume respirator. (Courtesy Chemetron Corp., Chicago, Ill.)

THE GILL 1 RESPIRATOR

The Gill 1[13] (Fig. 11-44) is an electrically powered and controlled, double-circuit, gravity-driven, weighted piston ventilator that can be an assistor, a controller, or an assistor/controller and is designed to volume limit. The control panel for the unit is seen in Fig. 11-45.

Referring to the diagrams of Fig. 11-46, the weighted piston, 5, is sealed in its cylinder by a rolling diaphragm, 6.[13] During *exhalation*, the piston is raised to the desired height by the vacuum side of a compressor, 9. Air and oxygen are drawn in below the piston through a one-way valve, 18. Once the piston has been raised to the set volume (tidal volume), solenoid 7 closes, and the piston is held suspended until inhalation begins.

Once an inspiratory signal, either from the rate control or the assist mechanism, is seen, a solenoid, 2, opens and allows a communication with atmospheric pressure above the piston. Gravity causes the weighted piston to fall, expelling its gases into the patient system through a one-way valve, 19, past an oxygen sensor, 23, through a filter, 22, a humidifier, 25, and to the patient outlet. The exhalation valve, 12, is inflated by the compressor, 9, by way of the open expiratory control solenoid, 11.

When the piston reaches bottom and its cylinder is empty, inhalation ends (volume limit). Solenoid 11 opens the exhalation valve to atmospheric pressure, causing it to decompress, and the patient is allowed to exhale. Meanwhile, solenoids 2 and 7 close and open, respectively, at the same time. Solenoid 2 provides a seal so that when the piston is exposed to the negative pressure of compressor 9 through open solenoid 7, it is lifted for refill.

Drive mechanism and flow characteristics. The drive mechanism for the Gill 1 is

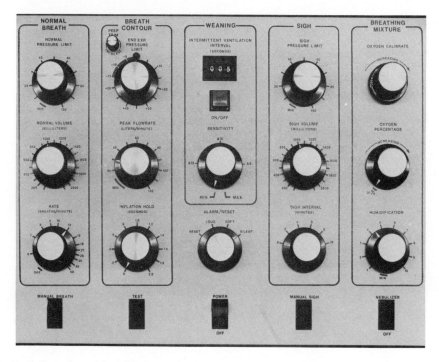

Fig. 11-45. Control panel for Gill 1 Respirator. (Courtesy Chemetron HealthCare Systems, St. Louis, Mo.)

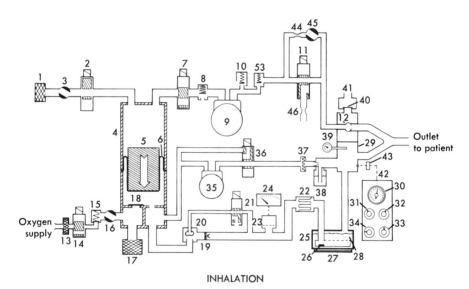

Fig. 11-46. Functional flow diagram for Gill 1 Respirator during expiratory mode and inhalation. *1*, Control air-intake filter; *2*, piston-delivery (drop) solenoid valve; *3*, peak flowrate control valve; *4*, cylinder assembly; *5*, weighted piston; *6*, rolling diaphragm; *7*, piston reset (lift) solenoid valve; *8*, vacuum-relief valve; *9*, vacuum/pressure pump; *10*, pressure-relief valve; *11*, expiratory control solenoid valve; *12*, patient manifold balloon valve; *13*, oxygen-intake filter; *14*, oxygen-control solenoid valve; *15*, oxygen pressure regulator; *16*, oxygen percentage control valve; *17*, patient air intake filter; *18*, breathing gas intake check valve; *19*, breathing gas outlet check valve; *20*, inspiration lockout valve; *21*, inspiration lockout control/solenoid valve; *22*, mainline bacterial filter; *23*, oxygen sensor; *24*, oxygen percentage display meter; *25*, humidifier assembly; *26*, check valve; *27*, humidifier heater; *28*, water reservoir; *29*, patient manifold assembly; *30*, patient air-pressure gauge; *31*, normal pressure-limit control; *32*, sigh pressure-limit control; *33*, end expiratory pressure limit control; *34*, sensitivity control; *35*, nebulizer pump; *36*, nebulizer control solenoid valve; *37*, nebulizer air bacterial filter, *38*, nebulizer (part of patient manifold assembly); *39*, thermometer; *40*, expired gas check valve; *41*, expired gas exhaust port; *42*, pressure-sensing line; *43*, pressure-sensing line isolator; *44*, fixed orifice; *45*, PEEP trim control; *46*, fixed orifice; *53*, control air pressure regulator. (Courtesy Chemetron HealthCare Systems, St. Louis, Mo.)

simply gravity's effect on the weighted piston.[13] It functions basically like a weighted concertina bag.[2]

Fig. 11-47 shows examples of flow and pressure patterns recorded while ventilating a lung simulator. Because of the relatively low driving force of the falling piston, the flow curve is slightly tapered in a *decelerating* fashion.

Peak inspiratory flow rate can be controlled by an independent control, 3 (Fig. 11-46; also see control panel in Fig. 11-45). Peak flows up to 120 L/min can be obtained. The control itself functions by restricting the inflow of ambient air *above* the piston as it falls during inhalation.

Volume control. The tidal volume adjustment is a *potentiometer* on the panel that sets a reference voltage to be matched by another potentiometer that senses the position of the piston.[13] As the piston rises, the piston potentiometer voltage changes until it matches the reference setting and causes solenoid 7 leading to the vacuum pump, 9, to close. The piston is then held in this position until inhalation.

When the piston reaches bottom during inhalation, *volume limit* occurs; that is, inhalation is terminated, and the piston refills to the preset volume again.

The amount of piston movement can be seen on the *inspiration volume* indicator arising from the back of the ventilator over the display and control panels (Fig. 11-44).

The compressibility factor is constant at approximately 3 to 3.5 cc/cm H_2O pressure. Different tubing circuit sizes and water level changes in the humidifier can change this value.

Rate mechanism. The rate control is a timing mechanism that divides each minute into equal parts. This single control sets how many times per minute the ventilator cycles on as a minimum value. The rate control can be set for 6 to 60 breaths/min.[13]

I:E ratio. Since the rate control establishes how long each complete ventilatory cycle may last, the inspiratory-to-expiratory ratio is primarily a function of set tidal volume, inspiratory flow rate, and rate controls. Since changes in the patient's airway resistance and lung compliance can change the inspiratory flow rate and, therefore, inspiratory time, these changes also affect the I:E ratio. Examples of the effects of these changes can be found in Chapter 8.

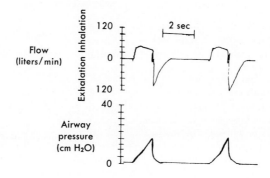

Fig. 11-47. Flow and pressure curves for Gill 1 Respirator applied to lung simulator set for compliance of 50 ml/cm H_2O and resistance of 5 cm H_2O/L/sec. (Modified from Chemetron HealthCare Systems, St. Louis, Mo.)

The Gill 1 has a feature that, during control mode, prevents inspiratory time from exceeding expiratory time. Once inhalation lasts for half of the ventilatory cycle time set by the rate control, an abort signal stops inhalation, and the I:E ratio alarm will be triggered. Therefore the I:E ratio cannot be less than 1:1 during control mode.[13]

Assist and sensitivity mechanism. The assist mechanism is a pressure transducer that is referenced to system pressure (pressure within the patient circuit). When the reference voltage set by the sensitivity control is reached, the appropriate solenoids are triggered, and inhalation begins. To make the unit more sensitive to the patient's effort, a reference voltage, which requires less movement by the transducer's diaphragm for the matching voltage, is set. The *lockout* solenoid (*21* in Fig. 11-46) closes the lockout diaphragm, *20*, so that the patient cannot breathe from the cylinder until the set level of differential pressure is achieved for an assist signal.

Assisted breaths when PEEP is being used are possible as the *end expiratory pressure* control references the sensitivity to the increased baseline pressure.

Oxygen system. As the piston rises during refill (expiratory phase), gas is drawn into the cylinder below through a one-way valve, *18*, through the air supply inlet filter, *17*, and the oxygen supply inlet filter, *13*. The proportion of the intake gases is adjusted by a variable restriction, *16*, in the oxygen supply line. The *greater* the restriction, the lower the flow of oxygen into the intake and the lower the oxygen concentration. The oxygen supply solenoid, *14*, closes when 21% is set, so all gas entering the bottom portion of the piston is drawn in through the air inlet filter only.

Oxygen levels are adjusted by changing the oxygen control, *16*, until the desired concentration is displayed on the analog meter, *24*, reading in oxygen percentages. This meter obtains its signal from a galvanic (fuel cell) analyzer probe, *23*, which senses oxygen within the patient circuit. An optional system allows for alarms at variable low and high oxygen values.

Sigh system. A timer for setting the number of minutes between sigh breaths (Fig. 11-45) can be set from 0 to 10 minutes in 2-minute increments. When this timer establishes that the next breath will be a sigh, the *normal volume* control setting is ignored, and another potentiometer (the *sigh volume*) is used to set the piston's volume for the next breath.

A *manual sigh switch* can also be used to initiate a sigh breath.

Pressure limit systems. Both the *normal pressure limit* and *sigh pressure limit* controls function in the same manner but are independent of one another. The controls are potentiometers that set a reference voltage to correspond with a certain amount of pressure. A master pressure transducer continuously senses pressure in the patient circuit. As pressure in the patient system changes, the voltage in the pressure transducer changes proportionately. If the reference pressure set on the pressure limit controls is ever reached, a signal to end inhalation (open solenoids *7* and *11* and close solenoid *2*) immediately occurs.

During normal tidal volumes, the normal pressure limit control is functional while the sigh pressure limit control setting is ignored, and during the sigh mode the reverse occurs.

Inflation hold control. The inflation hold control establishes a delay between the time the piston reaches bottom (end of active inhalation) and the time when exhala-

Specifications for Gill 1 Respirator

Tidal volume:	200 to 2100 cc
Rate:	6 to 60 breaths/min (or 5 to 199 seconds between IMV breaths)
Peak flow rate:	Up to 120 L/min
Sensitivity:	From approximately 0.15 cm H_2O to -20 cm H_2O pressure
Pressure limit:	20 to 100 cm H_2O pressure
Inflation hold:	0 to 2.0 seconds in 0.2 second intervals
Sigh intervals:	0 to 10 minutes
Oxygen percentage:	21% to 100% (noncalibrated)
End expiratory pressure:	-15 to $+50$ cm H_2O pressure
Visual indicators:	Pressure limit*
	Low pressure*
	Improper cycle* (set tidal volume not delivered in 20 seconds)
	I : E ratio (below 1 : 1)
	Power failure*
	Assist
	Control
	Oxygen added
	Improper oxygen percentage*
	Fill humidifier*
	Sigh
	Alarms silent

*Audible alarm also

tion can begin when the exhalation solenoid dumps the exhalation valve. The set volume is delivered into the patient system and held trapped there until inflation hold is over. Values from 0 to 2 seconds can be set.

This control *adds* to the inspiratory portion of the I : E ratio, and since the set rate will remain unchanged, the expiratory portion will decrease. Inflation hold can also sound the I : E ratio alarm system if its addition extends inhalation beyond half of the total cycle time established by the rate control.

PEEP and NEEP system. These systems are controlled by the *end expiratory pressure* control. The control is another potentiometer for establishing a reference voltage that is proportional to a given pressure level. Pressures from -15 cm H_2O to $+20$ cm H_2O can be allowed with this control, which also references the sensitivity control.[13] Pressures up to 50 cm H_2O for PEEP are available as an option.

For negative pressures, an optional attachment is needed. The device is basically a Venturi system added externally that is fed from the pressure side of the compressor, 9.

The *PEEP trim control, 45,* sets the amount of positive pressure held in the exhalation valve during exhalation. Once the pressure within the patient system (sensed by the master pressure transducer) is equal to the desired level set on the *end expiratory pressure limit control, 33,* solenoid *11* opens and seals the exhalation valve, ensuring that no further pressure drop will occur around the exhalation valve.

Nebulizer system. Again referring to Fig. 11-46, during the inspiratory mode, compressor 35 draws some gases from the piston's cylinder, compresses them, and forces them through the filter, 37, and the nebulizer, 38, in the patient circuit by way of the open solenoid, 36. During the expiratory mode, solenoid 36 closes the patient circuit from the compressor and opens another line so that the compressor simply recirculates gases from its intake until inhalation starts again.

The results are that the nebulizer is driven during inhalation only from premixed air and oxygen from the piston, and, therefore, the oxygen concentration and set volume are *unchanged* by the nebulizer's use.

Other systems. An *IMV system* is available on later models. When the *IMV switch* is on, the rate control is bypassed, and another timer sets the interval between

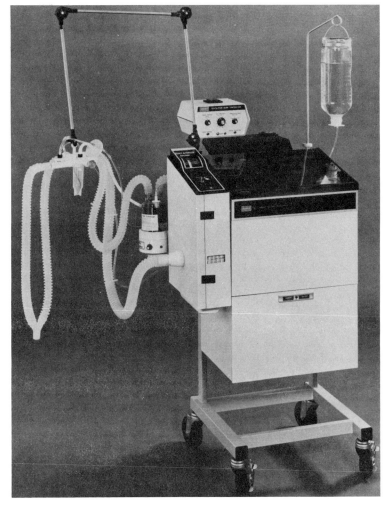

Fig. 11-48. Searle Volume Ventilator Adult (VVA). (Courtesy Searle Cardio-Pulmonary Systems, Inc., Hayward, Calif.)

IMV (control) breaths in seconds. It is adjustable up to 199 seconds.[13] Between these cycles, the patient may spontaneously breathe from an additional source of fresh gases, which must be connected to the patient circuit.

Visual signals for assist or control mode, sigh breaths, oxygen enrichment, and alarm silence are displayed above the control panel (Fig. 11-44). Visual and audible signals are available for indicating pressure limit, improper oxygen, low pressure, improper cycle, power failure, and empty humidifier conditions. An optional digital timing display can be selected to look at inspiratory and expiratory times, I : E ratio, and respiratory rates. The rate is a 30-second average recalculated every 10 seconds.

The box on p. 292 summarizes the Gill 1's specifications.

THE SEARLE VOLUME VENTILATOR ADULT (VVA)

The Searle Volume Ventilator Adult (VVA)[14] is an electrically powered and controlled spring-driven piston ventilator designed to be volume limited (Fig. 11-48). The unit can be patient- or time-cycled on so as to be used as a controller or an assistor-controller. The primary control panel is for the ventilator as seen in Fig. 11-49.

Referring to the diagram in Fig. 11-50, air from the *main compressor, 1,* and oxygen from the *oxygen regulator, 20,* is used to depress the piston in the *volume control chamber, 3,* to the desired tidal volume and oxygen percentage during the piston's filling phase (exhalation). During inhalation, gases from the piston are pushed out of the chamber by the springs. Gases pass through the *flow control valve, 9,* and the *variable orifice valve, 8,* and out to the patient circuit.

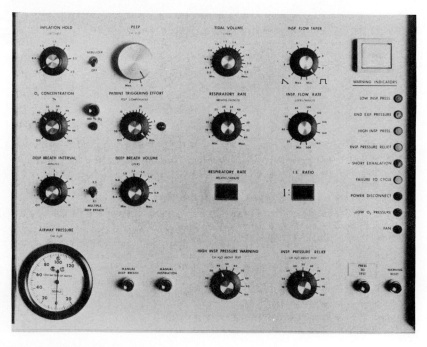

Fig. 11-49. Control panel for Searle VVA. (Courtesy Searle Cardio-Pulmonary Systems, Inc., Hayward, Calif.)

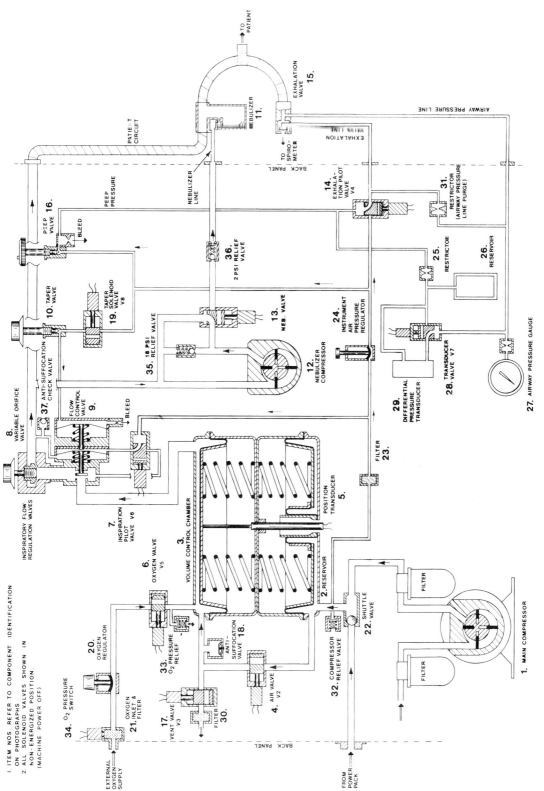

Fig. 11-50. Functional flow diagram for Searle VVA. All solenoid valves are shown in nonenergized position (machine power off). (Courtesy Searle Cardio-Pulmonary Systems, Inc., Hayward, Calif.)

Drive mechanism and flow characteristics. The drive mechanism for the VVA consists of four springs that maintain a pressure within the piston's chamber of above 100 cm H_2O, regardless of the chamber's gas volume.[14]

The *flow rate control valve* (Fig. 11-51) and the *taper valve* work together to produce either square or tapered flow patterns. The flow control valve is separated into two chambers. During inhalation, pressure from the patient circuit system is referenced back to the left chamber. As pressure increases, the diaphragm in this chamber is forced to the right and opens the outflow tract from the piston chamber more. Because of this feedback system, back pressure in the patient system does not decrease flow from the piston but rather is used to maintain a square wave or constant flow pattern. If the inspiratory flow taper valve is set toward the maximum taper level, then the right chamber of the flow control valve is used to override the left chamber. When the taper valve is open, the taper solenoid also opens to allow gases from the compressor *(instrument air)* to move against the right side of the diaphragm in the right chamber of the flow control valve during inhalation. The more open the taper valve, the more force exerted against the diaphragm, causing it to be pushed to the left. The spring-and-plunger mechanism in this chamber then pushes on the diaphragm in the left chamber, which causes the size of the outflow tract from the volume control chamber to be decreased. The *bleed* in the right chamber prevents pressure from the taper valve from ever becoming enough to completely close off the outflow tract. The minimum amount of flow allowed when maximum taper is set is 15 L/min.[14]

Examples of flow and pressure patterns for both square wave and taper are shown in Fig. 11-52.

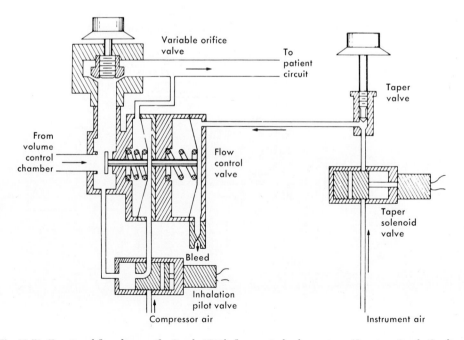

Fig. 11-51. Functional flow diagram for Searle VVA's flow control valve system. (Courtesy Searle Cardio-Pulmonary Systems, Inc., Hayward, Calif.)

Volume control and oxygen system. The tidal volume and oxygen concentration are determined by electronic logic according to the settings of the corresponding controls. Referring to Fig. 11-50, at the beginning of the refilling phase for the piston, the *oxygen valve, 6,* which is a solenoid valve, opens and begins pushing the piston downward. When the appropriate volume of oxygen is in the volume control chamber, the oxygen solenoid valve closes, and the *air valve, 4,* opens and fills the remaining volume needed. The *position transducer, 5,* is a linear potentiometer[14] that senses the position of the piston and therefore the volume above the piston.

Once the air valve closes, the piston is ready to expel the volume of air and oxygen within it for the next inhalation. The air from the main compressor now enters the *reservoir, 2,* depressing the springs there until this chamber is full. This system allows the air used for filling the piston chamber to come from the reservoir and the compressor if needed.

At end inhalation, the position transducer senses that the cylinder is empty, and volume limit occurs. Since the piston reaches the same position each time volume limit occurs, the compressibility factor is a nearly constant one, varying primarily with different tubing circuit sizes. The factor is about 2.5 cc/cm H_2O.

Rate mechanism. The rate control is a timing mechanism that divides each minute into equal parts. This single control sets how many times per minute the ventilator cycles on as a minimum value. The rate control is calibrated from 5 to 60 breaths/min.[14]

I:E ratio. The respiratory rate, tidal volume, inspiratory flow rate, and inspiratory flow taper controls all influence the I:E ratio, which is digitally displayed on the front of the machine.

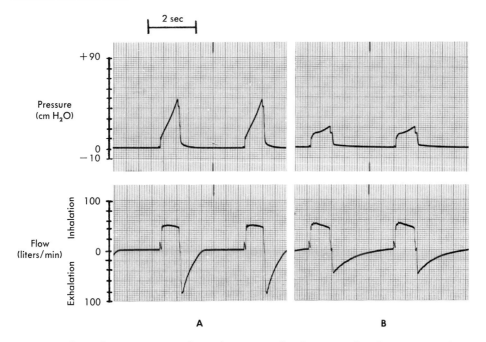

Fig. 11-52. Flow and pressure patterns for Searle VVA. Graph **A** shows unit when flow taper control is set for square wave and **B** when that control is set on maximum taper. Both graphs were made with VVA ventilated lung simulator set for compliance of 50 ml/cm H_2O and resistance of 5 cm H_2O/L/sec.

Assist and sensitivity mechanisms. The sensitivity adjusts the amount of patient effort required to trigger an assist breath. It functions as a reference to the pressure transducer. When positive end expiratory pressure, PEEP, is utilized, the sensitivity is compensated for this increase in baseline pressure. Therefore assist mode is available even when PEEP is applied. Sensitivity is adjustable so that patient effort causing pressures from -0.2 to -20 cm H_2O will cycle inhalation on.[14]

Pressure limit system. The inspiratory phase can end before volume delivery if the pressure set on the *inspiratory pressure relief* control is reached. The patient's circuit is depressurized by the *exhalation pilot valve, 14,* opening to atmosphere and allowing the exhalation valve to vent. The gases still in the volume control chamber, *3,* are simultaneously relieved or vented through a solenoid valve called the *vent valve, 17.* The pressure relief control and the *high inspiratory pressure warning* control (Fig. 11-49) both function at pressures above end expiratory. Therefore, if PEEP is used, the set pressures on these controls represent that amount *above* the PEEP level.

Inflation hold control. Inflation hold is adjustable from 0 to 3 seconds. When on, the exhalation valve is maintained in an inflated state after tidal volume delivery for the set time period by delaying the exhalation pilot (solenoid) valve from opening. Once this time elapses, the exhalation valve is allowed to vent, and exhalation occurs as usual.

Sigh system. The sigh volume control supplies a new reference for the piston's position transducer. Volumes and oxygen mixtures during a sigh breath are com-

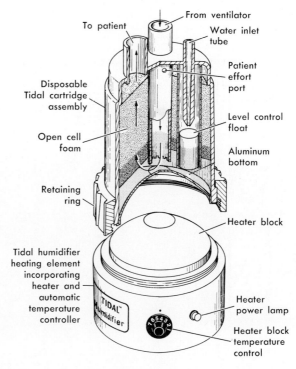

Fig. 11-53. Functional diagram of Searle's Tidal Humidifier system. (Courtesy Searle Cardio-Pulmonary Systems, Inc., Hayward, Calif.)

puted in the same fashion as for the normal tidal volume. The sigh rate controls can be set to deliver one, two, or three consecutive sighs every 1 to 10 minutes, or they can be off.[14] Ventilatory cycle times as set by the respiratory rate control are *unchanged* during the sigh breaths.

PEEP system. The PEEP control (*16* in Fig. 11-50) adjusts the amount of leak from the compressor against a bleed to the patient circuit's exhalation valve, thus maintaining a set pressure in that valve and therefore the patient's circuit. This pressure is referenced to the pressure transducer so that PEEP assist is available through the sensitivity control.

Nebulizer system. The nebulizer system uses a compressor (*12* in Fig. 11-50) to pump gases from the tidal volume through the nebulizer in the patient's circuit. Because the unit functions only during inhalation and draws from gases available only from the volume control chamber, oxygen concentration or tidal volume are *not* changed.[14] The nebulizer's only control is an on/off switch located on the control panel (Fig. 11-49).

Humidity system. The Searle VVA utilizes a heated humidifier system. The *tidal humidifier* system (Fig. 11-53) functions in a pulsatile fashion. During inhalation, gases from the ventilator push heated water into the *open cell foam* and pass on through it to the patient.[15] The foam provides a high surface area contact between the ventilator gases and the water. The water level in the tidal cartridge is maintained by the *level control float* built in and is fed by a continuous feed system. Because the water level is relatively constant and because the space above the water is small, the humidifier contributes only about 0.3 ml/cm H_2O to the circuit's compressibility factor.[15]

Intermittent Demand Ventilation (IDV) system. IDV can be set on the Searle's optional Ventilation Mode Controller[16] (VMC) shown in Fig. 11-54. On the IDV setting, the unit is set to deliver one pressurized volume preset breath out of *x* spontaneous breaths. Spontaneous breaths are accomplished by the ventilator sensing a patient effort and the piston expelling its volume into a special circuit with a reser-

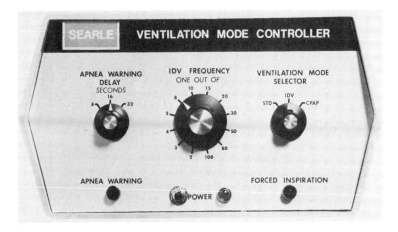

Fig. 11-54. Searle's Ventilation Mode Controller (VMC). (Courtesy Searle Cardio-Pulmonary Systems, Inc., Hayward, Calif.)

voir and extra valves inline. During this spontaneous breath, however, the exhalation valves are not closed. Therefore the gases from the piston may be inhaled or just vented according to the patient's inspiratory efforts.

The IDV system works on assist signals only,[17] and if the patient's rate falls below that set on the respiration rate control, the ventilator takes over to breathe for the patient with pressurized, volume preset ventilation. An apnea alarm will sound if no *assist* efforts are seen for 8, 16, or 32 seconds as set on the delay switch.

On CPAP mode all breaths are unpressurized spontaneous breaths with the same backup (control) rate and alarm capabilities. Standard (STD) mode allows the VVA to operate in assist/control or control modes as usual even though the VMC is connected.

Expiratory spirometer system. The Searle VVA utilizes the Autowedge Spirometer[18] system (Fig. 11-55). This unit is a wedge that collects the expired gases. The expansion position of the wedge is electronically monitored and converted to volume on the meter found on the top of the unit. The next inhalation causes a motorized *pusher plate* to exhaust the wedge, making it ready for another expiratory volume.

The accompanying box summarizes the various specifications of the Searle VVA.[14]

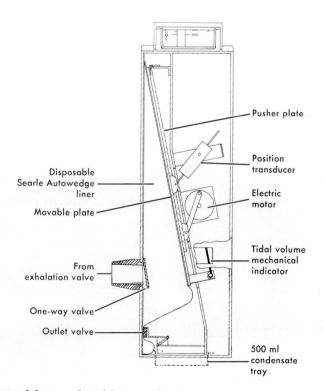

Fig. 11-55. Functional diagram of Searle's Autowedge Spirometer. (Courtesy Searle Cardio-Pulmonary Systems, Inc., Hayward, Calif.)

Specifications for Searle Volume Ventilator Adult (VVA)

Controls

Tidal volume:	0.3 to 2.2 liters
Respiratory rate:	5 to 60 breaths/min
Inspiratory flow rate:	20 to 200 L/min
Inspiratory pressure relief:	10 to 100 cm H_2O
High inspiratory pressure warning:	10 to 100 cm H_2O
Oxygen concentration:	21% or 24% to 100% oxygen
Positive end expiratory pressure:	0 to 20 cm H_2O
Inflation hold:	0 to 3 seconds
Deep-breath interval:	1 to 10 minutes
Deep-breath volume:	0.4 to 2.2 liters
Multiple deep breaths:	1, 2, or 3
Patient triggering effort:	−0.2 to −20 cm H_2O for patient-initiated cycling
Manual starts:	Inhalation and deep breath
Inspiratory flow taper:	Adjustable flow pattern, square to tapered curve

Displays

Airway pressure:	−20 to 100 cm H_2O
Respiratory rate (digital):	5 to 60 breaths/min
I:E ratio (digital):	1:0.5 to 1:9.9

Outputs for remote monitoring

Patient triggering
Inhalation
Airway pressure
Warning signal
Spirometer volume

Warning systems*

Low inspiratory pressure†:	Airway pressures less than 8 cm H_2O at end of inhalation
High end expiratory pressure† (visual only):	Airway pressure greater than 5 cm H_2O at end of exhalation (visual only)
High inspiratory pressure†:	Selected value 10 to 100 cm H_2O
Inspiratory pressure relief†:	Selected value 10 to 100 cm H_2O
Short exhalation (visual only):	1 greater than E (visual only)
Failure to cycle:	After 15 seconds
Power disconnect:	Power switch *on* without AC power
Low oxygen pressure:	Oxygen supply pressure less than 10 psi
Fan:	Activated when cooling fan flow is insufficient

*Audible and visual indicators
†PEEP compensated

REFERENCES

1. McPherson, S. P., and Roads, J. S.: History of respiratory therapy. (To be published.)
2. Mushin, W. W., et al.: Automatic ventilation of the lungs, ed. 2, Philadelphia, 1969, F. A. Davis Co.
3. Detailed instruction manual for the AS-18000 Mueller-Mörch Piston Ventilator, Chicago, V. Mueller & Co.
4. Mörch, E. T., et al.: Artificial respiration via the uncuffed tracheostomy tube, J.A.M.A. **160**:864, 1956.
5. Emerson Post Operative Ventilator operating instructions, Form 3-PV-1, Cambridge, Mass., 1969, J. H. Emerson Co.
6. Conlee, K.: Control of oxygen concentration during the sigh mode with the Emerson Post-Op Ventilator, Respir. Care **20**:268, 1975.
7. Engström Respirator System ER-300 service manuals, Rockville, Md., LKB Medical, Inc.
8. Instruction manual, Bourns Infant Ventilator, Model LS104-150 with PEEP System, 4-21, 2-74, Riverside, Calif., Bourns, Inc., Life Systems Division.
9. Instruction manual, Bourns O_2 Blender model LS145, Riverside, Calf., 1974, Bourns, Inc., Life Systems Division.
10. Rogers, E. J.: Physics versus physiology in infant ventilation, Respir. Ther. vol. 2, no. 5, 1972.
11. Epstein, R. A.: The sensitivities and response times of ventilatory assistors, Anesthesiology **34**:321, 1971.
12. McPherson, S. P.: New products reports; Bourns Pediatric Ventilator with PEEP assist, Respir. Care **19**:474, 1974.
13. Gill 1 Volume Controlled Respirator operations manual, Form No. 102300-89, St. Louis, March, 1975, Chemetron HealthCare Systems.
14. VVA Volume Ventilator Adult operating manual, OM1-4, Form no. 12125-B, Hayward, Calif., 1976, Searle Cardio-Pulmonary Systems, Inc.
15. Searle Tidal Humidifier operating manual, Form no. 11852 A (6-75), Hayward, Calif., 1975, Searle Cardio-Pulmonary Systems, Inc.
16. Searle Ventilation Mode Controller operating manual, Form no. 12594-A (2-76), Hayward, Calif., Searle Cardio-Pulmonary Systems, Inc.
17. Shapiro, B. A., et al.: Intermittent demand ventilation (IDV): a new technique for supporting ventilation in critically ill patients, Respir. Care **21**:521, 1976.
18. Searle Autowedge Spirometer Operating Manual, Form no. 12123-A (3/76), Hayward, Calif., 1975, Searle Cardio-Pulmonary Systems, Inc.

12 Bellows and other ventilators

THE AIR SHIELDS ICV-10 VENTILATOR

The ICV-10 Ventilator, formerly the Air Shields 10,000 (Fig. 12-1), is an electrically powered and controlled, low-pressure blower-driven bellows, time- and/or patient-cycled, time-limited, double-circuit ventilator.[1-3] Referring to Fig. 12-2, during inhalation a *centrifugal blower* sends gases past the *solenoid valve*, through the *flow control* and into the *cylinder*, which surrounds the *bellows*. These gases push the bellows upward, and the gases within the bellows move into the patient circuit, past the *centrifugal nebulizer* (or heated humidifier on later units) and to the *patient connection*. The *exhalation valve* is inflated by pressure from the driving circuit created by the blower.

In the expiratory phase, the solenoid valve closes, the bellows cylinder and the exhalation valve exhaust their pressure into the atmosphere, and the patient exhales. The bellows falls and fills with gases from the *air* and *oxygen inlets*.

Drive mechanism, flow, and volume characteristics. The primary drive mechanism for the ICV-10 is a centrifugal blower. It is capable of providing pressures of up to about 55 cm H_2O.[1,2] Flow and pressure patterns are consistent with those described in Chapter 8 for bellows ventilators driven with a relatively low pressure. Fig. 12-3 shows examples of curves for the ICV-10 under different clinical settings.

A peak flow is set with the *flow control* (Figs. 12-2 and 12-4). The flow control is a variable-sized restriction in the line from the blower.[1] The smaller the restriction, the lower the peak flow. Even when inspiratory flow is maximum and as pressure builds in the circuit, the flow tapers (Fig. 12-3) because of the decreasing pressure gradient. The *inspiratory time control* (Fig. 12-4) establishes the time duration of flow. If the flow were constant, the volume could be calculated. However, *flow is not constant*, and changes in the patient's resistance and compliance will affect the pressure gradient, the flow, and therefore the *volume* delivered during the set inspiratory time.[2]

Basically, then, the Air Shields provides a timed, nonconstant flow. The factors controlling *volume* delivery are (1) the flow rate set on the machine, (2) the inspiratory time allowed, and (3) the resistance and compliance of the patient system. As an example, increased flow during a set inspiratory time would cause an increased tidal volume. Increased inspiratory time at a set peak flow setting would also achieve an increased tidal volume. Decreased patient compliance or increased airway resistance would cause a *drop* in a delivered tidal volume.

Rate and I:E ratio. Rate is a function of (1) the inspiratory time control and (2)

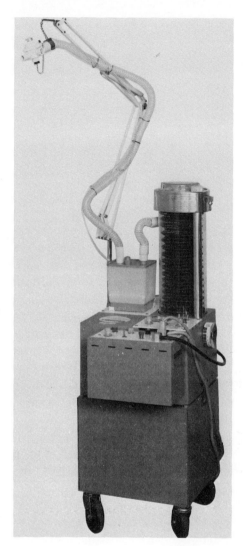

Fig. 12-1. ICV-10 Ventilator. (Courtesy Isolette, Warminster, Pa.)

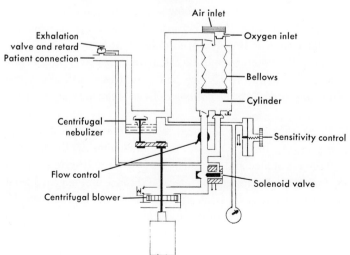

Fig. 12-2. ICV-10 (Air Shields 10,000) schematic. (Modified from Mushin, W. W., et al.: Automatic ventilation of the lungs, ed. 2, Philadelphia, 1969, F. A. Davis Co.)

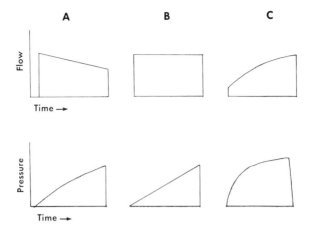

Fig. 12-3. Typical flow and pressure curves for ICV-10 Ventilator under different clinical situations. **A,** Curves against lungs having low compliance and low airway resistance. **B,** Curves against normal lungs with high compliance and low airway resistance. **C,** Curves against lungs with high compliance and high airway resistance.

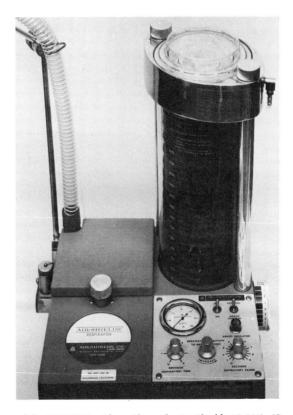

Fig. 12-4. Control panel for ICV-10 Ventilator (formerly Air Shields 10,000). (Courtesy Isolette, Warminster, Pa.)

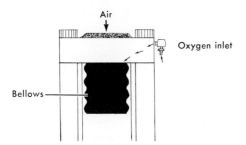

Fig. 12-5. Oxygen mixing system for ICV-10 Ventilator. When bellows falls during expiratory phase, it refills with filtered air and oxygen is added through oxygen inlet, increasing oxygen concentration inside bellows.

the expiratory time control setting (another electric timer) or (3) in the case of patient assist, the patient establishes his own rate and decreases the set I:E ratio.

The compressibility factor is variable from about 3 to 6 cc/cm H_2O, depending primarily on the bellows position at the end of each inhalation. Each inhalation begins with the bellows completely full and ends with generally only *part* of the 2400 cc maximum volume emptied.

Assist and sensitivity mechanism. The solenoid is activated by either the expiratory time control when the preset time has elapsed or by the *sensitivity mechanism*, if the patient assists. When the patient takes a breath, the subatmospheric pressure in the circuit pulls the sensitivity diaphragm (Fig. 12-2) to the left, making an electric contact that sends current to the solenoid. The sensitivity adjustment is threaded, and movement of the sensitivity control changes spring force applied to the diaphragm at the contacts.[1] The more sensitive the setting, the more the spring tension. This requires minimal effort on the part of the patient to move the diaphragm enough to cause contact.

Oxygen system. Oxygen control is a simple addition mechanism where a reservoir can be attached. As the bellows drops, it draws in air as well as any oxygen in the vicinity of the air intake (Fig. 12-5). A modification of this system (not shown) provides an increased-volume reservoir supplied by a high flow from an oxygen controller. The oxygen concentration achieved may vary as changing inspiratory pressures cause changing inspiratory volumes. If the patient is assisting and thus changing the minute volume delivered from the bellows, the oxygen concentration may also change.

Humidity system. Early models of this ventilator utilized a centrifugal nebulizer to provide humidification (Fig. 12-2). Later models used heated bubble-cascade type humidifiers as pictured in Fig. 12-1.

The accompanying box summarizes the specifications for the Air Shields ICV-10.

Specifications for Air Shields ICV-10 Ventilator

Tidal volume:	Up to 2400 cc
Flow rate:	Up to 120 L/min
Inspiratory time:	0.5 to 3 seconds
Expiratory time:	0.5 to 10 seconds
Functional rate:	From about 5 to 60 breaths/min
Sensitivity:	Adjustable from 0.5 to 2 cm H_2O
Pressure manometer:	0 to 60 cm H_2O

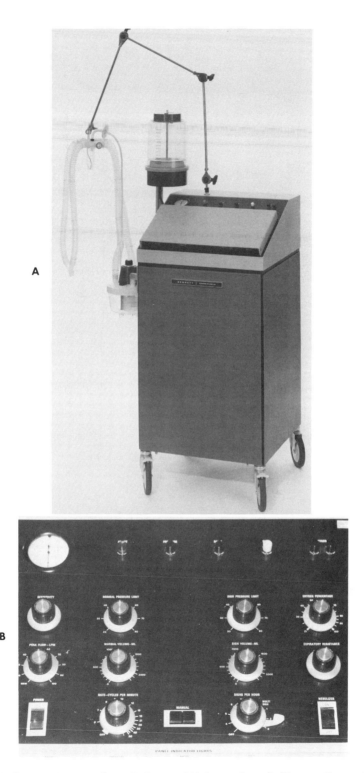

Fig. 12-6. A, Bennett MA-1 ventilator. **B,** Bennett MA-1 control panel. (Courtesy Bennett Respiration Products, Inc., Santa Monica, Calif.)

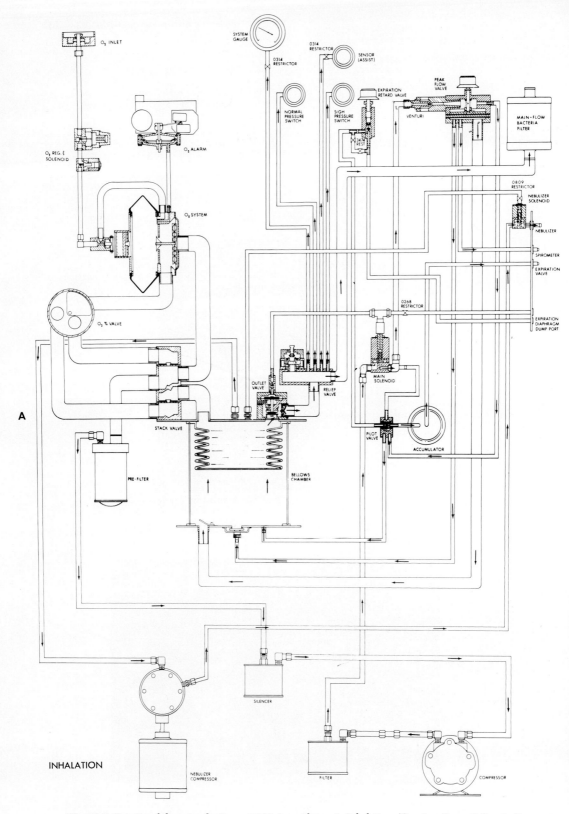

Fig. 12-7. Functional diagrams for Bennett MA-1 ventilator. **A,** Inhalation. (Courtesy Bennett Respiration Products, Inc., Santa Monica, Calif.)

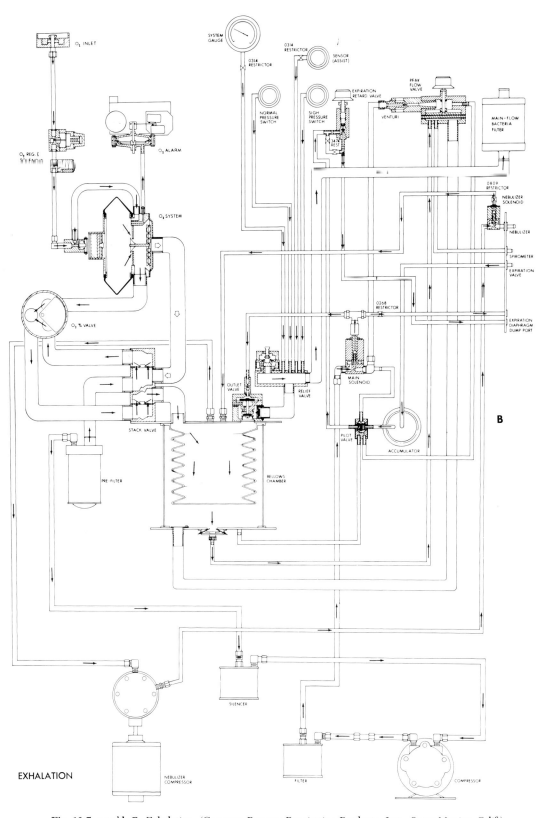

Fig. 12-7, cont'd. B, Exhalation. (Courtesy Bennett Respiration Products, Inc., Santa Monica, Calif.)

THE BENNETT MA-1 VENTILATOR

The MA-1 (Fig. 12-6) is an electrically powered, low-pressure drive, double-circuit, compressor-powered bellows ventilator and is designed to be volume limited.[4] The unit can be patient cycled or time cycled, which provides for assist, assist-control, or control modes.[4]

Referring to the diagram in Fig. 12-7, *A*, during inhalation gas from a *compressor* flows through the *main solenoid* and is directed from there up to the *Venturi* and *peak flow* system. The main flow of gas leaving the Venturi is directed to the *bellows* chamber (cylinder) by a large-bore tube and through a one-way valve. The bellows contains the gases that the patient will receive. Pressure from the Venturi compresses the bellows upward. Gases from the bellows flow out of the ventilator through the *bacteria filter* to the patient tubing circuit (not shown).

During exhalation (Fig. 12-7, *B*), the main solenoid switches the gas from the compressor away from the Venturi. Now the compressor pressurizes the *outlet valve* on top of the bellows as well as vents out the side of the ventilator.

The bellows falls and refills, pulling gases from the *stack valve* of the oxygen system. When the main solenoid receives a signal from either the rate control, the assist mechanism, or the manual breath button, the main solenoid will once again switch the compressor's gas flow to the Venturi to begin inhalation.

Drive mechanism and flow characteristics. The power drive mechanism (Fig. 12-8) of the MA-1 consists of a *compressor* that delivers about 7 psig peak pressure and a *master solenoid* that directs gas flow to or away from the Venturi. The Venturi is fairly effective in that it can take the incoming gas pressure, which is about 6 psi because of the resistance to flow through the circuitry and drops to about 1.8 psi after air entrainment[5] (Fig. 12-9). The gas leaving the Venturi travels to the bellows chamber, compressing the bellows upward. The main solenoid either sends gas to

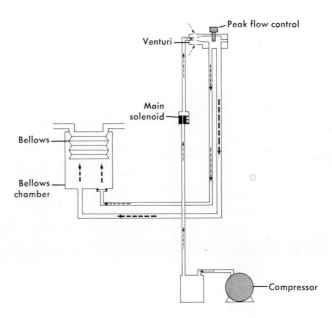

Fig. 12-8. MA-1 drive circuit. (Modified from Bennett Respiration Products, Inc., Santa Monica, Calif.)

the Venturi, causing inhalation, or sends flow out the side of the MA-1, which is either dumped into the atmosphere or is used to power expiratory controls.

Gas from the Venturi enters during initial inhalation at peak flow, and the bellows correspondingly delivers that flow to the patient circuit. From that point on the flow of gas *tapers* as resistance causes increased pressure in the patient's machine circuitry and as the pressure gradient drops (Fig. 12-10).[4] The peak flow delivery of the unit is preset with the peak flow control, and the flow then tapers toward zero as the peak pressure of the master Venturi is approached. Normally, the volume is delivered *much sooner* than peak pressure is reached where the flow would drop to zero. Functionally, the peak pressure of the driving system is never reached because the maximum pressure is limited to 80 cm H_2O by the pressure limit control.

As mentioned in Chapter 8, other resistance/compliance situations for this type of ventilator can cause altered flow patterns.[4] Examples of flow and pressure curves taken while ventilating a lung simulator are shown in Fig. 12-11.

Volume control. The volume control (Fig. 12-12) is actually a *reference potentiometer* that sets a reference electric potential.[5] There is another potentiometer connected to the bellows bottom by a *pulley wheel* that senses the position of the bellows by changing its voltage as the bellows rises. Once the bellows potentiometer has reached the *same* voltage as the reference voltage set on the volume control, the main solenoid is switched to the expiratory phase. Gas flow to the bellows canister then stops from the Venturi, and the bellows returns to the bottom.

Because the bellows always starts inhalation from its full position (2200 ml) and only empties part (set tidal volume) way, the compressibility factor is variable with each tidal volume set. The factor is usually about 4 to 5 cc/cm H_2O subtracted from

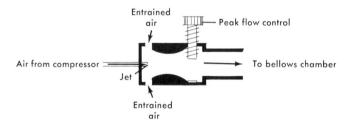

Fig. 12-9. MA-1 functional diagram of Venturi and peak flow control for MA-1.

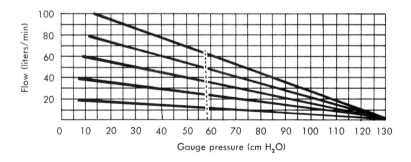

Fig. 12-10. MA-1 tapering flow. Flow will normally taper from peak flow until preset volume is delivered and then drop to zero (as indicated by dotted line). (Courtesy Bennett Respiration Products, Inc., Santa Monica, Calif.)

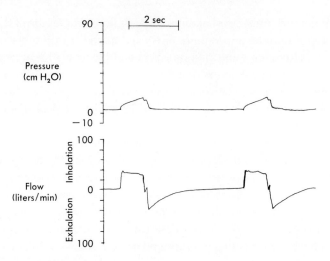

Fig. 12-11. Pressure and flow patterns redrawn from actual tracings for MA-1 ventilator while ventilating lung simulator set for compliance of 50 ml/cm H_2O and a resistance of 5 cm H_2O/L/sec.

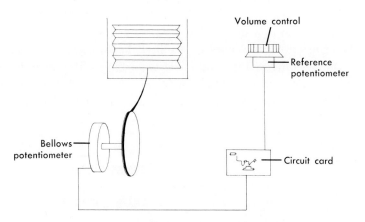

Fig. 12-12. Functional diagram of MA-1 volume control system.

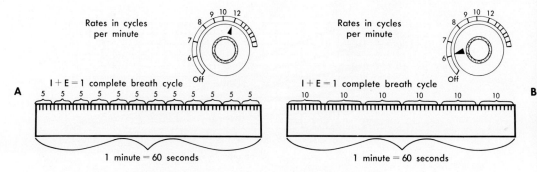

Fig. 12-13. Rate control for MA-1 divides each minute into individual ventilatory cycle times. **A,** With rate set at 12 breaths/min, ventilator starts every 5 seconds. **B,** With rate decreased to 6 breaths/min, ventilator starts every 10 seconds. (Courtesy Bennett Respiration Products, Inc., Santa Monica, Calif.)

the *set* tidal volume. Approximately 3 cc/cm H_2O can be used when subtracting this value from the exhaled volume observed on the expiratory spirometer.[4]

Rate mechanism. The rate control is an *electric timer*. It sets how often inhalation is to occur and sends an impulse to the main solenoid, causing a flow of gas to go to the Venturi.[6] Basically (Fig. 12-13), the rate control divides a minute up into *x* number of parts. When the allotted ventilatory-cycle period is over, the control establishes the next inspiratory phase by activating the main solenoid.

I:E ratio. The I:E ratio for the MA-1 is a function of (1) the *rate control,* which sets the allotted time for each ventilatory cycle, (2) the set *tidal volume,* and (3) the *peak flow setting;* (2) and (3) together establish the time required for inhalation. Changes in the patient's resistance and compliance can also alter the time of inhalation by affecting flow rate. The remainder of the ventilatory cycle, as established by the rate control, becomes the expiratory portion of the cycle. If the I:E ratio should drop *below 1:1* during control mode, the ratio light displays this condition.

Assist and sensitivity mechanism. The sensitivity control adjusts the relationship of an electric contact to a contact on a diaphragm (Fig. 12-14). When the patient removes gas from the circuitry, generating a negative pressure, the diaphragm will collapse and break contact. This broken contact causes the master solenoid to switch to the inspiratory position. The farther the contact is moved down by the control, the more negative pressure has to be exerted by the patient, making the machine less sensitive. If the control is moved all the way down, the patient cannot generate sufficient effort to move the contacts apart, and ventilation is strictly controlled. Because of the adjustable capabilities of the sensitivity unit to positive pressure values, PEEP can be compensated for achieving positive triggering values. Therefore PEEP assist up to about 8 to 12 cm H_2O can be acquired by raising the contact points high within the sensitivity mechanism. The patient assisting will always decrease the I:E ratio from a controlled value.

Oxygen system. The *oxygen system* of the MA-1 is adjusted on the face of the unit. It consists of a reducing valve for incoming gas that drops line pressure to a lower value before it enters the series of balance valves (Fig. 12-15). Gas is supplied to the bellows reservoir of the oxygen system at between 1.8 and 2.1 cm H_2O pressure.[6] The balance line provides a feedback so that air and oxygen enter the precision metering device at the same pressure. On the oxygen side of the balance

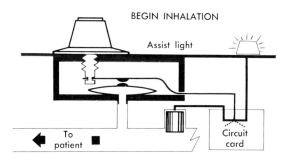

Fig. 12-14. Functional diagram for MA-1 assist and sensitivity mechanism. (Courtesy Bennett Respiration Products, Inc., Santa Monica, Calif.)

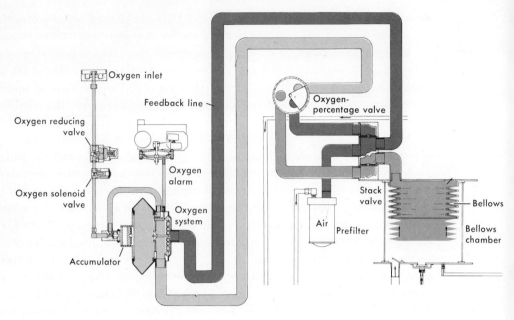

Fig. 12-15. Functional diagram for MA-1 oxygen system. (Courtesy Bennett Respiration Products, Inc., Santa Monica, Calif.)

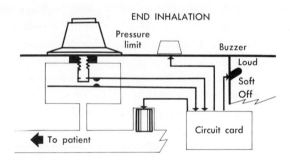

Fig. 12-16. Functional diagram of pressure limit mechanism for MA-1 ventilator. (Courtesy Bennett Respiration Products, Inc., Santa Monica, Calif.)

line is a small reducing valve. It is a simple diaphragm and poppet assembly. If the oxygen pressure is higher than the air pressure in the balance line, the diaphragm is pushed to the right, closing oxygen's access to the precision metering device. When the air system pressure is higher than oxygen system pressure, the diaphragm is pushed to the left, allowing oxygen's access to the precision metering device. So the balance line provides oxygen and air at the same pressures to enter the precision metering device. The precision metering device is the dial on the face of the machine and *occludes* one gas orifice as it *opens* the other. For example, as the dial is turned to higher oxygen concentrations, the air line is occluded to a greater degree and the oxygen line is opened more.

The alarm system on the oxygen control unit is a pressure sensor.[6] If the pressure in the oxygen bellows should exceed about 3 to 6 cm H_2O pressure or if it should drop below 1 cm H_2O pressure, the pressure alarm senses that there is a lack of delivery pressure gas and, therefore, a malfunction.[6] This is reflected by the alarm light switching from green to red and by an audible alarm sounding. The pressure-sensing unit for the alarm is shut out of the system when the unit is turned to 21%, and neither the red nor the green light is functional.[4]

Pressure limit system. The pressure limit is another diaphragm and electric contact mechanism (Fig. 12-16). The level at which contact is to be made by the diaphragm is set by the control. The higher the control is set, the greater the pressure required within the diaphragm to force it up and make contact with the control contact. Once the contact is made, the main solenoid is switched immediately to the expiratory position, the bellows returns to the bottom, and inhalation ends before *volume* limit is reached. Concurrent with the pressure limit signal to the main solenoid, signals are sent to the alarm light and to an audible buzzer to indicate that the set pressure limit has been reached.

A secondary safety feature for the MA-1's pressure limit system is a valve that sits atop the bellows in the relief valve (Fig. 12-7). This is a relief valve set to open at 85 cm H_2O and exhaust pressure within the patient system to atmospheric levels. It serves two primary functions: (1) if the electric pressure limit fails, this valve is a back-up system; (2) if the patient were to cough spontaneously during inhalation and cause a sudden increase in pressure to 85 cm H_2O, not only would the normal pressure limit be reached and the exhalation valve opened, but this valve, too, would open. Thus the pressure created in the circuit by the high flows of a cough could be vented more quickly out both systems.

Sigh system. The sigh controls work similarly to the rate, normal tidal volume, and normal pressure limit controls. The sigh timer sets the *frequency* and *number* in sequence that a sigh(s) will occur.[4] Once a sigh is established either by the timer or manually, the circuit cards switch to the sigh control system. The sigh volume potentiometer is now the reference for the bellows potentiometer. The bellows will rise until that voltage is reached. The sigh pressure limit is structurally the same as the normal pressure limit. When the machine switches to the sigh mode, the normal pressure limit is electrically ignored, and the sigh pressure limit becomes functional. During each sigh interval, the ventilatory time set on the rate control is automatically doubled (rate setting halved) to allow for exhalation of the larger volumes delivered.

Nebulizer system. The nebulizer control is actually an on/off switch for a small compressor.[6] This compressor draws gas from the bellows and, on the expiratory phase, simply returns it back to the bellows. On inhalation (Fig. 12-17), the solenoid leading to the bellows closes, and gas drawn from the bellows by the nebulizer pump goes to the jet of the nebulizer. This system accomplishes basically two things. First, it does not alter the delivered volume from the bellows. Second, it does not alter the oxygen concentration delivered.

PEEP and NEEP systems. There are two expiratory attachments for the MA-1, and each can be attached to the expiratory gas-flow port of the main compressor. This flow of gas goes either (1) to the jet of the master Venturi on inhalation or (2) out the side of the MA-1, as dictated by the main solenoid. Part of this gas pressure is then supplied to the control attachments on the expiratory phase.

The PEEP attachment (Fig. 12-18) functions as a reducing valve using a spring

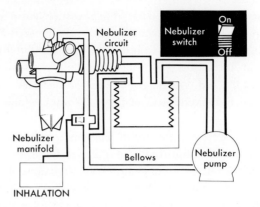

Fig. 12-17. Functional diagram for nebulizer system of MA-1. (Courtesy Bennett Respiration Products, Inc., Santa Monica, Calif.)

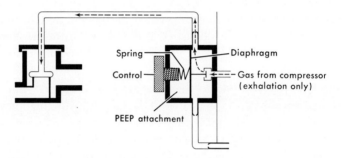

Fig. 12-18. Functional diagram of PEEP attachment for MA-1 ventilator.

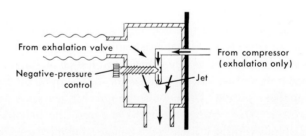

Fig. 12-19. Functional diagram of NEEP attachment for MA-1 ventilator.

and diaphragm. It takes about 2 psi from the compressor and reduces it down to the level of pressure set by the spring and maintains that pressure in the exhalation diaphragm. The exhalation diaphragm, in turn, does not allow the patient's exhaled gas to leave the tubing circuit once pressure after inhalation is dropped to the level contained in the diaphragm. Pressures up to about 15 cm H_2O can be achieved.[4]

The *negative-pressure* attachment's control (Fig. 12-19) is a needle valve that adjusts the flow of gas from the compressor to the jet of a Venturi.[4] This Venturi then attempts to entrain the gases from the patient's circuit. The higher the flow to the jet through the needle valve, the lower the negative pressure generated in the circuitry by the attachment. Pressures to about -9 cm H_2O can be generated.[4]

Expiratory resistance system. The expiratory retard or *expiratory resistance control* consists of an accumulator and a needle valve in the exhalation valve line (Fig. 12-20).[6] As the expiratory resistance control is turned toward *increase,* the needle valve restricts the outflow tract from the exhalation diaphragm's accumulator. The accumulator is simply a pneumatic reservoir inline to provide increased volume and, therefore, accentuate the resistance to flow out of the exhalation diaphragm. As the restriction is increased, the diaphragm deflates more slowly, causing expiratory resistance or retard. In the fully occluded position, gas can no longer pass through the needle valve and must bypass the needle valve assembly itself through a bypass line containing two restrictions. Since gas must (1) flow across the first restriction, due to the pressure gradient from pressurized gas in the exhalation valve line to atmospheric past the restriction, it will then (2) establish the second pressure gradient to travel across the second restriction. This provides a time lag before the exhalation valve can dump its gas, acquiring a *short volume hold* and then maximum expiratory resistance.

Humidity and monitoring systems. The MA-1 utilizes the heated cascade humidifier described in Chapter 4.

The *spirometer* collects *expired* gas volumes in a bellows and provides a visual *readout* based on the height of excursion of the bellows itself within the cylinder (Chapter 7).

On top of the spirometer is a *spirometer alarm,* which is a *timing mechanism* that is reset by a metal plug in the spirometer stick. The lowest allowable volume is set on the stick. If the stick does not transverse the spirometer alarm sensing unit within 20 seconds, it will not be reset, and an alarm will sound.

The accompanying box summarizes the specifications for the MA-1 ventilator.

Specifications for Bennett MA-1 ventilator

Tidal volume (normal and sigh):	Up to 2200 ml
Rate:	Calibrated from 6 to 60 breaths/min
	Uncalibrated from 60 to 100+ breaths/min
	Modified for IMV rate from less than 1 to 60 breaths/min
Peak flow rate:	Approximately 15 to 100 L/min
Pressure limit (normal and sigh):	20 to 80 cm H_2O
Sigh rate:	1, 2, or 3 sighs, 4, 6, 8, 10, or 15 times per hour or off
Oxygen percentage:	Continuously variable from 21% to 100%
Nebulizer:	Inhalation only
PEEP:	Approximately 0 to 15 cm H_2O
NEEP:	Approximately 0 to -9 cm H_2O
Pressure manometer:	-10 to $+80$ cm H_2O
Sensitivity:	Stable from -0.1 to -10 cm H_2O or self-cycle (+ pressure level)

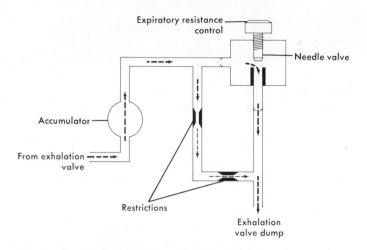

Fig. 12-20. Functional diagram of MA-1's expiratory resistance system.

THE OHIO 560 VENTILATOR

The Ohio 560 (Fig. 12-21) is an electrically powered and controlled, low-pressure drive, rotary-blower, double-circuit bellows ventilator that is designed to be volume limited.[7] It can be time or patient cycled, providing an assistor-controller or controller mode of operation is available.[7] A prototype of this device manufactured by J. J. Monaghan Company was described in 1968.[8]

Referring to the diagram in Fig. 12-22, the 560 contains two bellows systems from which patient gases are delivered. During a normal inhalation the *turbine* (a rotary compressor or blower) pressurizes the *TV canister* and collapses the bellows. The volume within the bellows (set tidal volume) is expelled into the patient circuit by way of a one-way valve and through the *flow control*. These gases pass by the *pressure relief* valve through the *ultrasonic humidifier* (nebulizer) and out to the *patient manifold*. The exhalation valve within the manifold is inflated by pressure from the driving circuit (tidal volume canister pressure).

During a sigh or deep breath, both bellows are emptied into the patient circuit together.

During exhalation, the canister(s) and exhalation valve are vented to atmospheric pressure, and the bellows fall. As the bellows fall they refill from the *reservoir* containing premixed air and oxygen or from the *air inlet filter* when the oxygen control is on the *20% setting*.

Drive mechanism and flow characteristics. The main drive system of the unit is a four-stage *rotary compressor* or turbine (Fig. 12-23). The pressure developed by this compressor is about *100 cm H$_2$O pressure*.[7-9] Gas from the blower enters the *main valve assembly*, which is controlled by solenoids (Fig. 12-24).

There are two halves of the main valve assembly. One activates tidal volume bellows, and the other activates the additional sigh volume bellows. Normally the *solenoid valve vent* is closed, the pressures above and below the diaphragm of the pressurizing half are equal, and gas cannot enter the bellows chamber. If the solenoid is activated, the bottom portion of the diaphragm can dump. Pressure above the

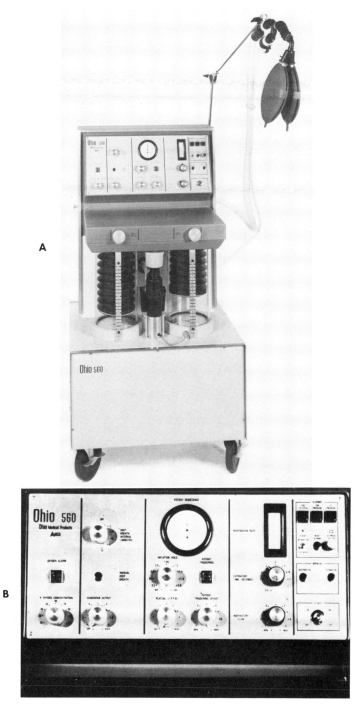

Fig. 12-21. A, Ohio 560 volume ventilator. **B,** Control panel for Ohio 560 ventilator. (Courtesy Ohio Medical Products, Inc., Madison, Wis.)

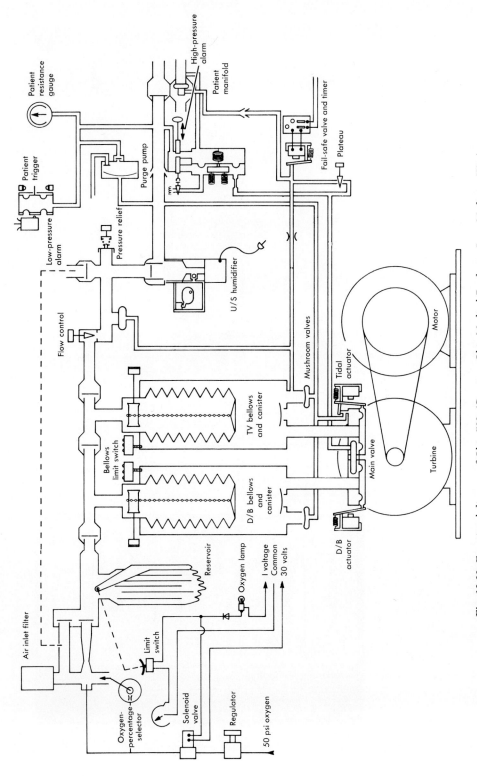

Fig. 12-22. Functional diagram of Ohio 560. (Courtesy Ohio Medical Products, Inc., Madison, Wis.)

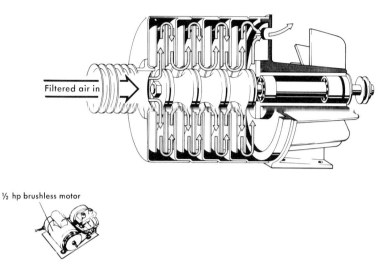

Filtered air in

½ hp brushless motor

Fig. 12-23. Functional diagram of Ohio 560's rotary compressor. (Courtesy Ohio Medical Products, Inc., Madison, Wis.)

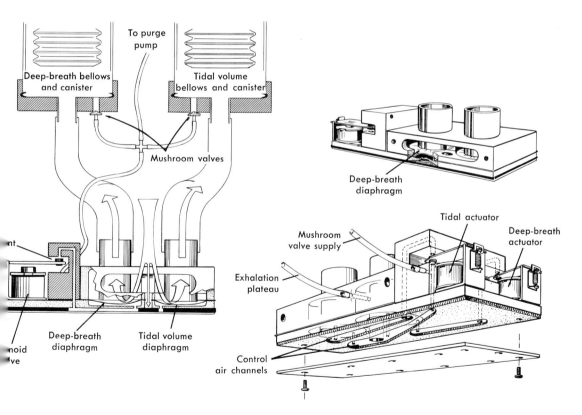

Fig. 12-24. Main valve assembly for Ohio 560. (Courtesy Ohio Medical Products, Inc., Madison, Wis.)

diaphragm pushes it downward and sends gas flow to the bellows cylinder. This flow of gas into the bellows cylinder compresses the bellows *upward*, delivering the bellows volume. On normal tidal volumes, only the tidal volume solenoid is activated, and when the sigh volume is delivered, both solenoids are activated, delivering the gas volume from *both* bellows canisters.

The *peak inspiratory flow control* is a variable-sized restriction to gas flow from the bellows (Fig. 12-25). Therefore it limits the maximum flow out of the 560 unit into the patient system.

Flows of up to 180 L/min are obtainable with the 560, and 100 L/min can be maintained against 40 cm H_2O back pressure.[7,9]

Flow patterns for this ventilator are generally fairly constant or square-wave-like under normal conditions. However, when extremely low compliances are encountered, causing high delivery pressures (80 to 100 cm H_2O), flow will in fact taper in a decelerating fashion, somewhat consistent with low-pressure–driven bellows ventilators described in Chapter 8.

Examples of flow and pressure patterns obtained for the 560 while ventilating a lung simulator are shown in Fig. 12-26.

Volume control. *Tidal volume* is set (Fig. 12-27) on the 560 by adjusting the distance the tidal volume bellows can fall during refill (exhalation). This is accomplished by the *bellows rope* attached to the *volume control* and to the *bellows weight*. Volume *limit* (end inhalation) is accomplished when the bellows reaches the top of its canister and triggers the *volume limit switch*, which electrically cycles the ventilator into the expiratory phase.

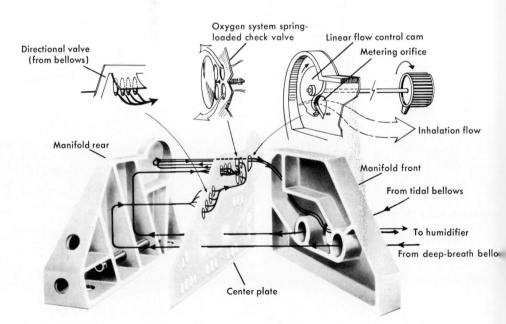

Fig. 12-25. Peak inspiratory flow control for Ohio 560. (Courtesy Ohio Medical Products, Inc., Madison, Wis.)

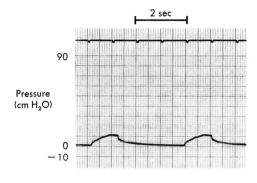

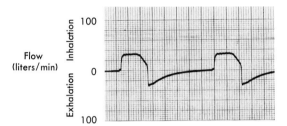

Fig. 12-26. Pressure and flow curves taken for Ohio 560 ventilator while ventilating lung simulator set for compliance of 50 ml/cm H_2O and resistance of 5 cm H_2O/L/sec.

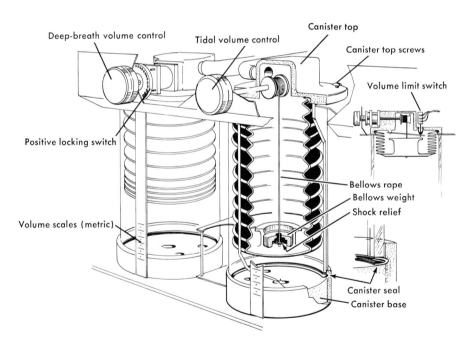

Fig. 12-27. Cutaway of tidal volume bellows and canister system for Ohio 560 ventilator. (Courtesy Ohio Medical Products, Inc., Madison, Wis.)

The typical compressibility factor is constant at about 2.0 cc/cm H_2O pressure, primarily dependent on the patient's tubing circuit size.

The volume control of the deep breath or sigh bellows functions in the same manner. The *additional* volume desired for a sigh is set on the sigh bellows rather than the entire sigh volume (Fig. 12-28). For example, if the tidal volume were set at

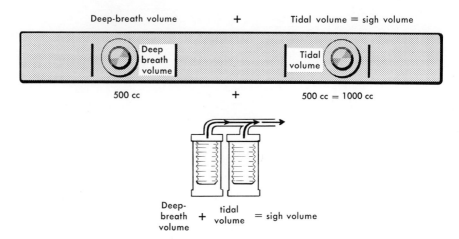

Fig. 12-28. Example of sigh volume delivery for Ohio 560 ventilator. (Modified from Ohio Medical Products, Inc., Madison, Wis.)

500 cc, and a sigh volume of 1000 cc were to be delivered, the sigh bellows setting would be 500 cc. The two bellows would be activated *simultaneously* for a sigh delivering 500 cc from the tidal volume bellows plus 500 cc from the sigh volume bellows for a total of 1000 cc.

Rate mechanism and I:E ratio. The control rate system is generally set by three controls: (1) the expiratory time control, (2) the tidal volume control, and (3) the inspiratory flow control. The tidal volume set and the flow rate primarily determine the duration of inhalation with the influence from the patient's compliance and resistance factors. The expiratory timer (Fig. 12-29, *A*) sets the duration of time elapsing from the beginning of exhalation until the next control breath begins. If the assist mechanism is functional, the patient may interrupt this timer and cycle the ventilator on.

The results of the above factors influencing the number of breaths per minute are displayed on the analog rate meter (Fig. 12-29, *B*). However, this meter really reflects the time between the beginning on one inhalation and the beginning of the next inhalation, that is, the ventilatory cycle time. The meter then displays the rate in breaths per minute if that ventilatory cycle time continued for a minute. During control mode this feature is helpful in establishing the control rate, but during assist-control mode the patient who breathes at an erratic rate will cause the meter to jump from one value to another with each breath.

The I:E ratio is a result of the inspiratory time factors (set tidal volume, inspiratory flow, and patient conditions) and the expiratory timer setting. Any change of tidal volume, inspiratory flow, or expiratory time will change not only the I:E ratio but the set control rate as well.

Assist and sensitivity mechanism. The assist and sensitivity mechanism (Fig. 12-30) uses a *photoelectric* light and sensor cell blocked by a flap connected to a diaphragm. As the patient generates the negative pressure by evacuating gas volume from the tubing circuitry, the diaphragm moves *up*, bringing with it the small flap between the photoelectric bulb and the photoelectric receiving cell. As the dia-

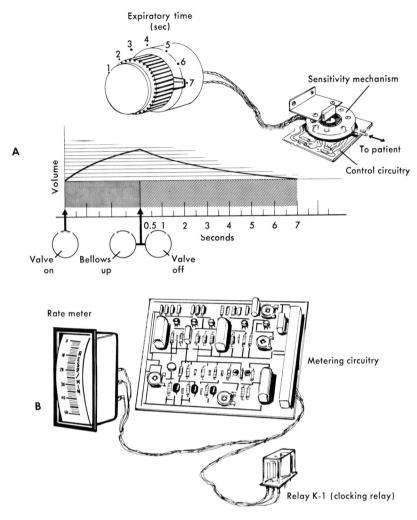

Fig. 12-29. **A,** Ohio 560 expiratory time control. **B,** Ohio 560 rate meter. (Courtesy Ohio Medical Products, Inc., Madison, Wis.)

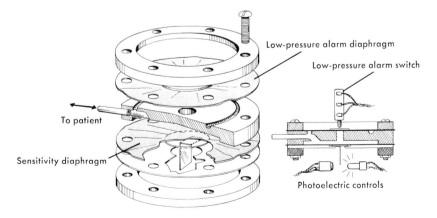

Fig. 12-30. Cutaway and side view of sensitivity mechanism for Ohio 560 ventilator. Low-pressure alarm switch is also shown. (Courtesy Ohio Medical Products, Inc., Madison, Wis.)

phragm and flap move upward, increased quantities of light are received by the cell, and increased quantities of electric current are generated. Once the current has reached a specific level, the main valve solenoid of the 560 is triggered into the inspiratory phase. The sensitivity *adjustment* (patient triggering effort control) itself is an additional current flow to the circuit card. The photoelectric unit cannot generate sufficient current by itself to cause the unit to trigger. With no reference current from the sensitivity control, the ventilator would be in the control mode. However, by increasing the current flow from the sensitivity control, less photoelectric current is required to cause the unit to trigger. Therefore less effort is required on the part of the patient, making the unit more sensitive. The sensitivity mechanism on the Ohio 560 is *not* compensated for PEEP. Therefore assisting when PEEP is used requires a significant increase in patient effort.

Oxygen system. Oxygen percentage control (Fig. 12-31) is obtained in the 560 through a *Venturi* mechanism.[7,9] When on, oxygen comes into the unit through a solenoid valve and then is attached by a **T** connector in the *proportioning block* before it reaches the jet of the Venturi. Oxygen powers the jet of the Venturi and is also supplied to the oxygen percentage control, which functions like a *needle valve*, providing variable openings. When in operation, the Venturi entrains air by drawing gas through the preinlet filter of the machine. To increase the oxygen concentration above about 27% to 30%, the oxygen percentage control is turned above 30%, which opens the needle valve–like mechanism, allowing more oxygen to enter the entrainment compartment around the jet of the Venturi. Finally, as the 100% setting is reached, the entrainment needs of the Venturi system are met nearly exclusively by the incoming oxygen flows from the percentage control. The alarm system of the unit depends on whether the *oxygen reservoir* (accumulator bag) for premixed per-

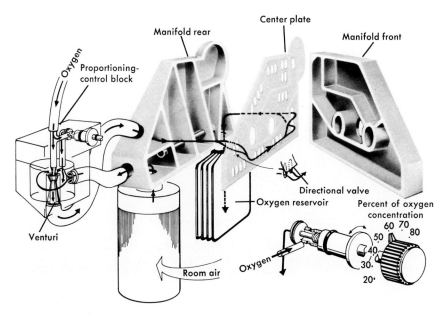

Fig. 12-31. Functional diagram for Ohio 560's oxygen system. (Courtesy Ohio Medical Products, Inc., Madison, Wis.)

centage gases collapses. If the bag ever collapses, an indicator will light. This alarm is deactivated on the 20% setting. Any compressed gas source that can keep the bag inflated, however, will deactivate the visual alarm system, meaning that oxygen concentration per se is *not* monitored.

Sigh system. The mechanism for sigh volume setting is described on pp. 323 and 324. The *deep-breath interval minutes* control (Fig. 12-21, *B*) establishes the time duration between single sigh breath deliveries. It is calibrated from *off* to a sigh delivery once every 2, 4, 6, 8, or 10 minutes.[7] The preset value on the expiratory timer is automatically doubled to allow for exhalation of the additional volume as well as to more closely mimic a natural sigh.

PEEP system. The control marked *plateau (CPPB)* actually establishes the level of PEEP if desired. It is a needle valve that adjusts the flow of gas to both the exhalation diaphragm and a bleed into the bellows chamber (Fig. 12-32). The higher the flow to the diaphragm and restriction, the higher the PEEP level that is maintained.

Inflation hold system. The *inflation hold* control provides an electronic delay in the electric circuitry that results in the bellows remaining at the top of the canister, holding the volume delivered for a period of 0 to 2 seconds (Fig. 12-33).[7] Normally, when the bellows reaches the top, a switch is depressed and deactivates the main valve solenoid of the drive circuit. Once the solenoid is deactivated, the bellows drops, and exhalation occurs. When the inflation hold is activated, the signal from the

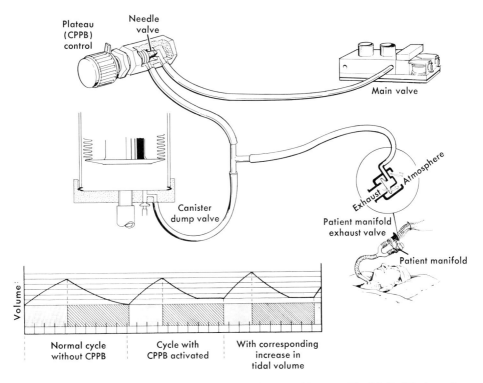

Fig. 12-32. Functional diagram of Ohio 560 PEEP (CPPB) system. (Courtesy Ohio Medical Products, Inc., Madison, Wis.)

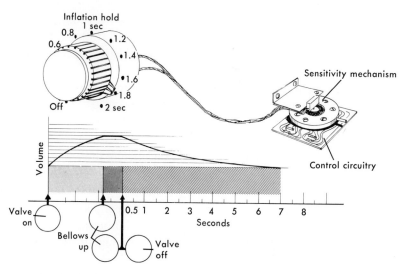

Fig. 12-33. Ohio 560 inflation hold control. (Courtesy Ohio Medical Products, Inc., Madison, Wis.)

top of the canister switch is delayed, and the main valve solenoid remains activated during the delay period. The result is that the volume from the bellows is held in the patient circuit for this same delay period.

NEEP system. The *negative-pressure* attachment for the 560 is a *Venturi*.[7] The Venturi jet receives gas from the high-pressure oxygen inlet on the *expiratory* phase of the ventilator (Fig. 12-34). The level of negative pressure is adjusted by the negative-pressure control, which sets the amount of air that the unit is allowed to entrain directly from the room. The *larger* the opening provided by the needle valve for entrainment, the *lower* the negative pressure actually exerted on the patient circuit. The negative expiratory pressure range is from -20 cm H_2O pressure (control closed) to about zero (control wide open).

Pressure relief system. Under the silver ledge on the front of the machine is the spring-loaded disk that acts as a *pressure pop off* for the machine (Fig. 12-35). The pressure relief level is established by the threaded adjustment of the control knob, compressing the spring to a specific degree. Gas pressure is required to move the disk away from its seat against the spring. If circuit pressure reaches the spring tension force, excess gas pressure will be exhausted into the room for the remainder of inhalation unless the pressure within the circuit again is less than spring tension. There is also an *independent, high-pressure alarm* that can be set at a specific value (Fig. 12-36).[9] Normally, this unit would be set *under* the actual pressure release value so that the release would not be functional at a lower level than the high-pressure alarm. If the pressure release were *lower* than the alarm-activation pressure, those clinicians at the patient's side might not immediately sense the basic problem of decreased volume delivery. The high-pressure alarm control (Fig. 12-36) is an adjustable bleed out of the left side of the diaphragm. System pressure is exposed to the right side. If system pressure becomes *higher* than the pressure on the left, the diaphragm is pushed to the left and the microswitch is depressed, activating the high-pressure alarm. The greater the leak out of the left side set by the alarm-control

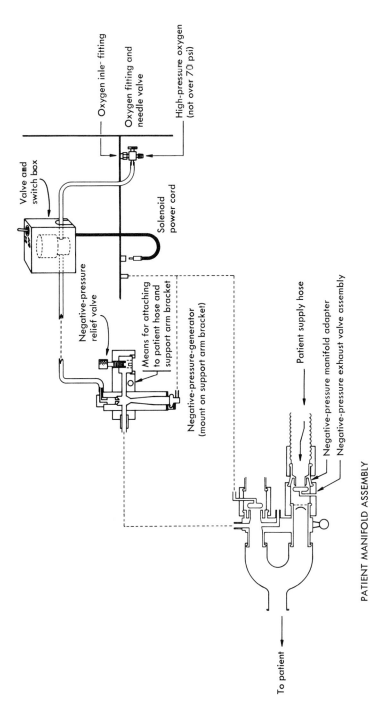

Oxygen inle* fitting

Oxygen fitting and needle valve

High-pressure oxygen (not over 70 psi)

Valve and switch box

Solenoid power cord

Negative-pressure relief valve

Means for attaching to patient hose and support arm bracket

Negative-pressure-generator (mount on support arm bracket)

Patient supply hose

Negative-pressure manifold adapter

Negative-pressure exhaust valve assembly

PATIENT MANIFOLD ASSEMBLY

To patient

Fig. 12-34. Diagram of negative-pressure attachment for Ohio 560 ventilator. (Courtesy Ohio Medical Products, Inc., Madison, Wis.)

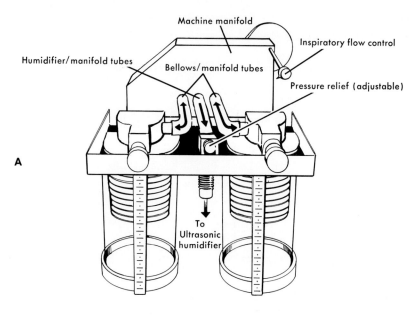

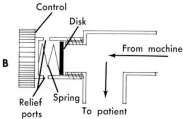

Fig. 12-35. A, Manifold system for Ohio 560 showing pressure relief. **B,** Ohio 560 spring-loaded pressure-relief valve. (**A** courtesy Ohio Medical Products, Inc., Madison, Wis.)

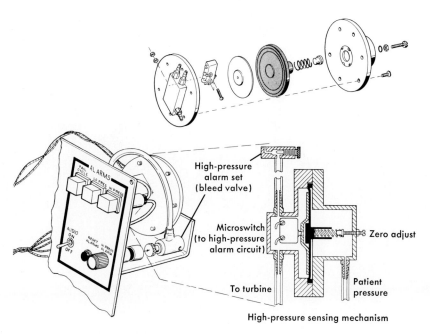

Fig. 12-36. Ohio 560 high-pressure alarm. Bleed valve adjusts pressure on left side of diaphragm by varying leak out of left as gas travels from turbine. (Courtesy Ohio Medical Products, Inc., Madison, Wis.)

needle valve, the lower the pressure on the left, requiring a *lower* system pressure to activate the alarm.

Humidification system. Normally, the 560 is supplied with an ultrasonic nebulizer (Fig. 12-37) that has its output control on the control panel of the ventilator. However, a heated humidifier can also be adapted to the unit (Fig. 12-38).

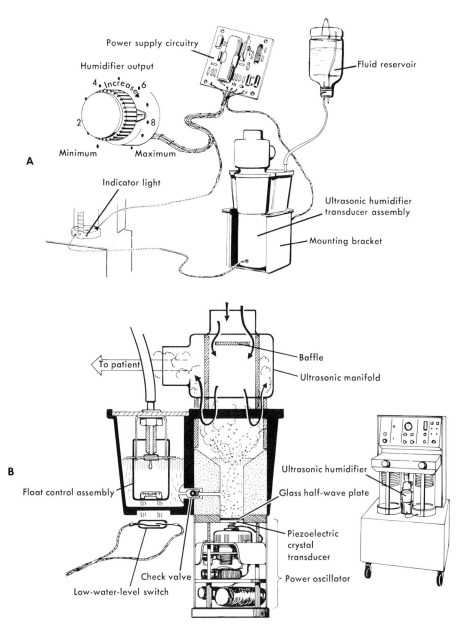

Fig. 12-37. A, Ohio 560 ultrasonic nebulizer system showing fluid reservoir and nebulizer output control. **B,** Ohio 560 ultrasonic nebulizer system showing cutaway of system as well as its position on ventilator. (Courtesy Ohio Medical Products, Inc., Madison, Wis.)

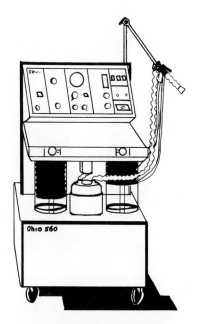

Fig. 12-38. Ohio 560 with heated humidifier adapted.

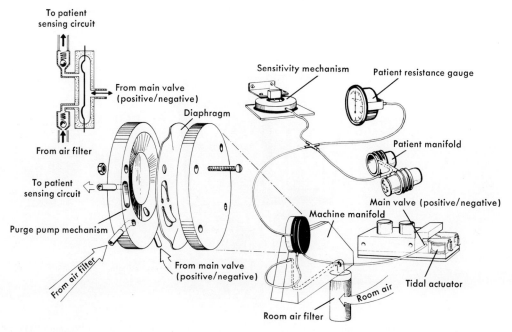

Fig. 12-39. Functional diagram of Ohio 560's purge system. (Courtesy Ohio Medical Products, Inc., Madison, Wis.)

Other systems. The *purge system* is a small *diaphragm pump* (Fig. 12-39) acti- vated by system pressure.[7] The pump sends a small flow of air through the sensing line to remove any *moisture* present, thus keeping the assist mechanism, the low- pressure alarm system, and the pressure manometer dry.

A *low-pressure* alarm system, located in the sensitivity mechanism (Fig. 12-30), will cause an audible and visible alarm if the 8 cm H_2O required to deactivate the switch is not developed in the patient circuit each breath.

A *failure-to-cycle* alarm (audible and visible) is activated when inhalation lasts longer than about 8 seconds or exhalation lasts longer than about 14 seconds.[7] Each of these may be tested by depressing either the *manual inspiration* or the *manual expiration* button and holding it down until the allotted time has passed. If the system is functioning properly, the alarm will activate.

If electric power fails, an audible battery-powered *loss of power* alarm will sound.

The accompanying box summarizes the specifications for the Ohio 560.

Specifications for Ohio 560 ventilator

Tidal volume:	Up to 2000 ml
Flow rate:	Up to 180 L/min (100 L/min against 40 cm H_2O back pressure)
Expiratory time:	0.5 to 7 seconds approximately (doubled during sigh mode automatically)
Rate:	From about 6 or 7 to 60 breaths/min
Pressure relief:	10 to 100 cm H_2O
Sigh rate:	One sigh every 2, 4, 6, 8, or 10 minutes or off
Sigh volume:	Up to 4000 ml
Oxygen percentage:	20% or 30% to 100% (calibrated in 10% increments)
Inflation hold:	0 to 2 seconds
PEEP (CPPB):	Up to about 12 cm H_2O
NEEP:	Adjustable to about −20 cm H_2O
Sensitivity:	From *approximately* −0.5 to 2 cm H_2O or lockout (control)
Pressure manometer:	−20 to +100 cm H_2O

Alarms

Low pressure:	Audiovisual; activated if 8 cm H_2O pressure in patient circuit not exceeded *each breath*
High pressure:	Audiovisual; activated if set pressure is reached dur- ing inhalation
	Audiovisual; activated if set pressure is reached dur- ing inhalation
Failure to cycle:	Audiovisual; activated if inhalation lasts over about 8 seconds or if exhalation lasts over about 14 seconds
Loss of power:	Audio; activated if electric power failure or disconnect occurs; battery operated
Oxygen failure:	Visual; activated if accumulator (oxygen reservoir) bag cannot maintain minimal inflation level

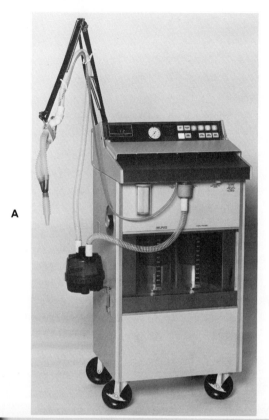

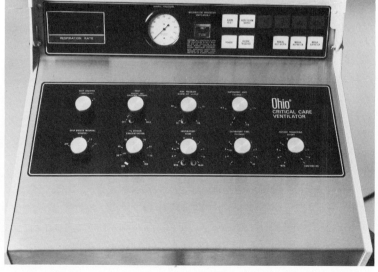

Fig. 12-40. A, Ohio Critical Care Ventilator (CCV). **B,** Ohio CCV's control and display panels. (Courtesy Ohio Medical Products, Inc., Madison, Wis.)

THE OHIO CRITICAL CARE VENTILATOR (CCV)

Generally, the description for the Ohio 560 is adequate for the Critical Care Ventilator (CCV) (Fig. 12-40). Since the two ventilators are similar, the emphasis here will be aimed at the primary differences between them.

Flow characteristics. Because the turbine in the CCV is somewhat more efficient, the maximum flow capabilities are higher than those of the 560. Flow from 10 to 250 L/min is available with the ability to maintain 200 L/min against 40 cm H_2O back pressure.[10,11]

Examples of flow and pressure patterns for the CCV are shown in Fig. 12-41.

Assist and sensitivity mechanism. The mechanism for patient triggering itself is similar to that of the 560. However, the unit (Fig. 12-42) has been encased so that the side of the diaphragm opposite the patient circuit side is referenced to PEEP pressure. Thus PEEP assist can be achieved easily. The unit is automatically compensated so that *no* change in the patient triggering effort control is needed when PEEP is added. If the sensitivity were set for −1 cm H_2O, for example, and if 10 cm H_2O PEEP were applied, then the patient would need only to drop the pressure to 9 cm H_2O to trigger the ventilator. An advantage to the CCV's method of PEEP compensation is that there will be no continuous self-cycling of the ventilator when the patient is temporarily disconnected as happens with some other ventilators when PEEP assist is used.

Oxygen system. Oxygen is controlled in the CCV by means of a precision metering device. Fig. 12-43 shows a functional diagram of the system. Oxygen enters and passes through a *regulator* and on to the *oxygen reservoir*. Pressure in the reservoir is nearly atmospheric. When the bellows fall for refilling (exhalation), air and oxygen are pulled through the *oxygen mix valve* (precision metering device). The valve functions so that when it is turned on the control panel, it opens one side (air or oxygen) as it *proportionately* closes the other side (air or oxygen).

This system allows for continuous control of oxygen percentage from 21% to 100%.[10,11]

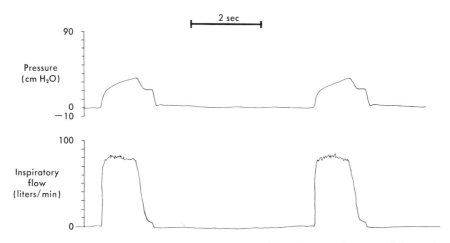

Fig. 12-41. Waveforms for pressure and flow for Ohio CCV redrawn from actual tracings while ventilating lung simulator set for compliance of 40.3 ml/cm H_2O and resistance of 7 cm H_2O/L/sec.

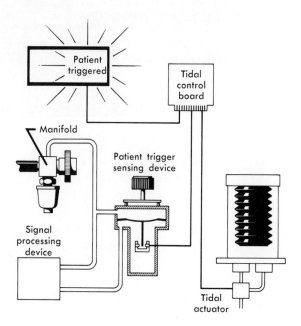

Fig. 12-42. Functional diagram of sensitivity system for Ohio CCV. (Courtesy Ohio Medical Products, Inc., Madison, Wis.)

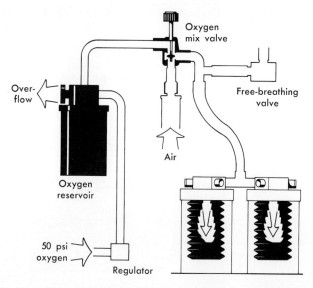

Fig. 12-43. Functional diagram of oxygen control system for Ohio CCV.

Sigh system. The sigh system (Fig. 12-44) for the CCV also utilizes both bellows as does the 560. The *deep-breath intervals* control can be set for 3, 5, 7.5, or 15 minutes between sigh cycles or *off*. In addition, another control, the *deep breaths (consecutive)* for 1, 2, or 3 sighs in a row is provided.

Humidification system. The Ohio CCV utilizes a heated bubble-through humidifier (Fig. 12-45).[10,11] Water temperatures are adjustable from 90° F to 160° F.[11] A

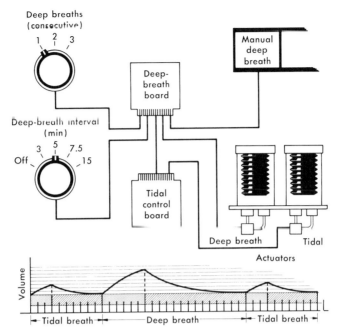

Fig. 12-44. Functional diagram for sigh mechanisms for Ohio CCV. (Courtesy Ohio Medical Products, Inc., Madison, Wis.)

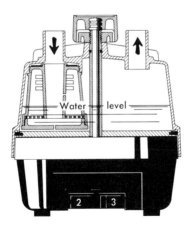

Fig. 12-45. Ohio Heated Humidifier. (Courtesy Ohio Medical Products, Inc., Madison, Wis.)

thermometer is supplied with the patient tubing circuit for monitoring gas mixture temperatures.

IMV system. When the *IMV* button (Fig. 12-46) is depressed, several functions change. First, the expiratory timer settings are multiplied by 10 so that the range is 5 to 100 seconds. Second, a free-breathing valve is opened so that the patient may withdraw blended gases from the oxygen system spontaneously through the humid-

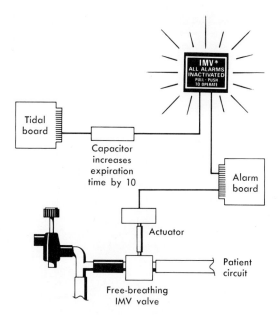

Fig. 12-46. Diagram of IMV system for Ohio CCV. (Courtesy Ohio Medical Products, Inc., Madison, Wis.)

ifier. Third, all alarm systems, including the loss-of-power alarm, are *deactivated*. To use this system the assist mechanism must be turned to *off*, and it is suggested that the sigh system also be in the *off* position.[11]

Fig. 12-40, *B*, shows the control and display panels for the CCV. The accompanying box and Fig. 12-40, *B*, can be used to compare the other minor differences between the Ohio 560 and the Ohio Critical Care Ventilator.

THE MONAGHAN 225 VOLUME VENTILATOR

The Monaghan 225 Volume Ventilator (Fig. 12-47) is a pneumatically driven unit with *fluidic* control.[13,14] It can be volume, pressure, or time limited, and it can operate as an assistor, assistor-controller, or controller. It is a bellows unit with a high-pressure driving force.[13,14]

The incoming source gas of 50 psig oxygen is reduced by a preset reducing valve to 5 to 7 psig, which powers the fluidic and pneumatic components of the 225 (Fig. 12-48).[13] The master fluidic flip-flop (mini-fluid amp in diagram) element is *bistable* and controls the phase of the ventilator. Pneumatic pressure signals entering from the left cause the flip-flop's main stream to switch to the right, starting inhalation. Input signals for the master flip-flop for starting inhalation are (1) manual inhalation, (2) patient trigger, and (3) the exhalation timing bellows. Those for starting exhalation are (1) volume limit signal, (2) pressure limit and (3) the inhalation timing bellows.

Once inhalation begins, 50 psig source gas passes through the *flow control* (Fig. 12-50) and into the *canister*, which houses the *bellows*. This causes the bellows to expel its contents into the patient circuit. During exhalation, pressure is relieved from the canister and the bellows falls, refilling with gases from the oxygen mixing system.

Specifications for Ohio CCV

Tidal volume:	Up to 2000 ml
Flow rate:	Up to 240 L/min (up to 200 L/min against 40 cm H_2O back pressure)
Expiratory time:	From about 1 to 10 seconds (doubled during sigh mode automatically)
Rate:	From about 5 to 40 breaths/min
IMV:	Changes expiratory time to about 5 to 100 seconds (deactivates all alarms)
Pressure relief:	About 10 to 100 cm H_2O
Sigh rate:	1, 2, or 3 sighs every 3, 5, 7.5, or 15 minutes
Sigh volume:	Up to 4000 ml
Oxygen percentage:	Continuously variable from 21% to 100%
Inspiratory hold:	0 to 2 seconds
PEEP:	Up to 15 cm H_2O
Sensitivity:	As low as 0.5 cm H_2O drop (PEEP compensated)
Pressure manometer:	0 to 100 cm H_2O

Alarms

Low pressure:	Audiovisual if pressure in tubing does not exceed either 8 or 12 cm H_2O (depending on model) at least once every 15 seconds
High pressure:	Audiovisual; activated if set pressure is exceeded for two consecutive breaths
Failure to cycle:	Audiovisual; activated if inhalation exceeds 5 seconds or if exhalation exceeds 22 seconds
Loss of power:	Audio; activated if electric power failure or disconnect occurs; battery operated
Oxygen failure:	Audiovisual; activated if oxygen fails while control is turned on

A mode selector switch (Fig. 12-47, *B*) provides for dialing control mode, assist mode (*no* backup rate), or assist-control mode.

Drive mechanism and flow characteristics. The driving source for the bellows is source gas, usually 50 psig.[13] This high driving force potential causes the flow pattern for the 225 to be a constant one or square wave, even against substantial back pressure.[14] This 50 psig source pressure is not allowed to be reached, however, due to a diaphragm-like vent valve located between the oxygen percentage control and the flow control in Fig. 12-48. This valve is powered by gases from line 6 of the *dual OR/NOR* fluidic switch and clinically has been observed to vent and hold the pressure against the bellows at 105 to 110 cm H_2O. Examples of pressure and flow curves for the 225 are shown in Fig. 12-49.

The flow control (Fig. 12-50) is a needle that provides a variable restriction within the source gas line leading to the bellows canister.[13] Flows from near 0 to 100 L/min are available[14] at pressures up to 100 cm H_2O.[15]

Volume control. The *volume control* is a threaded screw adjustment that moves a *sealed platform* (Fig. 12-50).[13] The platform determines the depth to which the

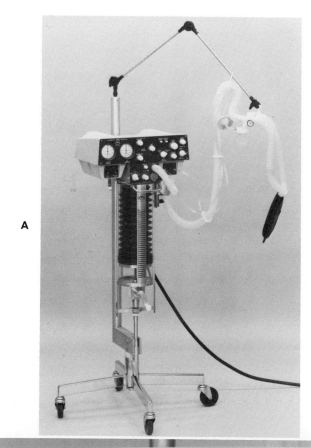

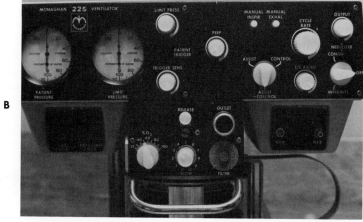

Fig. 12-47. A, Monaghan 225 Volume Ventilator. **B,** Control panel. (Courtesy Monaghan, Littleton, Colo.)

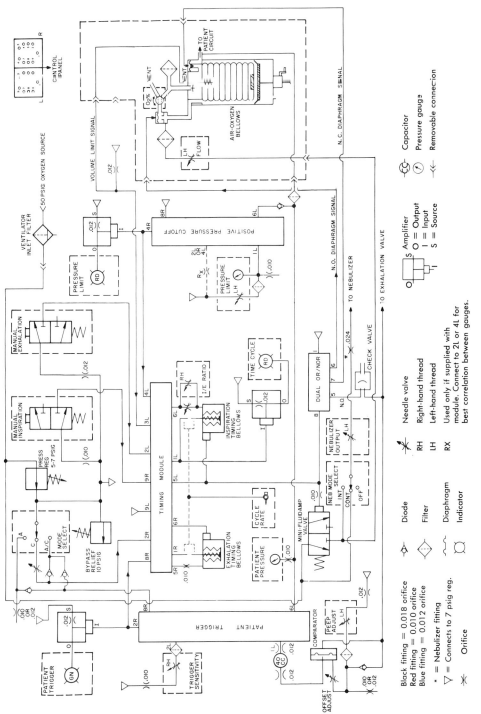

Fig. 12-48. Functional diagram for Monaghan 225. (Courtesy Monaghan, Littleton, Colo.)

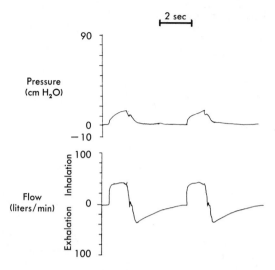

Fig. 12-49. Pressure and flow curves for Monaghan 225 Volume Ventilator redrawn from actual tracings taken while ventilating lung simulator set for compliance of 50 ml/cm H_2O and resistance of 5 cm H_2O/L/sec.

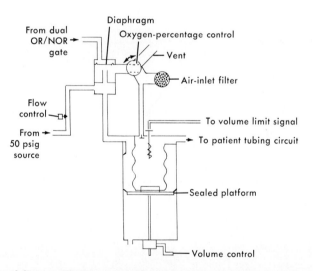

Fig. 12-50. Functional diagram of bellows system for Monaghan 225 Volume Ventilator including volume control, flow, and oxygen mixing systems. (Modified from Monaghan, Littleton, Colo.)

bellows can fall and, therefore, the volume delivered during the next bellows deflation. Volume limit occurs when the bellows reaches the top of the canister and a pneumatic signal causes the ventilator to switch to the expiratory phase.[13] Since the bellows deflates *completely* with any volume setting under volume-limiting situations, the circuit compressibility is about a constant 2.5 cc/cm H_2O pressure,[15] varying only with humidifier water level changes and circuit size variances.

Rate mechanism. Rate is a function of various controls: the tidal volume, the flow control, and the cycle rate control, which is really an expiratory timer.

The exhalation timer is a pneumatic accumulator that receives flow of gas during exhalation from the master flip-flop (Fig. 12-48).[13] A fixed orifice controls the amount of gas flow the accumulator receives and, therefore, controls *how fast* the accumulator will inflate. Once the accumulator has inflated completely, it closes a line leading from the low-pressure manifold to the left side of the master flip-flop. The increased pressure causes the master flip-flop to switch its main flow to inhalation.

Once the master flip-flop has switched into the inspiratory phase, flow travels to three different places.

First, a line travels to the *inspiratory timer* through a needle valve (I:E ratio control) and inflates an accumulator, as described for the expiratory timer (Fig. 12-48). Once the accumulator is inflated, gas flow from the low-pressure manifold is cut off, providing an input pressure on the right side of the master flip-flop. The more the I:E needle valve is closed, the slower the accumulator inflates and the *longer* inhalation time allowed. During volume limiting, inhalation ends before this timing mechanism completes its cycle.

The second line from the master flip-flop outflow provides a signal to the *power valve*. Once the power valve is activated by the signal, flow of gas from the 50 psig source travels through it. This gas is usually 100% oxygen and is utilized to drive the bellows upward. The flow control is located in this line.

The third flow line from the master flip-flop outflow supplies a switching signal to the *dual OR/NOR gate*. Once this valve is closed, the gas from the power valve can pressurize the bellows cylinder and drive the bellows upward. Once the bellows reaches the top, a signal line orifice is closed so that a pressure signal is sent to the right side of the master flip-flop, which switches it to the left. With no flow leaving the right side of the master flip-flop, the bellows drops, and a new exhalation cycle begins.

When the unit is in use, any change of tidal volume, flow, or the cycle rate control will change the number of breaths per minute delivered.

I:E ratio. As mentioned above, the I:E ratio control establishes the maximum inspiratory time available. The control is servo-controlled by the cycle rate control as well, so that if the cycle rate control is changed, the I:E ratio system is also changed *proportionately*. This keeps the *ratio* of the cycle rate control (expiratory timer) to the I:E ratio control (inspiratory timer) the same although their actual *time* settings change.

During time limiting, a desired I:E ratio from 1:1 to about 1:4[13,15] can be set on the I:E ratio control. Then a desired breathing rate can be established by the cycle rate control.

During volume or pressure limiting the I:E ratio functions primarily as a safety feature that establishes the maximum available inspiratory time.

Assist and sensitivity mechanisms. The *patient trigger* mechanism is a high-gain fluidic amplifier (Fig. 12-48).[16] The flow of gas out of the trigger will normally take the straight path to the left. When the patient generates sufficient subatmospheric pressure in the circuit by way of an input at the right (6L), the flow of gas is switched to the right outflow tract (8R), providing a pressure signal to the master flip-flop. This signal causes the master flip-flop to switch to inhalation. The *trigger sensitivity* adjustment control is a needle valve that adjusts an input-flow reference signal to the left side of the patient triggering mechanism.[16] The greater the flow from the sensitivity control, the more reference pressure exerted on the trigger, making the main flow *tend* to move to the right. The higher the sensitivity control flow is, then the *less* negative pressure is needed to be exerted by the patient to switch the patient trigger module main flow to the right (8R).

Sensitivity levels from about +1 to −5 cm H_2O can be established,[13] and the system is somewhat PEEP compensated. That is, if the maximum PEEP level of 20 cm H_2O, for example, is set on the PEEP control, the unit will trigger when the pressure is dropped to about 16 cm H_2O when the maximum level of sensitivity is used.

Oxygen system. The *oxygen system* uses a balance, or proportioning, valve (precision metering device). 100% oxygen from the mini-fluid amp valve is employed to drive the bellows on inhalation (Fig. 12-50). On exhalation, the gas for refilling the bellows comes from (1) the bellows canister (100% oxygen) as it vents to the atmosphere and from (2) the room through the air inlet filter. The *oxygen control* is a variable-sized restriction on the bellows intake line from the canister. Since each of these gases is at or close to atmospheric pressure, the amount of each that fills the falling bellows will be a function of the oxygen control's opening for each gas. The wider the oxygen opening is, the higher the volume of oxygen that will be drawn into the bellows as it drops. Finally, on the 100% setting, the restriction is wide open, and nearly all gas entering the bellows chamber comes from the cylinder.

This system efficiently uses oxygen twice: first to *drive* the bellows on one breath, then to help *fill* the bellows for the next breath.

Oxygen concentration settings are continuously variable from about 21% to near 100% with an accuracy range of about ±5% when the nebulizer is off. Clinical experience has shown the range commonly obtainable with the 225's oxygen system to be from about 23% to 97%.

Nebulizer system. The *nebulizer controls* are supplied by 100% source gas at 50 psig.[13] The nebulizer mode setting provides an *off* setting on which no gas travels to the patient nebulizer. On *continuous*, the gas source is 50 psig from the main source gas inlet at a flow regulated by the needle valve of the output control. On *intermittent*, the nebulizer flow is supplied by the mini-fluid amp valve on inhalation only. Both the continuous and intermittent settings add to the oxygen percentage and the tidal volume delivered by the 225. If a long period of medication delivery is necessary and the increased oxygen percentages may be considered undesirable clinically in certain situations, this problem can be alleviated by powering the 225 with an oxygen controller and setting the 225 oxygen percentage control on 100%. In this fashion, all nebulizer and bellows gas delivered to the patient is premixed by the controller. The tidal volume control could also be adjusted to compensate for the extra volume added by the nebulizer's gas flow. Flows up to 10 L/min can be added with the nebulizer output control.[13,15]

PEEP mechanism. The PEEP mechanism receives gas from the preset reducing valve (*Press. reg.* in Fig. 12-48). The PEEP adjustment is a needle valve that adjusts the flow of gas into the PEEP mechanism, which has a constant leak (Fig. 12-48). The *higher* the flow into the system is, the higher the PEEP pressure that is developed and held in the exhalation valve diaphragm in the patient circuit and the PEEP comparator. The pressure is transmitted through the comparator to the sensi-

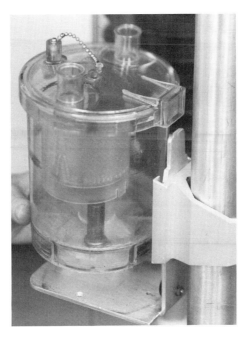

Fig. 12-51. Monaghan model 610 humidifier. (Courtesy Monaghan, Littleton, Colo.)

tivity element to offset the PEEP pressure supplying input to the right side of the patient trigger device. The result is PEEP compensation of the patient trigger so that an assist mode of operation with PEEP is possible.[13,15] As mentioned earlier, the compensation for the PEEP level is not complete but is generally clinically adequate to provide relatively low levels of patient effort required. PEEP levels of up to 20 cm H_2O can be set.[13,15]

Humidification system. Humidity is supplied by a bubble-cascade type humidifier (Fig. 12-51), the Monaghan model 610. A heater with a variable thermostat control can be used for setting elevated water temperatures. Gas temperatures are monitored in the patient tubing circuit's manifold by a thermometer.

THE MONAGHAN 225/SIMV VOLUME VENTILATOR

Recently Monaghan has produced an updated version of the 225. The ventilator is fundamentally the same except that a system for providing Synchronized Intermittent Mandatory Ventilation (SIMV) has been added.[17] A 225 modified for this system is shown in Fig. 12-52 along with the Monaghan 700 ventilation monitor (see Chapter 7 for a description of the monitor).

SIMV system. Functionally, the SIMV system allows the patient to breathe spontaneously with relatively *unpressurized* breaths from the ventilator inbetween mandatory *pressurized* breaths. The unit must be set to the *assist-control* position on the mode switch. The IMV (pressurized) breaths are set by the *respiration rate* control and the *BPM* (breaths per minute) control (Fig. 12-52). The BPM control establishes an approximate *range* for the respiration rate control to function within, either 0.3 to 5 or 4 to 16. Once either range is selected, the SIMV system is in opera-

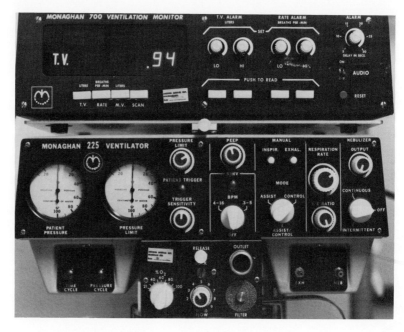

Fig. 12-52. Monaghan 225 modified for SIMV shown with Model 700 ventilation monitor attached.

tion. Then the desired mandatory rate is set primarily by the respiration rate control.

A red fluidic eye appears on the panel in between the mandatory volume-limited, pressurized breaths. During this time, any patient effort enough to trigger the assist mechanism results in the bellows being deflated in the normal fashion. However, the exhalation valve remains *deflated* so that the bellows gases are pushed through the circuit in a blow-by fashion, allowing the patient to inhale from them as desired.[17] In this way, the device provides somewhat of a blow-by-on-demand system.

When the red light is out, the ventilator is ready for a mandatory volume-, pressure-, or time-limited (pressurized) breath to occur and the exhalation valve will *inflate*. Any assist signal during a 4-second period (2 seconds at the highest rate setting) will result in a normal tidal volume delivery and reset the BPM timer.[17]

If no assist efforts are made by the end of that time period (4-second window), then the ventilator delivers a control breath and resets the BPM timer.

Oxygen concentrations and PEEP levels established are relatively unaffected by the SIMV system.[17] Because the gases during a blow-by breath are being pushed through the circuit and out the exhalation valve, a spirometer or monitor on a typical tubing circuit will sense this as a patient exhalation and therefore provide erroneous results. Using the CFV circuit mentioned in Chapter 8 and described elsewhere[18] will eliminate this problem.

Other changes. On early modified 225 ventilators such as shown in Fig. 12-52, the panel of controls still have an I:E ratio control. On new units with SIMV, the I:E ratio is preset so as not to allow inhalation to last longer than the value set by the respiration rate (expiratory timer) control. Otherwise, the volume, flow, sensitivity, PEEP, and oxygen system function as described for the Monaghan 225.

Specifications for Monaghan 225 and 225/SIMV ventilators

Tidal volume:	100 to 3300 ml
Flow rate:	Near 0 to 100 L/min
Expiratory time (*Cycle rate* control on 225 and *respiration rate* control on 225/SIMV):	0.5 to 7.5 seconds
Rate:	About 4 to 60 breaths/min
SIMV (225/SIMV only):	Sets rates of either about 4 to 16 or 0.3 to 5 breaths/min or *off*
Pressure limit:	Up to 100 cm H_2O
I:E ratio:	Maximum available from 1:1 to 1:4 (approximate) on 225; preset at 1:1 on 225/SIMV units
Oxygen percentage:	Continuously variable from 21% to 100%
PEEP:	Adjustable to about 20 cm H_2O (Referenced to trigger sensitivty for *PEEP assist*)
Sensitivity:	About +1 to −5 cm H_2O for 225 and from from autocycling to more than −10 cm H_2O for 225/SIMV
Pressure manometer:	−20 to 100 cm H_2O

Indicators

Time cycle:	Flashing red indicator when time limit ends inhalation
Pressure cycle:	Flashing indicator when pressure limit ends inhalation
Patient trigger:	Flashing green indicator when sensitivity mechanism starts inhalation
SIMV (225/SIMV only):	Red indicator shows during SIMV between mandatory breaths

---

The accompanying box summarizes the specifications for the Monaghan 225 and 225/SIMV ventilators.

THE OHIO 550 VENTILATOR

The Ohio 550 (Fig. 12-53) is a pneumatically driven, fluidically controlled, low-pressure drive, volume-limited, double-circuit bellows ventilator that is a time- or patient-cycled controller or assistor-controller.[19-21]

Referring to the diagram in Fig. 12-54, driving gas from a 50 psig oxygen source enters the system and divides (1) to power the fluidic logics by a *filter* and a *regulator* and (2) to an *interface valve* and Venturi system.

During inhalation, oxygen powers a Venturi system, and 100% oxygen enters the canister holding the *bellows*, driving it upward. The bellows gases enter the patient tubing circuit, flowing through the *humidifier*. The *exhaust* (or exhalation) *valve* is held closed by gases from the *diaphragm amplifier*.

On exhalation, the exhaust valve (exhalation valve) is deflated as well as the canister holding the bellows. The bellows falls, refilling with gases from the *oxygen mixer*.

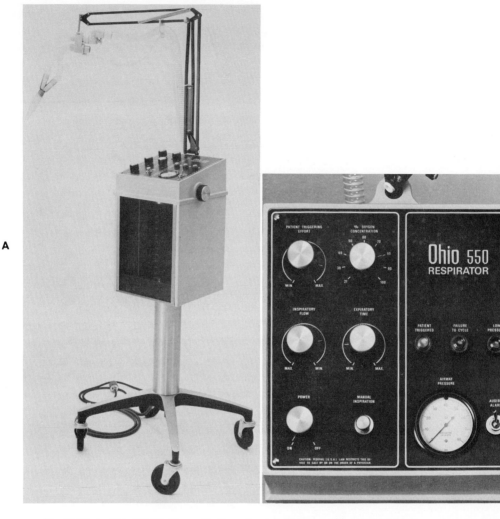

Fig. 12-53. A, Ohio 550 Ventilator. **B,** Control panel. (Courtesy Ohio Medical Products, Inc., Madison, Wis.)

Drive mechanism and flow characteristics. Because a Venturi system is used, the driving force for the 550 is relatively low. With a 50 psig source gas, the maximum pressure available is about 70 to 75 cm H_2O on early models.[19,20] Newer units will have a maximum pressure of about 90 cm H_2O pressure with a source pressure of 50 psig.[21] Flow characteristics are basically similar to those described for low-pressure-driven bellows units in Chapter 8, and drawings for common curves are shown in Fig. 12-55.

Supply pressure will affect the available driving potential. For example, if the oxygen system falls to 45 psig instead of 50 psig, the maximum driving force will probably be below 50 cm H_2O in earlier units and near 85 cm H_2O pressure in later units.[19,21]

The flow control valve (Fig. 12-54) adjusts the available source gas to be *added* to the flow of the Venturi jet. When this control is *closed*, peak flow to the bellows sys-

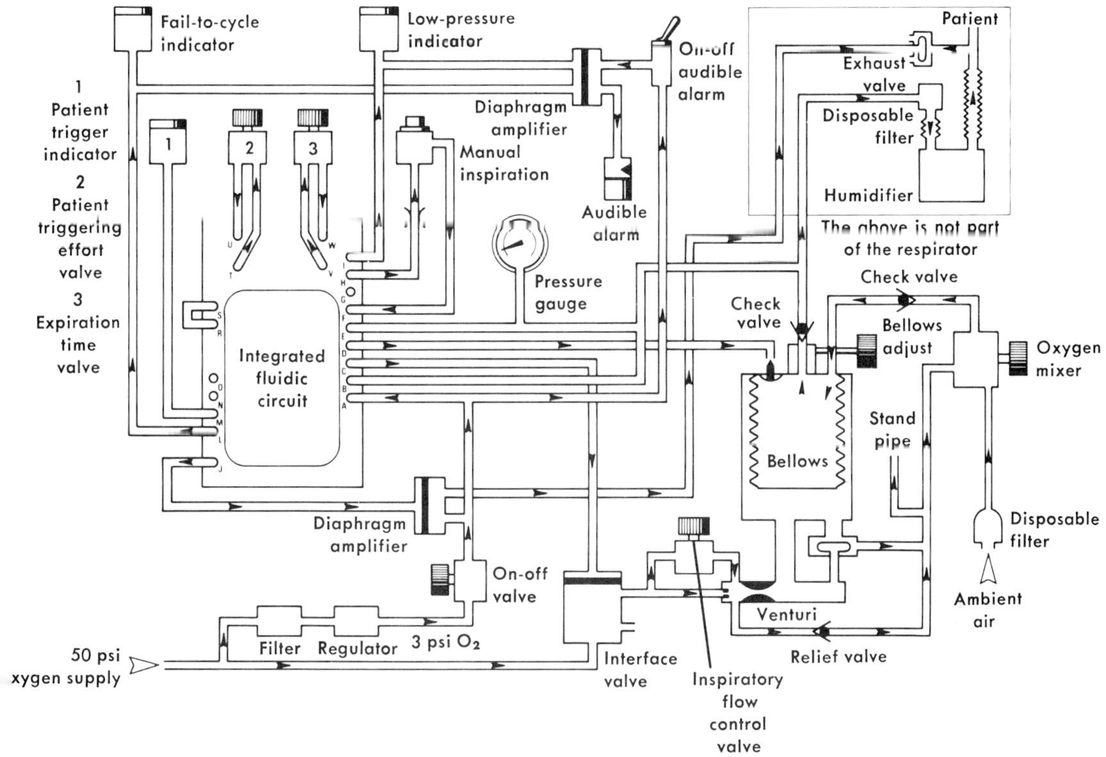

Fig. 12-54. Functional flow diagram for Ohio 550 Ventilator. (Courtesy Ohio Medical Products, Inc., Madison, Wis.)

tem is only from the Venturi jet, which is fixed at 30 L/min.[20] As the flow control is opened, more source gas is added, and the available peak flow is increased. Maximum flow is about 90 to 95 L/min against 20 cm H_2O back pressure on early units and up to 100 to 110 L/min on later units.[19-21]

Volume control. Tidal volume is set by adjusting a rope that limits the fall of the bellows during exhalation. The system is similar to that of the 560 and CCV volume controls. When the bellows reaches the top, a sensing port from the *integrated fluidic logic circuit* (Fig. 12-54) is occluded. This pneumatic signal causes the ventilator to cycle into exhalation (volume limit).

The bellows empties completely each breath, and therefore the compressibility factor is constant and dependent primarily on tubing circuit size and humidifier water level. A typical factor is about 2.5 cc/cm H_2O.

Rate and I : E ratio mechanism. Control breathing rate is a function of inspiratory time and expiratory time for the 550. Inspiratory time is a result of the tidal volume set, the flow rate set, and the patient's resistance and compliance conditions. Expiratory time is a result of an expiratory timer control. A change in any of these controls or the patient's resistance and compliance will change the breathing rate achieved. The assist mechanism can also influence the rate.

Assist and sensitivity mechanism. During *exhalation*, gas from the main flip-flop flows from port T (Fig. 12-54) to the sensitivity adjustment needle valve. If the

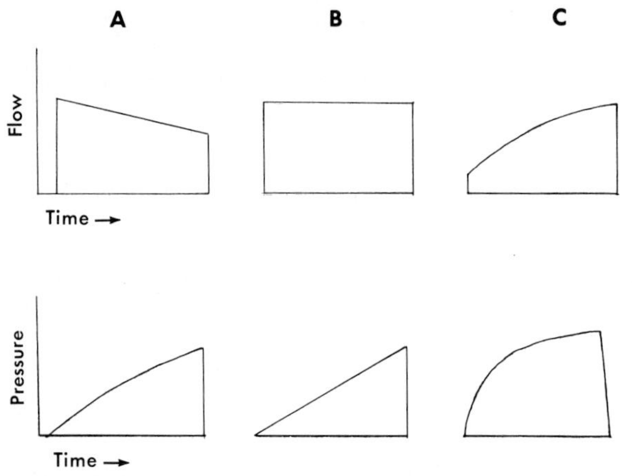

Fig. 12-55. Typical flow and pressure curves for Ohio 550 Ventilator. **A,** Curves against lungs having low compliance and low airway resistance. **B,** Curves against normal lungs with high compliance and low airway resistance. **C,** Curves against lungs with high compliance and high airway resistance.

patient tries to inhale, he will create a slight negative pressure in the breathing circuit. This pressure will be directed through port *B* to a *Schmidt trigger* in the fluidic circuit. If enough negative pressure is generated, the Schmidt trigger will be activated and switch the main flip-flop to the inspiratory side. To *increase* the amount of effort needed to trigger the ventilator, gas is allowed to flow through a Venturi, creating a negative pressure on the *reference side* of the Schmidt trigger. This negative pressure must be exceeded by the patient. The amount of flow through the Venturi, and thus the reference negative pressure, is controlled by a needle valve. Flow from the *expiratory time* control passes to an accumulator. Once sufficient pressure is generated in the accumulator by incoming flow from the needle valve, the main flip-flop switches to the inspiratory side. As the needle valve is opened, more flow will pass through it, and sufficient pressure will be generated in less time to switch the flip-flop to inhalation.

Manual inhalation is accomplished with an on-off push-button valve (Fig. 12-53, *B*). When activated, the valve provides a signal pressure to switch the flip-flop to the inspiratory position.

Oxygen system. The oxygen that pushed the bellows upward is also utilized to supply a portion of the bellows gas to be delivered to the patient. When the bellows drops, it creates a subatmospheric pressure at the oxygen-mixing valve (precision metering device). Air is drawn in through a filter, and oxygen is drawn from the bellows cylinder (Fig. 12-54). The oxygen-*mixing valve* allows the correct proportion of air and oxygen to be drawn into the bellows. The *stand pipe* serves to allow excess oxygen from the bellows to be exhausted.

Humidification system. The same heated humidifier that was mentioned for the Ohio Critical Care Ventilator is supplied with the 550.

Pressure relief. An optional adjustable pressure relief valve is available for external attachment.[19] It is a spring-loaded valve and functions in the same way the pressure relief on the 560 works (Fig. 12-35, *B*).

The accompanying box summarizes the specifications for the Ohio 550 Ventilator.

Specifications for Ohio 550 Ventilator

Tidal volume:	200 to 2000 ml
Flow rate, early models:	30-90 L/min peak flows (60 L/min against 40 cm H$_2$O back pressure)
Flow rate, later models:	Up to about 110 L/min (80 L/min against 40 cm H$_2$O back pressure)
Expiratory time:	Variable from 1 to 15 seconds
Rate:	From about 4 to 60 breaths/min
Pressure relief:	Up to about 100 cm H$_2$O
Oxygen percentage:	Continuously variable from 21% to 100%
Sensitivity:	From -0.5 to -5 cm H$_2$O
Pressure manometer:	0 to 80 cm H$_2$O

Alarms

Low pressure:	Audiovisual; activated when at least 8 cm H$_2$O is not generated once every 15 seconds
Failure to cycle:	Audiovisual; activated when inhalation lasts longer than 5 seconds or exhalation lasts longer than 15 seconds
Patient trigger:	Visual; activated when sensitivity starts inhalation
Audible alarm switch:	On/off

THE SIEMENS SERVO VENTILATOR 900B

The Servo Ventilator 900B by Siemens[22,23] (Fig. 12-56) is a pneumatically powered, electrically controlled, low-pressure drive, single-circuit, spring-driven bellows ventilator designed to be time limited and minute volume preset. The unit can be patient- or time-cycled on as an assistor/controller and can be set to end inhalation at a preset pressure limit. The driving pressure can be adjusted to produce a pressure hold before time ends inhalation.

Referring to Fig. 12-57, compressed gases enter through one or more of the inlets containing *nonreturn* (one-way) *valves*, pass through the *filter* and into the spring-loaded bellows, called the *gas pressure stabilizer* in the diagram. During inhalation, the *servo valve inspiratory*, a scissor-like valve (Fig. 12-58), opens and gases flow from the bellows, past the inspiratory *flow transducer* and out to the patient tubing circuit. Simultaneously, the *expiratory servo valve* is closed. During exhalation, these scissor valves reverse operation so that the inspiratory side closes while the expiratory side opens, allowing patient gases to flow past the expiratory *flow transducer* and out to the atmosphere.

Drive mechanism and flow characteristics. The drive mechanism for the 900B is a spring-driven bellows capable of delivering pressures up to 100 cm H$_2$O[22] into the patient circuit. The spring tension against the bellows can be adjusted to alter the driving force below 100 cm H$_2$O pressure.

Flow patterns can be set by two primary mechanisms. One is an electronic switch that can be set for either a square wave pattern or a sine-wave–like pattern. The

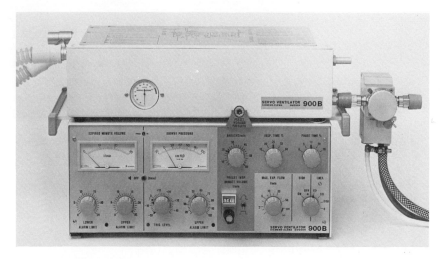

Fig. 12-56. Siemens-Elema Servo Ventilator 900B. (Courtesy Siemens Corp., Union, N.J.)

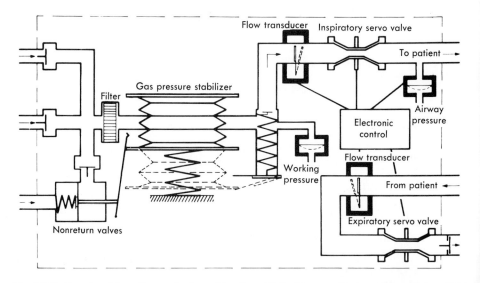

Fig. 12-57. Functional flow diagram for Servo Ventilator 900B. (Courtesy Siemens Corp., Union, N.J.)

other means of setting a flow pattern is adjustment of the driving pressure of the springs. This is done by changing the spring tension with the *preset working pressure* control (Fig. 12-56).

Along with the set rate, minute volume, and inspiratory time percentage controls, the flow pattern switch electronically calculates and controls the inspiratory scissor valve, with input from the inspiratory flow transducer, during inhalation so that the desired flow pattern is produced. The working pressure is generally set toward the higher values so that enough pressure reserve is available to maintain the desired flow pattern.

A decelerating flow pattern can be established by reducing the working pressure toward the patient's peak inspiratory pressure. In this mode the inspiratory time (set

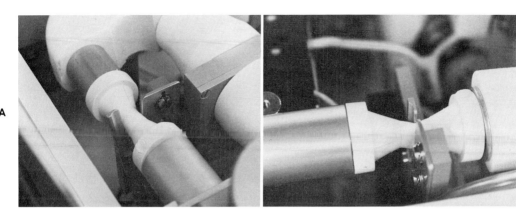

Fig. 12-58. Scissor-like valves used in Servo Ventilator 900B. **A,** Expiratory scissor valve open. **B,** Inspiratory scissor valve closed.

by the inspiratory time percentage control) will remain the same while flows, and therefore delivered volumes, lessen. If the patient's pressure equilibrates with the working pressure before end inhalation, a pressure hold will occur until exhalation begins.

Examples of flow and pressure patterns are shown for the Servo 900B in Fig. 12-59.

Volume control and rate system. The Servo 900B utilizes a preset minute volume system. The rate control value then divides the minute volume setting into individual tidal volumes. If the patient triggers assist breaths faster than the value set on the rate control, *tidal* volumes remain constant, and the *minute* volume increases. That is, the preset minute volume is set as a minimum value. On control mode, if either the rate control or the minute volume control is changed, the result will be a changed tidal volume as well.

Volume limiting inhalation is caused by a combination of several controls and an electronic calcuating system. During inhalation, a flow transducer system is utilized to monitor gases going to the patient. This flow transducer (Fig. 12-60) has a large main-flow port containing a fine wire mesh. The wire mesh causes a linear resistance to gas flow through the main-flow port and directs proportionally increased flow through the small-flow port. The small port contains a flow-sensitive strain gauge, and the increased strain on this flag is sent to the electronic control module as increased flow.

The electronics of the 900B compute the necessary gas flow during inhalation and control the inspiratory scissor valve. The set minute volume, the set inspiratory time percentage, the set rate, and the flow pattern switch setting (Fig. 12-56) all affect the electronic determination of flow necessary during each portion of inhalation. As set minute volume is increased, the flow necessary to deliver the volume must be higher. As the percentage of inspiratory time is decreased, the flow necessary to deliver the volume is increased. The rate determines division of the minute volume into each tidal volume. As the rate decreases, the tidal volume increases at a set minute volume. If the flow curve is set on square wave, the flow during inhalation will be a constant value computed from minute volume and percent inspiratory time

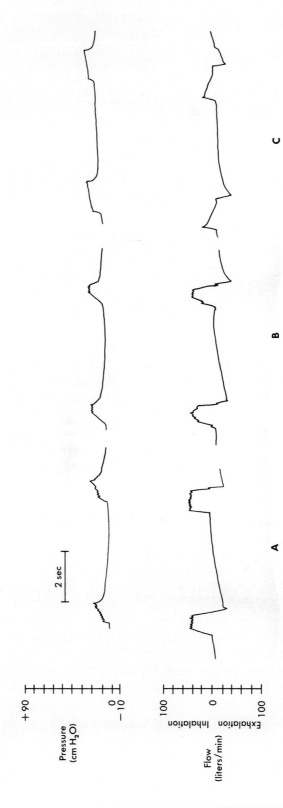

Fig. 12-59. Flow and pressure patterns for Servo Ventilator 900B redrawn from actual graphs. **A** and **B**, Unit ventilating lung simulator set for 50 ml/cm H_2O compliance and 5 cm H_2O/L/sec resistance. In **A** unit is set for square-wave flow curve, and in **B** it is set for sine-wave–like curve. **C**, 900B with working pressure reduced to 20 cm H_2O and lung simulator set for 10 ml/cm H_2O compliance and 5 cm H_2O/L/sec resistance. Note decelerating flow in **C**.

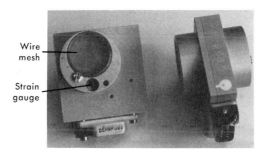

Wire
mesh

Strain
gauge

Fig. 12-60. Flow-sensing system for 900B. Unit on left shows end view, unit on right shows side view.

monitored by the inspiratory flow transducer. Once the control module has calculated the flow value, it monitors flow by the inspiratory flow transducer and adjusts the inspiratory scissor valve accordingly to maintain a constant flow throughout inhalation. Utilizing the same input factors, the accelerating/decelerating or sinewave–like curve setting makes the control module calculate the necessary flow during each portion of inhalation to produce this curve. The scissor valve is gradually opened more during the first portion of inhalation and then gradually closed during the last portion in response to electronic feedback from the inspiratory flow transducer.

A volume memory is built into the unit to compensate for resistance to flow that prevents an ideal or perfect square wave. After three breaths, the unit compensates by delivering a slightly higher flow to achieve the precise tidal volume.

I:E ratio. The I:E ratio is a function of the rate control, minute volume control, inspiratory time percentage control, and the inspiratory pause percentage control settings.

Assist and sensitivity system. The *trigger level* control (known as the *lower limit* on early models) adjusts a reference value for a pressure transducer. When the set pressure is established due to a patient's effort, inhalation is started. The control is calibrated from −20 cm H_2O to over +40 cm H_2O pressure, allowing for assist mode even if high levels of PEEP are applied.

Pressure limit system. During inhalation, pressures are monitored by an electric pressure transducer and displayed on a meter on the control panel (Fig. 12-56). The *upper alarm limit* control sets the maximum pressure allowed in the patient circuit. When this pressure is reached, inhalation ends immediately by the closing of the inspiratory scissor valve and the opening of the expiratory scissor valve. Simultaneously, an audible alarm is heard and a visual indicator lit.

Oxygen system. Oxygen concentrations can be set by an oxygen controller that attaches to the inlet of the 900B. This unit must be powered by compressed air and oxygen sources.

Sigh system. An *on/off* switch on the control panel provides for one sigh at twice the established tidal volume once every hundred breaths or no sigh at all.

Inspiratory pause percent control. On the front panel (Fig. 12-56) is a control for percent pause time. This value indicates the percentage of the ventilatory cycle that will be an inflation or volume hold and is additive to the percent inspiratory time control. This volume hold is accomplished by the inspiratory scissor valve closing after the delivery of the tidal volume and the expiratory scissor valve not opening for a time period based on percent pause setting and the ventilatory cycle time (set by the rate control).

Expiratory resistance system. A *maximum expiratory flow* control on the panel (Fig. 12-56) sets the peak expiratory flow from the patient and acts similar to an expiratory retard if expiratory flow attempts to exceed that value. The expiratory flow transducer is functionally the same as the inspiratory flow transducer with the addition of heat (60° C) to prevent condensation of water in the expired gases. The signals from the expiratory flow transducer are utilized by the control module to operate the expiratory scissor valve and maintain expiratory flow below the setting on the maximum expiratory flow control.

PEEP system. An external, spring-loaded device can be attached to the expiratory outflow tract for adjusting up to 50 cm H_2O PEEP. Since the sensitivity (trigger level) control can be adjusted into the positive pressure range, PEEP assist is available.

IMV system. The *IMV* control on the Servo 900B divides the rate setting by either 2, 5, or 10 (Fig. 12-56). When the IMV control is turned on, the combination of rate set and the division fraction set determines the frequency of mandatory breaths. In addition, the unit becomes pressure sensitive, allowing IMV/demand CPAP. The scissor valve is now controlled by pressure as set by the trigger level control and acts as a demand valve to deliver the gas required by the patient during the unpressurized breaths. When switched to IMV mode, the volume compensating memory is bypassed. Delivered mandatory breaths will, therefore, be slightly lower than expected, especially on the square wave setting. When the time comes for a mandatory breath, it is delivered in response to patient assist effort or is delivered at the predetermined time if the scissor valve is closed (that is, not delivered during a

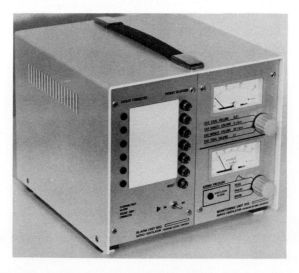

Fig. 12-61. Alarm Unit 920 and Monitoring Unit 910 combined for use with Servo Ventilator 900B. These devices provide parameters for monitoring tidal and minute volumes and peak, pause, and mean airway pressures. (Courtesy Siemens Corp., Union, N.J.)

spontaneous inhalation). The last setting, 0, provides the ability to allow totally spontaneous breathing through the machine with use of the demand gas source and expired volume monitoring and alarm systems.

Monitoring and alarm systems. Expired minute volumes are displayed on the control panel (Fig. 12-56). This volume is measured by the expiratory flow transducer and is displayed as an average value. The *lower alarm limit* and *upper alarm limit* controls can be set so that if the minute volume displayed is either lower or higher, respectively, than these set values, an audible and visual alarm occurs.

Additional monitoring systems can be added to the 900B. Electric outputs for pressure and for inspiratory and expiratory flows are available in the rear of the unit. Fig. 12-61 shows two devices that can be attached to the 900B for monitoring and displaying various pressure and volume parameters.

An infrared carbon dioxide analyzing system can also be added as shown in Fig. 12-62. This unit can calculate and digitally display such parameters as end tidal carbon dioxide percentage, effective and ineffective tidal volumes, effective minute volumes, and carbon dioxide production in milliliters per breath and milliliters per minute.

The accompanying box summarizes the specifications for the Servo 900B.[22]

Specifications for Siemens Servo Ventilator 900B

Minute volume:	0.5 to more than 25 L/min
Rate:	6 to 60 breaths/min on assist-control mode or 6 to 60 divided by 2, 5, or 10 on IMV
Inspiration percent:	15%, 20%, 25%, 33%, or 50% of set ventilatory cycle time established by rate control
Pause time percent:	0, 5%, 10%, 20%, or 30% of set ventilatory cycle time established by rate control
Sensitivity (patient triggering):	Variable from -20 to $+45$ cm H_2O pressure
Pressure limit:	Adjustable up to 100 cm H_2O pressure
Working pressure (driving force):	Adjustable up to 100 cm H_2O pressure
Flow pattern switch:	Square wave or sine wave
Sigh system:	One sigh every 100 breaths at double tidal volume or *off*

Displays

Pressure meter:	-20 to 100 cm H_2O
Expired minute volume meter:	0 to 30 L/min

Alarms

High and low minute volume:	Audio and visual
High-pressure limit:	Audio and visual
2-minute alarm silence:	Automatically reset
Electric power disconnect:	Approximately 1 min audio signal

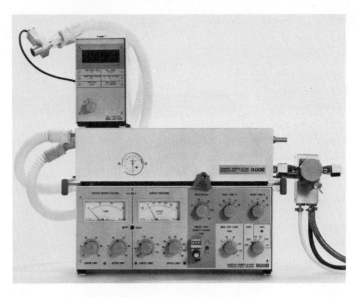

Fig. 12-62. Servo Ventilator 900B with carbon dioxide analyzer system attached. (Courtesy Siemens Corp., Union, N.J.)

THE BOURNS BEAR I VENTILATOR

The BEAR I[24] (Fig. 12-63) is a pneumatically and electrically powered, electrically controlled ventilator designed to be volume limited. It can be time- or patient-cycled on as an assistor-controller. The unit can also be time or pressure limited and has a built-in demand valve for spontaneous breathing during Synchronized Intermittent Mandatory Ventilation (SIMV) or CPAP modes.

Referring to the diagram in Fig. 12-64, external pressurized oxygen and either external compressed air or air from the internal *belt-drive rotary air compressor* are used to drive the ventilator. The oxygen pressure is regulated to match either the external air pressure after it passes through the *regulator* (reducing valve) or the compressor's air by way of the *relay valve* (gas-powered reducing valve). From there both gases move to the *oxygen concentration* control.

During positive pressure inhalation, the *main flow solenoid* opens, and oxygen and air are mixed passing through the oxygen concentration control. The gas mixture enters the *peak flow* and *waveform* controls section and exits the machine, passing through a *vortex flow sensor* and bacteria filter into the patient main tube. Simultaneously, the *three-way solenoid* sends gas to inflate the exhalation valve.

During exhalation, the main-flow solenoid closes, ending gas flow into the patient circuit, and the three-way solenoid blocks gas flow to the exhalation valve diaphragm, allowing the patient to exhale.

During assist-control, SIMV, or CPAP modes, gases leaving the oxygen concentration control feed the *demand valve* with blended gases. Spontaneous breathing from this source is available during SIMV or CPAP modes. The outlet of the demand valve sends gases, *demand flow*, to the same outlet to the patient circuit as the gases from the main-flow solenoid valve during pressurized breaths. Separate from the demand valve's outlet housing is a diaphragm sensing system that connects to the

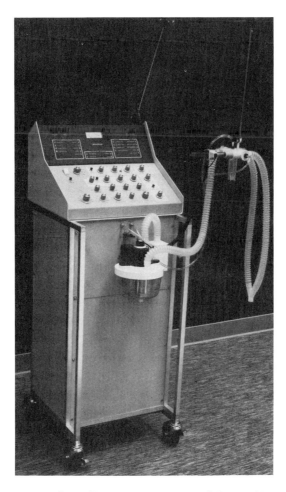

Fig. 12-63. Bourns BEAR I Ventilator. (Courtesy Bourns, Inc., Life Systems Division, Riverside, Calif.)

patient's circuit by way of the *pressure monitor* connection. When less than 1 cm H_2O drop is sensed by this line, the diaphragm moves such that the demand valve's outlet opens and gases are sent to the patient until pressures in the sensing line return to baseline again. If PEEP is applied, the opposite side of the diaphragm from the patient pressure sensing side is referenced to that new baseline pressure. Again, if the sensing line is subjected to less than 1 cm drop from the established baseline (PEEP) pressure, the demand valve opens. In this example, demand CPAP is being provided.

   Drive mechanism and flow characteristics. Compressed air and/or oxygen provide the driving force for the BEAR I. The two gas pressures are matched at about 11.5 psi by the regulator and relay valve previously mentioned or by the *relief valve* for the compressor. The compressor is automatically activated whenever the external air source is inadequate (below 30 psig) or absent. Once these gas sources are blended through the oxygen mixing system, their pressures are further reduced to an adjustable 1.8 to 3 psi range in the peak flow and taper flow control system (Fig. 12-65). The peak flow control is a variable restriction that limits the maximum flow that

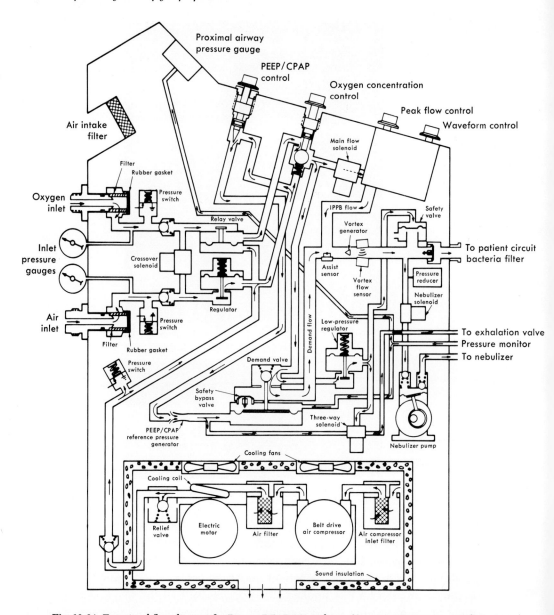

Fig. 12-64. Functional flow diagram for Bourns BEAR I Ventilator. (Courtesy Bourns, Inc., Life Systems Division, Riverside, Calif.)

can pass through it into the waveform control. The waveform control is an adjustable reducing valve that allows the reduction of driving pressure. On a constant wave setting, a maximum driving pressure of 3 psi is available, and the patient/circuit resistance is not sufficient to cause much flow taper within the allowable 100 cm H_2O pressure in the patient system. As taper is dialed, the reducing valve reduces the driving pressure toward the minimum 1.8 psi. As circuit pressure increases during inhalation, the decreasing pressure gradient causes flow to taper. Flow will not taper below 40 L/min.[24]

Theoretical flow and pressure patterns for the BEAR I are seen in Fig. 12-66.

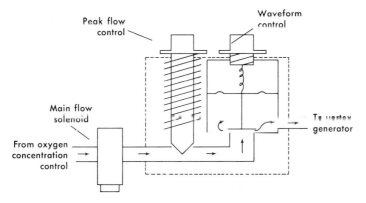

Fig. 12-65. Functional flow diagram of peak flow and waveform control system for BEAR I. Peak flow control provides variable restriction, and waveform control provides means for driving pressure reduction.

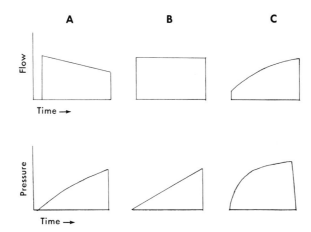

Fig. 12-66. Drawings of theoretical flow and pressure patterns for BEAR I Ventilator. **A,** Curves when some flow taper is set and reduced compliance is met. **B,** Curves when unit is set on square-wave flow pattern against low airway resistance and normal-to-low compliance. **C,** Unit set on square wave when ventilating system offering high resistance to air flow.

Volume control. Tidal volumes are determined by a vortex shedding sensor measuring gas flows during inhalation. The volume adjustment on the control panel (Fig. 12-67) sets a reference signal for the electronic logic in the BEAR. When the signals from the vortex sensor during inhalation match that of the reference (volume control) setting, inhalation is ended. Functionally this occurs by the main flow solenoid closing off gas flow from the oxygen control and the three-way solenoid opening the exhalation valve drive line.

Since there is little or no space internally for gas compression, the gas compressibility factor for the BEAR I is a relatively constant 3 cc/cm H_2O pressure,[24] dependent primarily on the size of the patient tubing system.

The *single-breath* button initiates a pressurized, volume-preset breath when depressed. However, if active exhalation is occurring, the breath will be delayed until 100 msec after expiratory gas flow cessation.[24]

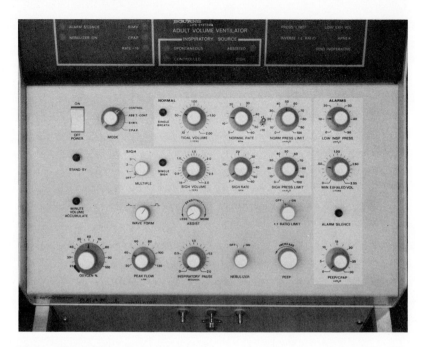

Fig. 12-67. Control panel for early model of BEAR I Ventilator. (Courtesy Bourns, Inc., Life Systems Division, Riverside, Calif.)

Rate mechanism and I:E ratio. The normal *rate* control (Fig. 12-67) is an electronic timer that sets the frequency at which the main flow solenoid opens starting inspiratory gas flow. Rates of 5 to 60 breaths/min can be set when a toggle switch next to the rate control is in its ×*1* position. When that same switch is in its *divide by 10* position, rates from 0.5 to 6 breaths/min can be set. The *I:E ratio limit* control is another electronic timer that measures the time allotted for inhalation and exhalation based on the time per ventilatory cycle set by the rate control. The actual I:E is displayed on an I:E ratio digital display. If inhalation becomes longer than half of the ventilatory cycle time, an indicator light flashes if the I:E ratio limit control is *off*. If the I:E ratio limit control is *on*, then inhalation ends (time limited) when it reaches half the allotted time available for each ventilatory cycle, that is, when the I:E ratio equals 1:1.

Assist and sensitivity mechanisms. During assist-control mode, when the patient creates less than 1 cm H_2O pressure drop, gases from the demand valve begin to flow out to the patient's circuit. These gases pass by the *assist sensor,* a heated thermistor bead, before flowing through the vortex flow sensor (Fig. 12-64). Flow passing this thermistor cools it, and an electric signal change is produced. This signal change, if great enough, can start inhalation by triggering the main flow solenoid open and by triggering the three-way solenoid such that it closes the exhalation valve.

Sensitivity changes are created by adjusting a reference adjustment so that more or less flow by the thermistor is needed to trigger inhalation. This adjustment is labeled the *assist* control on the control panel (Fig. 12-67).

During spontaneous breathing modes (SIMV and CPAP), in which the demand valve supplies the gases for the patient's breathing, this assist control also monitors when the demand valve opens so that an indicator light marked *spontaneous* can flash on and the BEAR's calculating logic can count that breath for the rate display.

Since the thermistor is flow sensitive, as opposed to pressure responsive, it is PEEP compensated. In the case of circuit leaks with PEEP, the demand valve will supply gas to compensate for the leak. The assist sensor will restabilize in the face of this constant flow level and remain functional.

Oxygen system. The oxygen concentration control system (Fig. 12-64) receives high-pressure oxygen and air and/or low-pressure air from the internal compressor. Both high-pressure gases are matched by a reducing valve system lowering their pressures to about 11.5 psi. The incoming air from the compressor is about 11.5 psi. There is an automatic switchover system that switches among the remaining gas sources should one or more of the required gas sources fail. This is accomplished by two electric pressure-sensing switches on the external gas sources inlets and by the *crossover solenoid* valve. The oxygen percentage control proportions oxygen and air by adjusting the position of the ball and therefore the openings from which oxygen and air flow to the patient. By changing the oxygen percentage control, the position of the ball is altered to open or close more of the oxygen and air ports proportionately.

Pressure limit system. A pressure transducer at the patient circuit outlet monitors the pressure generated within the machine during inhalation. If the measured pressure reaches that set on the pressure limit control, an audiovisual alarm is activated, and inhalation is ended by closing the main solenoid. Pressure settings are adjustable up to 100 cm H_2O.

A secondary safety feature is the *safety valve* (Fig. 12-64) located at the machine's main flow outlet. This valve will release at about 105 cm H_2O pressure, venting patient circuit gas in the event that the electric pressure limit system failed to prevent pressures from reaching this value. This safety valve is fed by gases from the *low-pressure regulator*, a preset reducing valve that supplies 3 psig gases to the three-way solenoid as well. The surface area of the safety valve's diaphragm, which seats on its outlet port, is responsible for the 3 psig to be functionally reduced to about 105 to 115 cm H_2O.

Sigh system. The *sigh rate* (Fig. 12-67) control works principally as the normal rate control in that it is a timer that establishes the frequency at which sighs are to occur. It works only in control and assist/control modes. The multiple sigh control sets the number of sigh breaths that occur in succession. The sigh module also has a separate pressure limit setting capabilities. When the sigh rate timer elapses, the next assist or control breath will be a sigh breath. The main solenoid and vortex monitor are then controlled by the sigh volume control. One, two, or three sighs in a row may be programed from two to sixty times each hour, or none may be programed.

The *single-sigh* button functions basically the same as the single-breath button except that tidal volumes and pressure limits during the resulting inhalation are controlled by the sigh volume and sigh pressure limit controls. Even when the *multiple* switch is *off*, the single sigh may be activated.

Nebulizer system. The nebulizer control is an on/off switch for a small compressor. When on, this pump (Fig. 12-64) runs constantly. During inhalation, the *nebulizer solenoid* opens and draws gas from the premixed gas volume to be delivered to the patient and utilizes it to power the nebulizer. Therefore oxygen percentage and tidal volume are not affected. During exhalation, the nebulizer solenoid closes, blocking flow into the pump and therefore to the nebulizer.

PEEP, CPAP, and SIMV. The PEEP or CPAP level to be utilized is established by the PEEP/CPAP control (Fig. 12-64). This control is a needle valve that adjusts air flow to the jet of a Venturi. The Venturi pressure developed is exerted on the exhalation diaphragm during exhalation and to the demand valve to servo it to this same positive pressure level. All spontaneous breaths on CPAP and SIMV are drawn from the demand valve. The demand valve also acts as a leak compensation unit to maintain PEEP and CPAP levels.

During SIMV spontaneous breath delivery, the assist sensor electronically ignores patient efforts and does not send a pressurized breath. Once the time has elapsed as determined by the normal rate control, it is time for a mandatory breath to be delivered. The next spontaneous effort from the patient will cause the assist sensor to deliver a pressurized breath. If the assist sensor does not receive an assist effort, the machine will deliver a control breath when the *next* time sequence occurs.

Inspiratory pause system. The control provides an adjustable delay for a volume hold at end inhalation adjustable from 0 to 2 seconds. When on, active inhalation ends by the main flow solenoid valve closing and the hold period occurring by the inspiratory pause timer delaying the three-way solenoid from releasing pressure in the exhalation valve for the set time period. During this inflation hold, the circuit pressures and the patient's lung pressure tend to equilibrate.

Humidity and monitoring systems. The BEAR I utilizes a heated cascade humidifier (described in Chapter 4).

A variety of visual displays are available and are shown in Fig. 12-68, some of which also have audio alarms.

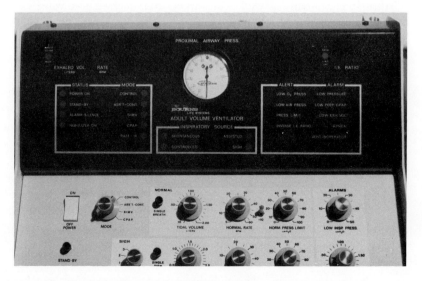

Fig. 12-68. Display panel for early model of BEAR I Ventilator. (Courtesy Bourns, Inc., Life Systems Division, Riverside, Calif.)

Exhaled volumes are monitored by another vortex shedding flow sensing device. This unit is basically similar to the Bourns LS-75 described in Chapter 7. Externally attached to the exhalation valve, this monitor detects expiratory gas flows, and each breath is displayed digitally on the display panel. When the *minute volume accumulate* button (Fig. 12-67) is depressed, all exhaled volumes are added together for the next 60 seconds while the digital numbers displayed reflect the ongoing total. After displaying the collected minute volume for 1 minute after collection, the display reverts back to tidal volume read-outs. During this second minute, the minute volume accumulate can be reset manually by depressing the button.

Adjustable alarms are found on the control panel's right side (Fig. 12-67). The *low-pressure* alarm, adjustable from 0 to 50 cm H_2O, sets the minimum pressure during pressurized breaths that must be sensed by the internal pressure transducer to avoid an audiovisual alarm.

Minimum exhaled volume, adjustable from 0 to 2 liters, sets the minimum measured exhaled volume that must be exceeded at least once out of every three exhaled (pressurized or spontaneous) breaths. When three exhaled breaths in a row are all lower than the value set, an audiovisual alarm is activated. Once an exhaled volume exceeds the set value again, the alarm is reset.

The *alarm silence* button allows for silencing the audible systems for 60 seconds. The silence button can be reset manually before the 60 seconds or it will reset automatically at the end of that time period.

The *PEEP/CPAP* alarm, adjustable from 0 to 30 cm H_2O, sets the minimum pressure that must be maintained during exhalation to avoid an audiovisual alarm condition. This alarm also resets when the pressure is once again exceeded.

The box on p. 366 summarizes the specifications for the BEAR I ventilator.[24]

THE BOURNS BP200 INFANT PRESSURE VENTILATOR

The Bourns BP200 Infant Pressure Ventilator[25] (Fig. 12-69) is a pneumatically powered, electrically controlled, time-cycled, time-limited, pressure-relief preset, continuous-flow ventilator. The unit functions in IPPB/IMV (control) or CPAP (no pressurized, mandatory breaths) modes.

Referring to the diagram in Fig. 12-70, compressed air and oxygen enter into the unit through their respective inlets and pass by *pressure switches* for detecting proper inlet pressures. The *regulators* (preset reducing valves) in each line drop and match the gas pressures to about 10 psig each. These gases, at their matched pressures, then flow through the *oxygen percent control*, the *flow control*, the *flowmeter*, past a *pressure limit* (relief) *control*, the *fail-safe valve*, and out to the patient's circuit. These gases are flowing continuously into the circuit. During a pressurized control breath, the *solenoid* valve closes against the *exhalation valve diaphragm*, and the continuous flow of gases is directed to the patient's airways. If the pressure increases during this time to match the pressure set on the pressure limit control, this pop-off valve opens and attempts to hold the pressure at the set level, resulting in a pressure hold (see Chapter 8 for description). The *PEEP Venturi*, powered by oxygen at its inlet pressure, allows for an elevated baseline pressure to be established.

During the ventilator's expiratory phase and during CPAP mode, the solenoid is

Specifications for BEAR I Ventilator

Modes:	Control, assist-control, Synchronized Intermittent Mandatory Ventilation (SIMV), and CPAP
Tidal volume:	100 to 2000 ml
Rate:	5 to 60 or 0.5 to 6 with divide by 10 switch
Pressure limits:	0 to 100 cm H_2O pressure separately adjustable for normal and sigh breaths
Sigh volume:	150 to 3000 ml
Sigh rate:	1, 2, or 3 consecutive sighs from 2 to 60 times per hour or off
Waveform:	Constant flow or decelerating flow taper
Peak flow:	20 to 120 L/min
PEEP:	0 to 30 cm H_2O pressure
Inspiratory pause:	0 to 2 seconds
Oxygen concentration:	21% to 100%
Assist:	Less to more sensitive (50 msec response time)
Nebulizer:	On or off, inspiratory phase only
Ratio limit:	On or off, stop inspiratory phase when half of ventilatory cycle time (set by rate control) is reached

Alarms

Low pressure:	Audiovisual, variable from 0 to 50 cm H_2O
Minimum exhaled volume:	Audiovisual, variable from 0 to 2 liters, must sense three consecutive low volumes exhaled
PEEP/CPAP:	Audiovisual, variable from 0 to 30 cm H_2O
Apnea:	Audiovisual, activates if inspiratory phases, pressurized or spontaneous, are not sensed for 20 seconds
Ventilator inoperative:	Audiovisual, indicates machine has electric failures or loss of gas supplies

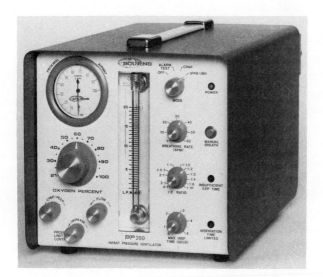

Fig. 12-69. Bourns BP200 Infant Pressure Ventilator. (Courtesy Bourns, Inc., Life Systems Division, Riverside, Calif.)

open. Both the patient's exhaled gases and the continuous flow gases exit through the *expiratory check leaf.* Throughout both phases, circuit pressures are monitored by the *proximal airway pressure gauge* (aneroid manometer).

Drive mechanism and flow characteristics. Because of the relatively high driving force from the regulators of air and oxygen, the flow pattern for the BP200 during pressurized breaths begins as a constant or square wave (Fig. 12-71, *A*), and then when or if the pressure relief is reached, some gases exit the circuit through the pressure limit valve. If pressure-relief pressure is reached, gas flows to the patient during

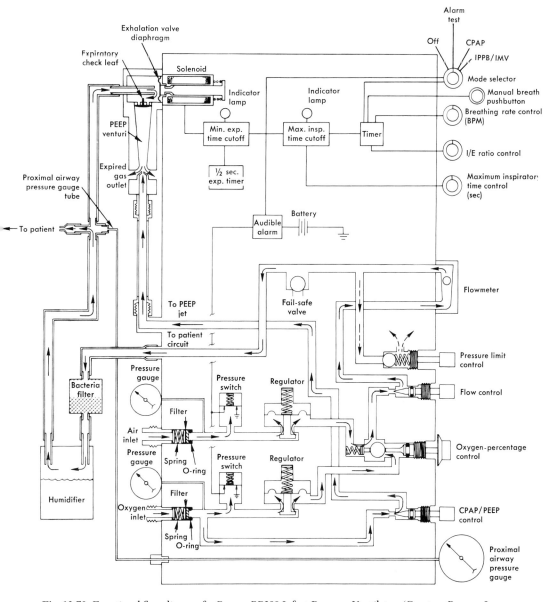

Fig. 12-70. Functional flow diagram for Bourns BP200 Infant Pressure Ventilator. (Courtesy Bourns, Inc., Life Systems Division, Riverside, Calif.)

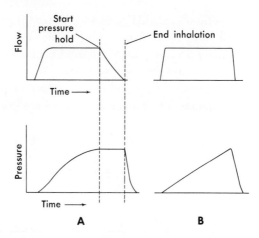

Fig. 12-71. Drawings of theoretical flow and pressure patterns for BP200 Infant Pressure Ventilator. **A,** Flow and pressure pattern when preset pressure limit (pop-off) is reached before end inhalation. **B,** Unit when pressure limit is not reached.

the rest of inhalation are primarily a function of the patient's airway resistance until the circuit pressure equilibrates with the patient's alveolar pressure or until time ends inhalation. If the preset pressure limit is not reached, the flow remains essentially constant, and a square-wave pattern results (Fig. 12-71, *B*).

Flow rates from 0 to 20 L/min can be set by the flow control and read on the calibrated scale of a non–back-pressure-compensated flowmeter. Because of the relatively high pressure gradient (10 psig) to ventilation pressure (less than 80 cm H_2O pressure) the flowmeter is relatively accurate.

Volume control system. The BP200 is basically designed to be used as a pressure-controlled rather than volume-controlled, time-limited ventilator. If the pressure limit set is in fact reached during inhalation, the delivered tidal volume will depend primarily on the flow, pressure limit and inspiratory time values, and the patient's resistance and compliance. However, the maximum *available* tidal volume can be estimated by the following formula:

$$\text{Tidal volume available} = \frac{\text{Inspiratory time (seconds)} \times \text{Flow (L/min)}}{60}$$

In this formula, inspiratory time is either that set on the *maximum inspiratory time* control (Fig. 12-69) or is a result of the *breathing rate* control's setting times the sum of the parts of the value set on the I:E ratio control divided into 60.

The results of those calculations do not indicate what the patient receives, especially if the preset pressure limit is reached before end inhalation. Rather they represent a set tidal volume, and only if the pressure limit is not reached can an estimated delivered tidal volume be calculated by subtracting the gases compressed in the circuit.

Compressibility factors calculated in the clinical setting vary from about 0.5 to 1 ml/cm H_2O pressure, depending primarily on the patient tubing and humidification system used.

Rate mechanisms and I:E ratio system. The breathing rate control (Figs. 12-69) is an electric timer adjustable from 1 to 60 begin inhalations per minute and there-

---

Specifications for Bourns BP200 Infant Pressure Ventilator

Rate control:	1 to 60 breaths per minute
I:E ratio control:	4:1 to 1:10
Inspiratory flow:	0 to 20 L/min
Maximum inspiratory time control:	0.5 to 5 seconds on early units and 0.2 to 5 seconds on newer units
Minimum expiratory time:	Internally preset for 0.5 second
PEEP:	Up to 20 cm H_2O pressure
Pressure limit:	10 to 80 cm H_2O
Oxygen concentrations:	21% to 100%
Pressure manometer:	0 to 100 cm H_2O
Audible alarms:	Electric power failure
	Inadequate air and/or oxygen pressures
Visual indicators:	Power pilot light—indicates electric power on
	Inspiration time limited—setting on maximum inspiratory time control reached
	Insufficient expiratory time—indicates preset internal time is not allowing exhalation to last over 0.5 second.
	Air inlet pressure gauge
	Oxygen inlet pressure gauge

---

fore establishes the length of each ventilatory cycle. The I:E ratio control then electrically divides each ventilatory cycle into inspiratory and expiratory times. This control is calibrated in inspiratory to expiratory ratios (rather than seconds) from 4:1 to 1:10.

The maximum inspiratory time control is adjustable from 0.5 to 5 seconds (newer units have a minimum setting of 0.2 second) as a safety mechanism during controlled breaths or as the primary time limit when slow respiratory (IMV) rates are used. Each time this mechanism ends inhalation, the *inspiration time limited* light flashes.

Pressure limit system. The pressure limit control (Fig. 12-70) is a spring-loaded relief valve that vents when its preset pressure is reached. Pressures from 10 to 80 cm H_2O are available.

Oxygen system. The oxygen percent control is a precision metering device that receives air and oxygen from their respective regulators and sets the outlet opening size for each gas. Similar to the Bourns LS-145 Oxygen Blender described in Chapter 11, the BP200's oxygen control opens one gas outlet while it proportionately closes the other when adjustments are made.

PEEP/CPAP system. The *PEEP/CPAP* control (Fig. 12-70) is a needle valve that adjusts the amount of oxygen from the oxygen inlet to be sent to the PEEP Venturi. The more gas sent to the jet of this Venturi, the greater forward pressure the Venturi exerts against the expiratory check leaf (one-way valve) and therefore the greater the PEEP or CPAP level maintained within the patient's circuit.

CPAP breathing with or without an IMV (control) rate is established by the mode switch. Spontaneous gases are available from the continuous flow set by the flow control. When the mode switch is set in the CPAP position, a pressurized breath may be initiated by the depression of the *manual breath* button.

Humidification and alarm systems. The humidifier supplied with the BP200 is a nebulizer modified to provide a heated blow-by humidifier. A thermometer at the humidifier displays the temperature of the gases leaving the unit.

An electronic pressure switch for each pressurized gas source monitors their inlet pressures and alarms if the pressures are inadequate. An audible alarm also can occur if an electric power failure occurs.

The box on p. 369 summarizes the specifications for the Bourns BP200 Infant Pressure Ventilator.[25]

REFERENCES

1. Mushin, W. W., et al.: Automatic ventilation of the lungs, ed. 2, Philadelphia, 1969, F. A. Davis Co.
2. Egan, D. F.: Fundamentals of respiratory therapy, ed. 3, St. Louis, 1977, The C. V. Mosby Co.
3. Air-Shields Respirator 10,000, 1969, Air-Shields, Inc., Hatboro, Pa.
4. Operating instructions, Bennett Model MA-1 Respiration Unit, Form 5030w, Santa Monica, Calif., 1975, Bennett Respiration Products, Inc.
5. Bevan, R.: Bennett Respiration Products, Inc., Kansas City: Personal communication, 1973.
6. Service and repair instructions, Bennett MA-1 Respiration Unit, Form 3190A, Santa Monica, Calif., 1974, Bennett Respiration Products, Inc.
7. Operation and repair manual, Model 560 Respirator, Form 1887, Madison, Wis., 1970, Ohio Medical Products, Inc.
8. Plut, H. G., Jr., and Miller, W. F.: New volume ventilator, Inhalation Ther. **13:**91, 1968.
9. Petty, T. L., Bigelow, D. B., and Broughton, J. O.: A new volume cycled ventilator, Respir. Ther. **2:**33, Nov.-Dec., 1972.
10. Ohio Critical Care Ventilator, Preliminary operation manual, Form 1937, Ohio Medical Products, Inc., Madison, Wis.
11. Ohio Critical Care Ventilator, In service outline, Form 631, Madison, Wis., 1975, Ohio Medical Products, Inc.
12. Ohio Products specification—Ohio Critical Care Ventilator, Form 630, Madison, Wis., 1974, Ohio Medical Products, Inc.
13. Monaghan 225 Volume Ventilator service Manual, Form 13914-02, Littleton, Colo., 1974, Monaghan.
14. Patterson, J. R., et al: Evaluation of a fluidic ventilator: a new approach to mechanical ventilation, Chest **66:**706, 1974.
15. Monaghan 225 Volume Ventilator operator's manual: questions and answers, Form 13929-01 5m, Monaghan, Littleton, Colo.
16. Brunner, D., Monaghan, Littleton, Colo.: Personal communication, 1975.
17. Addendum to 225 Volume Ventilator operator's manual, Littleton, Colo., 1975, Monaghan.
18. McPherson, S. P., et al.: A circuit that combines ventilator weaning methods using continuous flow ventilation (CFV), Respir. Care **20:**261, 1975.
19. Preliminary operation and maintenance manual, Model 550 Respirator, Form 1936, Ohio Medical Products, Inc., Madison, Wis.
20. Weill, H., et al.: Laboratory and clinical evaluation of a new volume ventilator, Chest **67:**14, 1975.
21. Ohio operation/maintenance, 550 Ventilator, Form 1936, 10/76-1M, Ohio Medical Products, Inc., Madison, Wis.
22. Siemens-Elema Servo Ventilator 900 operating manual ME 461/5098.101, 1974 and Servo Ventilator 900B preliminary supplement to operating manual, Solna, Sweden, 1975, Siemens-Elema AB.
23. Ingestedt, S., Jonson, B., Nordstrom, L., and Olsson, S.-G.: A servo-controlled ventilator measuring expired minute volume, airway flow and pressure, Acta Anaesthesiol. Scand. (Suppl.) **47:**9, 1972.
24. Instruction manual, Bourns Adult Volume Ventilator BEAR I, Form P/N 50000-10500, Bourns, Inc., Life Systems Division, Riverside, Calif.
25. Instruction manual, Bourns Infant Pressure Ventilator Model BP200, Form P/N 50000-10200, Bourns Inc., Life Systems Div., Riverside, Calif.

INDEX